Apples of Gold in Pictures of Silver

Apples of Gold in Pictures of Silver

Honoring the Work of Leon R. Kass

Yuval Levin, Thomas W. Merrill,
and Adam Schulman

LEXINGTON BOOKS
A division of
ROWMAN & LITTLEFIELD PUBLISHERS, INC.
Lanham • Boulder • New York • Toronto • Plymouth, UK

Published by Lexington Books
A division of Rowman & Littlefield Publishers, Inc.
A wholly owned subsidiary of The Rowman & Littlefield Publishing Group, Inc.
4501 Forbes Boulevard, Suite 200, Lanham, Maryland 20706
http://www.lexingtonbooks.com

Estover Road, Plymouth PL6 7PY, United Kingdom

British Library Cataloguing in Publication Information Available

Library of Congress Cataloging-in-Publication Data

Apples of gold in pictures of silver : honoring the work of Leon R. Kass / Yuval Levin, Thomas W. Merrill, and Adam Schulman.
p. cm.
ISBN 978-0-7391-4159-5 (cloth : alk. paper)
ISBN 978-0-7391-4160-1 (pbk. : alk. paper)
1. Philosophy. 2. Kass, Leon. I. Kass, Leon. II. Levin, Yuval. III. Merrill, Thomas W. (Thomas Westneat), 1974– IV. Schulman, Adam.
B29.K345 2010
191—dc22 2010008093

™ The paper used in this publication meets the minimum requirements of American National Standard for Information Sciences—Permanence of Paper for Printed Library Materials, ANSI/NISO Z39.48-1992.

Printed in the United States of America

A word fitly spoken is like apples of gold in pictures of silver.

–*Proverbs* 25:11

See how marvelously this saying describes a well-constructed parable. It says that, when a word has two meanings—an outer one and an inner one—the outer meaning must be as beautiful as silver, but the inner meaning must be still more beautiful, the inner being to the outer as gold is to silver. . . . In the parables of the prophets, their outer meaning contains wisdom useful in many respects, among which is the welfare of human societies. . . . But their inner meaning contains wisdom that is useful for knowing the truth as it is.

–Maimonides, *Guide of the Perplexed*, Introduction

The assertion of that principle ["Liberty to all"], at that time, was the word, "fitly spoken," which has proved an "apple of gold" to us. The Union, and the Constitution, are the picture of silver, subsequently framed around it. The picture was made, not to conceal, or destroy the apple; but to adorn, and preserve it. The picture was made for the apple—not the apple for the picture. So let us act, that neither picture, or apple, shall ever be blurred, or broken.

–Abraham Lincoln, fragment: The Constitution and the Union [1860?]

Contents

Introduction:
The Career of Leon Kass

Harvey Flaumenhaft

Attend to what a thinker thinks, rather than to where he may have come from. That is usually the better path to wisdom. But we learn from what Leon Kass has written—especially from his most philosophic work, *The Hungry Soul*, his learned meditation on the significance of eating in the lives of human beings—that our dignity as human beings depends upon our recognizing this twofold truth: that a living being does not simply outgrow what it grows out of, and that what a living being is is more than what it grows out of. Knowing Leon Kass means seeing how it is that soaring high and being rooted come together. Let us, then, consider how genesis and culmination unite in his career.

The preface to his first book, *Toward a More Natural Science*, gives a one-sentence *curriculum vitae*: "The author of this book," Leon says, "is by rearing a moralist, by education a generalist, by training a physician and biochemist, by vocation a teacher—and student—of philosophical texts, and by choice a lover of serious conversation, who thinks best when sharing thoughts and speeches with another."

In an acknowledgment of debts, he says that his parents first taught him by precept and example to put moral matters first. They pointed out that learning and schooling are no substitutes for character, he says, and they did so long before he read it in Rousseau. (Why Rousseau? We'll soon see.) His parents, poor unschooled Jewish immigrants who came from Eastern Europe between the wars, raised their children in a Yiddish-speaking home and sent them to Yiddish school after regular school hours. The home was decidedly non-religious. The place of Judaism was taken by morality—morality tinged with socialism, not so much on grounds of Marxist theory as out of zeal for human dignity and justice. Only years later did he come to think that the seemingly secular moral teaching of his home was, as he put it, parasitic on traditional Jewish religious thought. Before that thought occurred to him, he had moved on to college and to post-graduate work.

At the University of Chicago in the mid-fifties, Leon obtained the education that made him a generalist, as well as the beginning of the training that made him a physician and a biochemist. In moving from home to college, he had moved from a world where moral virtue had primacy into one where intellectual virtue did, primarily in a double manifestation: in great writings of Greek antiquity and in perplexing questions of modern natural science. He awakened philosophically, but his outlook remained that of a partisan of universalist enlightenment. He believed that religion was superstition and that the progress of science and the arts would ultimately lead to a world of peace and prosperity, which in turn would enable human beings to flourish morally too. In the thinking of his college years, unquestioning acceptance of scientific progress, along with fondness for the great books of ancient Greece, mingled with much that was derived from a mix of writers who were then considered most progressive—Marxists, Freudians, and existentialists. But where others found answers, Leon was, even then, eager to explore questions.

He and I first met when I entered the College of the University of Chicago, in the fall of 1956. What drew us almost immediately into close, long-lasting friendship was a taste for serious conversation. That taste led him to consider and to reconsider assumptions, whether casual or dearly held.

Leon had entered college early, and so it was only two years after I met him that he entered medical school, for which he stayed on at Chicago, and then went on to complete his training with an internship in medicine at a hospital in Boston. After that, he entered Harvard to earn a doctorate in biochemistry. There, from 1963 to 1967, he experienced the great excitement of the golden age of molecular biology—the discovery of messenger and transfer RNA, the search for the codons of the translational dictionary, and the race to find the repressor of gene transcription. But it was not inside the laboratory that his biggest discovery came.

What set him up for that discovery was an experience in the summer of 1965. Interrupting research for a month, he went with his wife to work in Mississippi with the Medical Committee for Human Rights. Living in rural Holmes County with a farming couple—in a house with no telephone, no hot water, and no indoor toilet—Leon and his wife visited many families in the community, participated in their activities, and helped with voter registration and other efforts to encourage people to organize themselves to defend their rights. The experience of that summer deeply moved Leon, but it did more than that: it provoked some fundamental questioning that changed his life. On returning to Cambridge, he could not stop asking himself why he had found more honor, decency, and dignity among the poor and uneducated black farmers in Mississippi than among his prosperous and well-schooled fellow graduate students at Harvard, whose progressive opinions he shared but whose self-absorption and self-indulgence put him off. As a man of the left and the enlightenment, he had unthinkingly held the view that education and progress in science and technology would allow humanity to become at last the society of morally superior creatures that only nature's stinginess, social oppression, and religious credulity had kept them from being. In Mississippi he had seen people, many of them illiterate, who lived in perilous and meager circumstances but were sustained by religion, by extended family, by attachment to community, and by pride in honest farming and homemaking. Around him back at Harvard, he saw all too many cocky young men on the make, filled with easy-going compassion for the unfortunate but looking out, in interpersonal relations, only for number one. How could this be explained if poverty, oppression, and superstition were the causes of bad character? This nagging question started Leon on a journey that would eventually lead him to study and reflect on the Hebrew Bible. Eventually—but not quite yet.

In the summer of 1966, I moved to Cambridge right next door to Leon and his wife, where I was preparing to begin teaching at a college in the area. Among the books that I planned to assign my classes that fall were Aldous Huxley's *Brave New World*, C. S. Lewis's *The Abolition of Man*, and Rousseau's *Discourse on the Sciences and Arts*. Knowing of Leon's wrestlings with the tension between intellectual and moral virtue, I urged him to read Huxley and Lewis, and we agreed to read Rousseau's *Discourse* together that summer. Reading those three books was a turning-point for him. The question that had nagged at him on returning to Harvard after his experience in Mississippi turned into a host of profound questions that challenged him more than any question about how genes are regulated. Those questions have occupied him ever since: What is the relation between scientific or technological progress and the moral health of a community? How can we reap the benefits of technology without eroding our freedom and our dignity? Does the scientific account of nature and human nature tell the whole, or even the best, story about us?

In Rousseau's *Discourse on the Sciences and Arts*, Leon encountered a powerful argument that progress in the arts and sciences debases taste and corrupts morals, leading not to human emancipation but to human servitude. Through reading Huxley's *Brave New World* and Lewis's *Abolition of Man*, he began to reflect on how the scientific project to master nature could, if we are not careful, lead to our dehumanization, via eugenics, drug-induced contentment, and other transformations of human nature—possibilities already foreseeable in the new biology. Here, Leon concluded, was the true challenge for the modern moralist: how to keep human life human, when the threat comes from powers arising out of the best thinking of humanity and wielded not by racists and gangsters but by philanthropic humanitarians. He gradually came to put the challenge this way:

Will man remain a creature made in the image of God, aspiring to align himself with the divine, or will he become an artifact created by man in the image of God-knows-what, fulfilling the aspirations only of human will? That was not the way he stated the challenge at first, but the terms in which it first made itself manifest did suffice to bring about a radical shift in his career. From doing science, he turned to thinking about its human meaning, worrying about upholding our humanity against possible technological degradation, and looking for a more natural science that would do justice to human life as lived.

The shift was not a slow one, but it did occur in stages. The following year, Leon moved to the Washington area to join the staff of the Laboratory of Molecular Biology at the National Institutes of Health. While there, in January of 1968, he published in the *Washington Post* "A Caveat on Transplants," the first product of the turn in his thinking. But although the pot had begun to boil, what the menu would contain was not yet clear—at least not to Leon.

He himself did not yet recognize where his true vocation lay. I remember his lamenting, while he was still in training for medicine, that he felt no strong inclination toward any medical specialty—but what on earth could he do if not be a physician? Teaching, I suggested. Deep down, I said, what he would really like to do was what a teacher does. He could not believe that I had said that. Him—teach? He had nothing to teach, he said, and no particular gift for teaching. I let it drop—and waited. Six months after Leon published his piece on transplants in the *Washington Post*, I moved to Annapolis to teach at St. John's College; and a year and a half after that, Leon left the laboratory to become for two years the Executive Secretary of the Committee on the Life Sciences and Social Policy of the National Research Council, National Academy of Sciences, where he was charged with writing a report on the shape of things to come and on what might be done about it. Leon and his family moved to Annapolis during that time, and my wife and I invited them to dinner with the Dean of St. John's College, which led to Leon's becoming a part-time member of the St. John's faculty for four years. During that time, he also held Guggenheim and NEH fellowships to do research on ancient and modern concepts of organism, species, and health, and he was a research professor in bioethics at Georgetown University.

Having found at St. John's College his vocation as that special kind of student called a teacher, Leon returned to the University of Chicago, now to teach in the College there and in the Committee on Social Thought, with some time away as a fellow at the National Humanities Center and at the American Enterprise Institute.

At Chicago, he won several awards for distinction as a teacher, and was a leader in the struggle to foster truly liberal education. He taught courses on such topics as the organism, the passions, courtship, science and morals, nature and custom, and human beginnings, and on such authors as Plato, Aristotle, Lucretius, Descartes, Rousseau, and Darwin, as well as on the beginning books of the Hebrew Bible. In addition to his scientific papers in molecular biology and his articles on bioethics, he wrote major books on the human significance of eating and on the Hebrew Bible as a path to wisdom.

His own path was not a straight one. At the time he turned to bioethics, in 1968, his orientation was still simply secular. It would take another ten years before he began looking for wisdom in the Hebrew Bible, for he continued to think that the answers to our moral dilemmas lay entirely in philosophy and liberal education and in the attempt to develop a philosophical ethic that would be able to hold the human fort against the coming danger. His discovery of the Bible as a possible source of wisdom, about human nature and about how to live, got under way in New Mexico in 1978, during a futile effort at digging for fossils in the company of his friend Robert Sacks. Sacks, who had just completed a full commentary on Genesis, regaled Leon with one after another of his discoveries. The previous year, Leon had taught Genesis in a new common-core course at the University of Chicago, but it had not then seemed to him a book worth studying as closely as the works of the great philosophers or poets; at that time he had thought it an edifying book that spoke only to believers. But as he listened to Sacks point out and interpret strange things in the text, he realized that he had badly underestimated the subtlety of the Bible and that he had yet to learn how to read it. He returned to Chicago eager to have another look. The stories of Genesis especially took hold of him. There was, it seemed, deep wisdom to be found in the Hebrew Bible: it belonged in conversation with all his favorite philosophical texts, where, he began to suspect, it could more than hold its own. Some twenty years of teaching it provided the most enjoyable and successful experiences of his nearly thirty years in the classroom. *The Beginning of Wisdom*, the book that resulted, was addressed especially to the children of skeptics, in the hope they might be able, more quickly than he, to benefit from the deep and profoundly humanizing teachings of a great but neglected ancient tradition that belonged to them.

It was by a wandering way that Leon came to deal with a double difficulty—that the Yiddishkeit in which he was rooted lacked a future and that he himself lacked a past containing a theologically grounded upbringing. His difficulty resembled that embodied in the paradoxical remark attributed to a prominent twentieth-century secular Zionist leader who, when asked for a religious credo, said: "I believe in the Jewish people, and the Jewish people believe in God." Leon confronted his own difficulties, and the threat to human dignity posed by immensely powerful know-how in combination with unlimited willfulness and appetite, by an ever more intense study of the book by which God and the Jewish people are linked, finding in it a deeply instructive source of humanizing wisdom.

The wisdom with which Leon has been concerned should not be called theology. It might be better characterized as anthropology, albeit of an unusual sort. Through careful reading of the Hebrew Bible he seeks to see, not the face of divinity, but moral humanity as the image of divinity. What he has made an effort to promote is not the propagation of correct doctrine but serious conversation as a means of living rightly.

In the summer of 2001, when Leon accepted the chairmanship of the newly created President's Council on Bioethics, he did so on the understanding that its work would go beyond scrutinizing stem cell research—that he would be presiding over a national forum to explore the relation between progress in modern technological science and the fostering of human dignity. "I esteem scientific discovery, and I treasure medical advance," he told the *Chicago Tribune*. "But it's very clear that the powers we are now acquiring to alter the human body and mind also pose a certain threat to the long-term future of the things that make us human." Viewing his work of leading the Council as very like his work of teaching in the university, he said that it would be fine, both for the president and for the country as a whole, if consensus were to emerge, "but what we really want is the clearest, deepest, most comprehensive presentation of the issues, perhaps even by advocates who disagree with each other." The fact that he was an outspoken man of firm convictions frightened those who expected his chairmanship to become a weapon in the hands of a zealot. But all who knew Leon knew better. Even those whose opinions do not agree with his have seen how much he values strong relentless efforts to test and clarify his views and statements. He has always welcomed vigorous dialogue, even and especially when it concerns the most important matters and provides challenges to his most cherished beliefs. To a remarkable degree, he delights in having pointed out to him any weaknesses in what he says—delights in being pressed, and forced to rethink his thoughts, and give reply. As he told the *Chicago Tribune*: "I'm a person who believes that . . . by living and reading and thinking . . . you can change your mind about important things. Speech is not just fighting by another name—it's a process of inquiry to try to understand things better."

He means what he says. His book *The Beginning of Wisdom* must set a record for generously exhibiting, through quoting his students by name, how much a teacher can learn from his students' words. No one could love serious conversation more than Leon Kass does, and no one I know makes it more central to true friendship.

1

The Homecoming of Penelope

By Amy A. Kass

There is a moment, in Book xxiii of *The Odyssey*,[1] toward which much of Homer's narrative seemingly tends. It is the moment when Penelope finally acknowledges and fully welcomes Odysseus. She runs to him, throws her arms around his neck, and together they submit to the passion for weeping (xxiii.205-208, 231-32). A small miracle is here achieved: this man and woman, husband and wife, separated for twenty years, are reunited on the threshold of old age. Their tears—sad yet joyful, melancholy yet hopeful—bespeak the many griefs they have suffered, the sorrows they have endured, but also the unspeakable joy they must feel, knowing that the promises of their youth may yet be realized. Even we, the readers or hearers of the poem, who have with Penelope waited and made trial of Odysseus, we too rejoice, relieved and assured that Odysseus is home safe.

In describing this climactic moment, Homer uses a surprising simile. He compares Penelope's running to embrace Odysseus to the landing of swimming, shipwrecked men setting foot on shore having barely escaped their doom:

> As when the land appears welcome to men who are swimming,/ after Poseidon has smashed their strong-built ship on the open/ water, pounding it with the weight of the wind and the heavy/ seas, and only a few escape the gray water landward/ by swimming, with a thick scurf of salt coated upon them,/ and gladly they set foot on the shore, escaping the evil;/ so welcome was her husband to her as she looked upon him,/ and she could not let him go from the embrace of her white arms. (xxiii.233-40)

Homer's image vividly reminds us of Odysseus's long journey home: his many encounters with monsters of the deep; his bitterness and terrible aloneness; his

1. All references to *The Odyssey* and *The Iliad* are to the following editions: Homer, *The Odyssey*, Richmond Lattimore, trans. (New York: Harper & Row, 1977); Homer, *The Iliad*, Richmond Lattimore, trans. (Chicago: University of Chicago Press, 1974). Book and line numbers follow quotes; upper case Roman numerals are used for references to books of *The Iliad*, lower case for *The Odyssey*.

wonder and gratitude to find himself in Ithaka, at last. But the image refers not to Odysseus but to Penelope. We are asked to imagine *her* as a shipwrecked one come home. We are taken by surprise, for Penelope has always been at home.

Invariably stationed beside a column, Penelope seemed almost to be a part of the structure of the house. Holding scores of raucous suitors at bay for more than three years, she seemed more a master than a victim. Openly sorrowing for Odysseus, she seemed ever faithful to her household and to her love for her husband. Prudently deliberating, she seemed steady and cautious, never disoriented or cut off.

But Homer's image suggests another story. By providing us access to the inner life of Penelope these many years, it gives voice to things otherwise silent and hidden. By explicitly inviting us to compare the fate of Penelope with that of the wandering Odysseus, it subtly suggests that, though Penelope never left Ithaka, she too was somehow at sea; she too had been shipwrecked—remote and suspended, severed from the relations and deeds that make a house a home. True, it is Odysseus's return that restores the household. True, everything in the narrative seems primarily to serve Odysseus's successful homecoming. But despite the well laid plans of some friendly gods and goddesses, despite the able assistance of the artful Phaiakians, despite Odysseus's own renowned wit and resourcefulness, Odysseus cannot return successfully unless Penelope does also. Odysseus's return ultimately depends on Penelope—*her* inner return, *her* homecoming. To understand why this is so, we need first to consider Homer's portraits of men and women.

HOMER ON MAN AND WOMAN

In the world as sung by Homer, polarity is an important organizing principle.[2] Basic dualities of the natural and human worlds inform everything that happens. If one were to ask Homer, for example, what he meant by human nature, he would offer us two "catalogues"—one male, one female. For him, the differences between men and women so override their sameness as human beings that to be an individual is to be either a man (*aner*) or a woman (*gyne*), never a human being (*anthropos*) as such. Let us collect some of the differences.

In *The Iliad*, Homer sings about heroes, manly-men, whose pride is in their manliness or martial virtue: their courage, strength, and swiftness. Both the Achaian and the Trojan heroes insist on being men as opposed to women.

2. See Norman Austin, *Archery at the Dark of the Moon: Poetic Problems in Homer's Odyssey* (California: University of California Press, 1975), Chapter 2, "Unity in Multiplicity: Homeric Modes of Thought."

So Menelaos, for example, reproaches the Achaians (also known as Danaans), when they remain seated and stricken to silence by Hektor's challenge, thus:

> Ah me! You brave in words, you women, not men, of Achaia./ This will be a defilement upon us, shame upon shame piled,/ if no one of the Danaans goes out to face Hektor./ No, may all of you turn to water and earth, all of you/ who sit by yourselves with no life in you, utterly dishonoured. (vii.96-100)

Women are garrulous, cowardly, sedentary, spiritless, weak-willed, and fameless.

Men live their lives publicly—on the battlefield, in the assembly, and in the arena; women privately—mostly indoors, at home. Men distinguish themselves by their brilliant and singular deeds; women by the care and regularity, the patience and fidelity, with which they perform their daily labors. Men are polygamous, women monogamous. Women who stray are regarded as weak-willed, that is, true to their sex; their wayward actions, though lamentable and regrettable, are therefore forgivable. Men differentiate themselves by their ancestral virtue, each differing from the next by virtue of his remarkable ancestors. Women differentiate themselves by their marriages—indeed, women, once married, abandon their linkages to their own lineages—and each woman differs from the next by the bride-price she brings her parents. Men are spurred by echoes from the distant past and hopes for the even more distant future; women, by the call of the immediate present. Women are far more concrete, seldom escaping from the dailiness of life, ever sensitive to the liveliness of today, always concerned about things here and now. In terms of brilliance, women seem altogether pale by comparison with men. Yet Homer's women are never nonentities.

Though *The Iliad* is a song about heroes, the men fight over women: the Achaians and the Trojans fight for the sake of Helen, Agamemnon and Achilles (the argument that informs the epic) for the sake of Briseis. The plot of *The Iliad* unfolds the sense in which Helen, and perhaps Briseis too, is more than a mere pretext: the abduction of Helen unleashed the war, and the love of Helen and what she represents somehow animates the warriors almost to the end. Though *The Odyssey* is the story of Odysseus, the *polytropos aner*, the man of many ways, throughout the poem it is women who direct, counsel, and protect this endlessly resourceful man. Moreover, home, the woman's domain, is not only not disdained, but it appears to be the *telos* (the prime "purpose") of the narrated action, perhaps even of Homer's tale.

As for the importance of women, take, for example, Nausikaa, the young princess of Phaiakia, whose courage and good sense, gentleness and loveliness, revive and restore Odysseus's ailing body and, even more important, his crushed spirit. He himself acknowledges this when he tells Nausikaa in parting, "You have given me [back] my [human] life" (viii.468).[3] Or, take Antikleia, Odysseus's mother, whose unexpected ghostly presence and speech, during his journey to Hades, makes Odysseus starkly confront his own mortality and drives home for him the price of his long absence. Or, Eurykleia, the loyal and trustworthy housekeeper in Ithaka, whose efficient keeping of accounts safeguards the family wealth. Or, the many goddesses, from Athene, who masterminds Odysseus's homecoming, to Ino, who, taking pity on Odysseus as he suffers on the open sea, gives him her veil, to the enchanting Calypso, or Circe, or any of the other mysterious females.

As for the primacy and significance of home, Odysseus's brief adventure with the Lotus-Eaters speaks volumes. The Lotus-Eaters gave Odysseus's men lotus, the food of oblivion, making them forget who they were, where they had been, and where they were headed. In his succinct description of this adventure, Odysseus says twice that the lotus made his men "forget the way home." To forget who you are and to forget home, it seems, are one and the same. One's human survival and, even more, one's very identity, depend on memory, principally memory of home. One's relations to home make one who and what one is.

Though women are neither his avowed subject nor his main concern, Homer's women are neither simply servile nor merely perfunctory. Though they are not obviously central in Homer's world, they appear to be central to Homer's thought. Indeed, one noted commentator, Samuel Butler, especially impressed by Homer's portraits of women and the importance he attaches to domestic life in *The Odyssey*, argued that the poem could only have been written by a woman.[4] But however much we may argue about the poet's gender, there is little doubt that Homer's women—like Homer himself—weave a subtle and not altogether invisible web through the action of both epics and seem ultimately to control and ensnare the whole.

But if Homer's women are indispensable for understanding Homer's thought, weaving is indispensable for understanding womanliness. Weaving is the only specifically female activity in both epics, and both women and goddesses weave. Weaving, both actually and symbolically, integrates and holds together the various strands and aspects of womanhood, and thereby also of home. So Hektor commands Andromache, "Go . . . back to our house, and take up your own work,/ the loom and the distaff . . . the men must see to the fighting" (vi.490-92).

3. The Greek word here translated "life" is *bios* which suggests human life, not *zoë* or animal life. Odysseus, in effect, credits her with giving him back his humanity.

4. See Samuel Butler, *The Authoress of The Odyssey* (Chicago: University of Chicago Press, 1967 [1897]).

Women's work is in the home, at the loom. If one's work reveals what one is essentially, then one suspects that it is in relation to weaving that a woman would show herself most fully. What then, according to Homer, is weaving?

WOMEN'S WORK: WEAVING

Homer alludes to many activities and instruments closely connected to weaving—shepherding, shearing and carding wool, collecting and refining dyes, to mention but a few. But two seem particularly important: spinning, an activity separable from but preparatory to weaving, and weaving proper.

In spinning, a bundle of unworked carded wool is held on a distaff from which it is drawn into a long and continuous, largely homogeneous, single thread, by means of a spindle. To spin (in Greek *klothein*, the root of our words "cloth" and "to clothe") requires patience and dexterity: one must carefully and laboriously draw out and carry through a strand, which is necessarily always delicate and weak.

Homer connects the activity of spinning with the work of the Spinners (*Klothes*) or Fates (*Moirai*), those dreaded women who spin the threads of human beings, allotting their portions or destinies (vii.197). When one is born, the Spinners spin out the thread or destiny of one's future life, which means, in the first instance, that they determine its length. They fix the time of one's death: one's "day of Fate" is, in Homer, the day of one's death. The Fates are restrictive; they enjoin a limit. Even the Olympian Deities, though themselves immortal and ageless, have their powers strictly limited by the Fates. What the Fates prescribe for human beings, not even Zeus can alter. As Athene tells Telemachos: "Not even the gods can fend it away from a man they love, when once the destructive doom of leveling death has fastened upon him" (iii.236-38).[5]

The spinning of woolen threads is thus like the merely natural activity of generation; the spun thread, an image of a naked, undifferentiated life in all its precariousness. While both convey the unavoidable fragility and vulnerability of embodied life simply, the solitary thread suggests the special weakness of a life lived cut off and isolated from others. By drawing together spinning and fate, Homer seems to suggest that a woman who spins is somehow akin to the goddesses of natural necessity.

But if spinning reminds one of the dark realm of necessity, weaving brings one to life and civilization. Weaving, in Homer, takes us to the realm of the Olympians. Here not the Fates but Athene holds sway.[6]

5. See Walter Otto, *The Homeric Gods* (London: Thames & Hudson, 1979), Chapter 7, "Fate."
6. Ibid., Chapter 3, Part 1, "Athena."

In weaving, a wooden loom or frame is erected and the warp, consisting of vertical threads, is stretched and immobilized upon it. A shuttle containing thread, the woof or the weft, is slid horizontally from side to side, backward and forward, between the warp threads to form the web. To weave is to bind together by interlacing threads in a steady and orderly way. Weaving integrates several strands into an articulated whole without doing violence to any of the parts. Unlike stitching, weaving creates form without violating matter, yet the woven whole does transform its parts. By being brought into union with other threads, each strand is made stronger and less vulnerable. Loose ends are tied in and protected. The web, a careful and sturdy yet delicate and intricate balance of many separate threads, assumes a character and texture of its own. By thus transforming the parts, the web not only preserves them but endows each one with a meaningful place in a patterned whole. Sometimes, the pattern becomes very elaborate and even articulate, as when variations of ordered sequences are used to weave a picture or a story into the web.

A woven web is thus a coming together of art and nature or, one might even say, of humanity and the cosmic order. For, ultimately, one weaves one's web out of the sun, which nourishes the grass, which nourishes the sheep, who grow the wool, which is spun into thread, which is preserved when it is patterned on a loom in weaving. Weaving is the very model of bringing nature under the artful use of intelligence and rational order.

No wonder Athene dowers weavers. For clear-sighted, bright-eyed Athene, the daughter of Zeus who most clearly resembles her father in intelligence and counsel, who kindles the courage of warriors but disdains their fury and rashness, inspirits human beings to meet necessity in a sensible or prudent way. She plots and contrives with an eye to the future, yet never loses sight of what is concretely before her, here and now. Her support of artfulness is matched by her deep concern for lawful arrangements, both evident in her patronage of weavers. For weaving is the orderly application of artful intelligence, guided by set rules and customs, which brings together disparate natural materials and forms them into harmonious union in the service of protection and perpetuation. Indeed, weaving is a wonderful image of marriage and homemaking, those paradigmatic human activities that preserve and perpetuate, and the woven web is a wonderful image of family.

In family—also a domain of Athene—otherwise solitary and fragile individuals take their place, find connections, gain support. Though each life, like each spun fiber, still has a beginning and an end, these ends are bound into a larger whole and related also to those that come before and after. The weaver, like the homemaker—or the statesman, also frequently compared to the weaver—is the unifier, the harmonizer, the ruler. She articulates the order that not only protects our vulnerable natures in the face of grim necessity, but that, given voice in shared speeches and conventions, humanizes and gives meaning to this particular web of interconnected lives.

Weaving is not only a metaphor for the ordering of a family. Most literally and concretely, weaving creates and adorns a household. The woman who weaves provides for its prosperity and perpetuation. For Homer, the loom, along with the hearth and bed, stands at the very center of a home. No loom, no home.

Women weave coverings for the body, the bed, the floor, the table, the wall, the grave—robes, blankets, rugs, cloths, tapestries, and shrouds. Such coverings not only protect the objects they cover; they also contribute to the wealth and substance of the household. Treasured tapestries and shining robes are passed from generation to generation; as we still say, we treasure our heirlooms. Some of the woven wealth begets more wealth: women weave sails that outfit ships that carry men abroad to increase their substance even further. Woven goods, used as guest gifts, also increase the influence of a household, through the ties they form with other households. It is no accident that Homer's Phaiakians, people who live in the greatest luxury, are the best weavers, the best sailors, and the best hosts—and, we note for later, also the best appreciators of stories.

Weavings not only protect us in the present and pile up wealth for the future. They also help us mark and render meaningful the passage of time. The daily and regular work of weaving punctuates, even as it flows along with, the regular stream of days. Seasons too are marked with the loom, by weaving different wear for winter and summer. Most important, weaving marks humanly significant times of life—the time of birth, the time of marriage, the time of death; it clothes the newborn, veils the bride, and enshrouds the departed. As weaving introduces patterns that cover over the homogeneity of unwoven thread, so woven garments commemorate and render visible the human patterns that cover over the otherwise undifferentiated and silent passage of the time of our lives. And for the weaver herself, as weaving is her work, so her weavings reveal much of the story of her life.

Thus we see why weaving is frequently a metaphor also for song and story. The Homeric word for story, *oime*, originally conveyed the imagery of weaving.[7] Through telling their stories, human beings try to hold together and give meaning to the various threads and times of their lives. Poets, inspired by that other daughter of Zeus, the Muse, are super-weavers; they bring together the story-threads of many lives to form a tapestry—in the grandest case, presenting the cosmic whole, showing us the relations not only of one life

7. Gregory Nagy, *The Best of the Achaians* (Baltimore: Johns Hopkins University Press, 1979), 18.

or household with another, but also of human beings to the immortal gods, above and below.

Remembering the gods reminds us that weaving, like other human arts in Homer, is not without its limits. On the one hand, though it confronts Fate, weaving cannot defeat it; it can anticipate change and decay, but it cannot thereby guarantee permanence. On the other hand, though dowered by Athene and the Olympians, weaving—human art generally—cannot make men godlike or independent. The arts tempt us to self-sufficiency, to rely only on our own cleverness; but weaving rightly understood requires remembering the gods and, generally, our dependence on things not of our own making. The goddess dowers weavers not because she likes them but because they need her. Good weavers acknowledge both these limits: the superior power of Fate or necessity, the superior wisdom of the divine. Expert weavers have knowledge akin to the Fates and a dowry from Athene. This does not enable them to predict the future or avoid suffering. It does, however, give them some understanding of how things stand between human life and the divine, and hence of what may be realistically possible within human experience.

Homer's weavers neither deny nor ignore human futility. But unlike the heroic warriors they do not meet necessity by going forth to beat it down. Weaving, a species of wealth-getting, symbolic of marriage and procreation, in the service of home, meets necessity by working harmoniously with the rhythms of nature. To weave is to live in time, to be ever aware of one's relation to those around one, as well as to those from the past and the future. Thus, by working in accordance with the permanently changing whole, weavers knit permanence into their own lives. Weavers seem, then, to embody the best possible relation between nature and human art. Womanly excellence points to the best human possibility.[8]

THE WANDERINGS OF PENELOPE

If weaving points to the right order of things, weaving gone astray signifies disorder. Homer gives us two conspicuous examples: Helen's weaving in *The Iliad*—weaving that is self-glorifying—and Penelope's weaving in *The Odyssey*—weaving that becomes self-denying. Both embody aspirations to timelessness: Helen's, the de-

8. Such understanding is displayed especially by the wife of King Alkinoos, Arete, an excellent weaver, whose name means "she who is prayed to or invoked." She is said to have been given "such pride of place as no other woman on earth is given." She is held high by her children, her husband, and by the people, "who look toward her as to a god when they see her,/ and speak in salutation as she walks about in her city. For there is no good intelligence that she herself lacks./ She dissolves quarrels, even among men, when she favors them" (vii.66-74).

sire to live forever, to have undying fame; Penelope's, the desire to hold on to the past, to freeze the moment and make time stand still. Both are signs of sterility and fruitlessness. Looking at Helen's weaving makes the problem with Penelope's all the clearer.

Everything about Helen reminds us of war. Even in *The Odyssey*, when she is back safely at home with Menelaos, the war remains prominent in her life: We first come upon her celebrating the marriage of her only child to the son of Achilles, warrior par excellence. Though not weaving, she is sitting beside her silver-wheeled wool basket, an object paralleled only by the wheeled tripods in *The Iliad* (xviii.375), and regaling her guests with stories about the war.

When we first meet Helen in *The Iliad*, she is in her chamber "weaving a great web, a red, folding robe, and working into it the numerous struggles/ of Trojans, breakers of horses, and bronze armoured Achaians,/ struggles that they endured for her sake at the hands of the war god" (iii.125-28). Helen, who is always associated with "shimmering garments" or "luminously spun" robes, is here weaving such a gown, but one that must always remain imperfect. For the story she is weaving into it can know no end.[9]

Helen is weaving into the robe the story that Homer follows. It is the pattern of heroic ambition, a pattern which she herself provokes. For Helen of Argos, divine among women, daughter of Zeus, beautiful and terrible Helen, both reflects and embodies the end of heroic ambition: to be forever young and beautiful, to be immortal and ageless, to be honored as the gods are honored (viii.538-40). To lift Helen's veil is to behold someone who is always young and beautiful, yet forever unattainable, beyond the reach of all men.[10] Though the warriors, in the course of *The Iliad*, become liberated from the immediate purpose of the war—the recovery of Helen and her possessions for Menelaos—they are never liberated from the desire to be united with immortal and ageless beauty. The love of fame and glory is essentially no different from the love of Helen.

Though Helen is often within a house, she is never of the home. She belongs neither to the home of Menelaos nor to the home of Paris. Her ability to imitate the voices of the wives of each of the Argives suggests her inability to be fully the wife of any one man. Similarly, her weaving, which records and anticipates struggles that men endure and will continue to endure for her sake, points to her abiding remoteness and elusiveness. Helen's beauty isolates her, elevates her, and

9. Of Helen's eleven epithets, four point to her divine origins, six to her appearance, and one to her horrible, accursed, or horrifying aspect, indicating her capacity to make one shudder.

10. For an interesting discussion of this idea see Kenneth J. Achity, *Homer's Iliad: The Shield of Memory* (Carbondale, Illinois: Southern Illinois University Press, 1978), Chapter 2, "Helen and Her Galaxy: 1," and Chapter 3, "Helen and Her Galaxy: 2."

finally transmutes her into an object; unwittingly, she even objectifies herself in her weaving. Not coincidentally, Helen is no longer fertile: She and Paris have no issue, and when she returns to Menelaos, "the gods gave no more children to Helen" (iv.12).

Helen's weaving, like Helen herself, can belong to no one, not now, not later. But like Homer's poem, it illuminates, as it commemorates, the futility of heroic ambition and the terrible human cost it exacts. Also like *The Iliad* itself, Helen's weaving makes clear the meaning of her prophetic remark, that Zeus set upon herself and Paris an evil fate so that they "shall be made into things of song for the men of the future" (vi.358). In short, Helen's unfinishable weaving shows us why men forever seek glory, and why its pursuit is forever a snare and a delusion.

Unlike Helen, very little about Penelope reminds us of the war. Penelope, whose name means "spinner" or "spinster," reminds us always of home. Praised for her steadiness, loyalty, self-restraint, discretion, and carefulness, and prized for her intelligence and beautiful handiwork, Penelope is always at home. Whether stationed at her loom, or in her upper chamber, or beside a stout column in the strongly built palace of Odysseus, she seems the very incarnation of the idea of home and Homer's ideal of womanhood. To lift Penelope's veil is to behold a living woman with hopes and joys and sorrows, someone essentially strong and enduring, prudent and thoughtful.

Penelope's endurance and cleverness are combined in her plot of weaving and unweaving. She strives, with the aid of her weaving, to save her home. Yet the clever device, notwithstanding—or perhaps because of—its success, contributes to the problems of her home. Perhaps worst of all, unbeknownst to herself, it even carries her away in spirit from hearth and home. Penelope's weavings are Penelope's wanderings.

The Odyssey begins at the end of things. It has been twenty years since Odysseus left Ithaka. For the last three, almost four of those years, Penelope has been besieged by suitors—more than a hundred haughty, arrogant, rapacious, overbearing, shameless young men who delight in games and gluttony. They while away the hours, as they eat away the substance of Odysseus. With their minds forever on pleasure, they are indifferent to the gods, ignoring both omens and strangers. They listen to sad songs—even the latest song of the sad return of the Danaans—but regard them only as pleasing distractions to fill the hours between eating and bedding down. These mindless and shallow pleasure-seekers remind us both of the Lotus-Eaters, for their pursuit of pleasure, and of the Cyclops, for their depthless vision, cannibalistic appetites, and singular indifference to the gods. Not only have they forgotten the gods; they seem even to have forgotten why they are where they are. Their siege is the completion of the decay in Ithaka that began when Odysseus left for Troy; the rot within Odysseus's home mirrors the corruption outside.

Antinoos (whose name means "hostile-minded") and Eurymachos ("wide-fighter") are the leaders of the pack, the sons, respectively, of Eupeithes ("compliant") and Polybos ("many oxen"). Their very names betoken what has happened in Ithaka: the elders, compliant and ignorant, have become indifferent and have withdrawn all claims to authority. The suitors go unchecked within the house of Odysseus because they have already subdued their parents, perhaps by the same contrariness and combativeness. There has been no assembly, no public governance in Ithaka, for twenty years. But perhaps nothing depicts the decadence of Ithaka as clearly as the sight that greets all guests, just before the entrance to the palace: a dunghill on top of which sits Odysseus's once splendid dog Argos, riddled with dog ticks, utterly neglected and long forgotten (xvii.290-323). Like Argos, Ithaka lacks both strength and substance. Ithaka has been abandoned.

Threatened from without and within, Penelope strove to make good Odysseus's charge: to care for his parents, Laertes and Antikleia; to rear and educate their son Telemachos; and to keep their home intact, ruling it until Telemachos came of age. Ever concerned that someone would come and deceive her, she actively sought to hold herself steady. The clever ruse she fashioned to deal with the suitors made manifest her effort of many years.

Penelope set up a great loom and for three years wove and unwove, undoing at night what she wove during the daytime. Allegedly weaving a shroud for her father-in-law Laertes, her loom ran empty day after day. Penelope wove emptiness to combat disorder, vacancy to guard against disorientation. Endlessly raveling and unraveling, weaving and unweaving, her efforts were productive of nothing.[11] Her weaving parodied weaving, or rather, it was more like an image of spinning. Threads were stretched out and twisted, only to be untwisted and rewound. Her threads, like her life, remained unconnected. By endlessly going round and round, covering and uncovering the same ground, she allowed her threads—like her life—to remain unmeasured, indeterminate, unfinished. In this activity, Penelope lived out her name: "Penelope, weaver" became "Penelope, spinner"; "Penelope, wife" became "Penelope, spinster."

Penelope's attitude toward the suitors mirrors her indeterminate weaving and unweaving. She holds them at bay, neither refusing nor accepting their proposals of marriage (i.249-50). She keeps her distance but sends them flattering

11. For a different, yet compelling, interpretation of Penelope's weaving, see Edwin Muir, "The Return of Odysseus," in *Collected Poems* (New York: Oxford University Press, 1965), and Mary Hannah Jones, "A First Reading of *The Odyssey*," in *St. John's College Prize Papers, 1977-78* (Annapolis: St. John's College Press, 1978).

messages (ii.90; xiii.379-81). She vacillates between active concern and passive withdrawal. She cries at night, but looks radiant by day. She tries to keep them away by holding them near, and her efforts to do so completely consume her attention and energies. Penelope's threads fail to ensnare her suitors, but they almost ensnare her. The emptiness she wove to deal with the emptiness she must have felt became habitual. Her attempts to leave room for Odysseus themselves almost replaced him. Her efforts to preserve her home attenuated her attachments to it.

Penelope's weaving and unweaving, her courting and uncourting, her habitual grieving and despair, show Penelope to be out of touch with time. In her desperate attempt to hold fast to what was, she ceases to live in a present that looks to the future, and thus acquires a false relation even to the past. She is suspended in time and place and becomes frozen within. Neither cutting nor weaving her threads, Penelope suspends herself from a single strand that becomes ever more fragile. She loses sight of the web of relations that make a house a home. She has forgotten Laertes and neglected her son Telemachos. She has become inhospitable to strangers, a sure sign (in Homer) of her estrangement from the gods. Her home is in shambles. The charge Odysseus gave her when he left for Troy seems to have been all but forgotten.

It should go without saying that none of this does Penelope intend. She is not guilty of willful wrong-doing; she faces terrible circumstances and seems rather to be pitied than blamed. Nevertheless, her attempts to beat back grief by making time stand still and to cope with despair by means of clever devices actually alienate her from her home and make her complicit in its decay.

Though *The Odyssey* begins with the council of Zeus that plots Odysseus's homecoming, Odysseus cannot return home unless Penelope does also. One cannot have a homecoming if there is no home. Reweaving the web of relations that comprise his home, however less prominent than Odysseus's many feats and defeats, is the deeper burden of much of the narrative. And this depends, most fundamentally, on Penelope.

If she is to restore life to her home, Penelope must again begin to weave. She must bring herself back into time. She must bring herself back into relation with her family and her gods. Only then will she be prepared to accept Odysseus, and to give him his home once again.

THE HOMECOMING OF PENELOPE

As the poem begins, Zeus, taking advantage of the absence of Poseidon (Odysseus's nemesis), calls a council and begins to reorder the affairs of men.

The time is right for Athene to make her appeal on behalf of Odysseus. In Ithaka, Penelope's ruse has been discovered, compelling her to finish the shroud. But what happens next depends on whether she is able, too, to reweave her unraveled life. Perhaps this is why it takes two councils of the gods to arrange the homecoming of Odysseus.

Of the many stages in Penelope's return, three appear to be decisive: the awakening and departure of Telemachos; the stories Penelope hears and tells as she sits beside the fire conversing with the "stranger," whom we know to be Odysseus disguised as a beggar; and finally, the test of the bed. Consider each in turn.

As we open the door to Odysseus's house, we find Telemachos, seated among the suitors, in the smoke-filled halls, grieving and daydreaming. Though aware of their malevolence, he knows not what he could or should do or even whether he could or should do anything. He consoles himself by imagining the great father, whom he has never seen, returning, scattering the suitors, and setting things right. Adorned in a foolproof disguise, Athene (as "Mentes" or "teacher") pays him a timely visit. Her questions are pointed: "Are you, big as you are, the very child of Odysseus? . . . What feast is this, what gathering? How does it concern you" (i.207, 225)? In responding, Telemachos promptly gets up and moves, physically but, more important, also psychically. He readily confesses his own ignorance, impotence, rage, and shame. Recognizing the able student that he is, Athene counters with some advice. She urges Telemachos to "consider some means by which [*he*] can force the suitors out" (i.269-70) but, leaving nothing to chance, she also makes specific suggestions: convene the assembly and travel abroad. Then, purposely dropping her disguise, she flies off.

Thus emboldened and inspirited, Telemachos straightway begins to act. But like many a young man, then and now, his first impulse—his own "considered means"—is to test his new powers against his mother, who now makes her first appearance in the poem, presumably for just this purpose. In no uncertain terms, Telemachos tells her to leave the hall of besotted suitors, to go back to her loom and distaff. Penelope retreats in "amazement," and, we imagine, Telemachos does too, even as he mulls over his next steps.

As instructed, the next morning Telemachos convenes the assembly, the first assembly held in Ithaka in twenty years. With the leader's scepter in hand, he publicly denounces the suitors for besetting his mother "against her will," warns them that things hitherto endured will "no longer" be so, and threatens to sue them for recompense. But in the midst of his speech, suddenly overwhelmed by his own bravado, Telemachos bursts into tears, and dashes the scepter to the ground. Antinoos's response in defense of the suitors turns out to strengthen his resolve. "You have no cause to blame the Achaian suitors," Antinoos retorts,

> it is your own dear mother and she is greatly resourceful./ And now it is the third year, and will be the fourth year presently,/ since she has been denying the Achaians./ For she holds out hope to all, and makes promises to each man,/ sending us messages, but her mind has other intentions./ And here is another stratagem of her heart's devising./ She set up a great loom in her palace, and set to weaving/ . . . a shroud, for the hero Laertes, . . ./ Thereafter in the daytime she would weave at her great loom,/ but in the night she would have torches set by, and undo it./ . . . but when the fourth year came . . . we found her in the act of undoing her glorious weaving./ So, against her will and by force, she had to finish it. (ii.87-110)

Telemachos had no doubt witnessed Penelope's weaving, and her behavior toward the suitors, but he apparently had made little or nothing of either. Antinoos forced his hand; concern for his mother's plight spurs him on, just as concern for his safety will soon rouse Penelope. As long as the weaving ruse held, Telemachos could remain a child. The success of Penelope's stratagem prevented him from growing up. Telemachos must now travel to serve his own pressing needs, but also for the sake of his mother and the restoration of the home. His journey not only launches Telemachos into adulthood, it brings into the open the criminal intentions of the suitors, and thus forces Penelope, now again weaving, also to awaken, to dislodge herself from her routinized and habitual attitude of grief. Note more closely her reaction.

Telemachos's departure was initially undetected by Penelope. She neither noticed he was missing nor heard any report of his journey for several days. Her earlier amazement at his sudden assertiveness did not suffice to overcome her habitual attitude. She is now most brutally tested. Penelope hears of Telemachos's departure only after the suitors do. Thus she learns of his journey and the suitors' plot to kill him at the same time. She collapses in utter despair; clouds of sorrow descend upon her; she falls to the floor and weeps pitifully; she refuses all food and drink. Homer compares Penelope, in her despair, to a besieged lion, who "caught in a crowd of men turns about/ in fear, when they have made a treacherous circle about him" (iv.787-94). She seems instinctively to understand that the plot against the life of her son is an attack on her own life. At last she sees that the fate of Telemachos cannot be separated from her own.

Penelope's fear and concern for Telemachos abruptly draw her back to the present and turn her attention to the future. Pondering what to do next, she not only thinks of Laertes but also recalls and prays to the gods (iv.735). She has a dream in which she contrasts the fame of her husband with the innocence of her son, the grief she has had for her husband with the even greater grief she now has for her son. Though just the beginning of her return, the poet underscores its importance. The narrative abruptly shifts to Ogygia, an island in the midst of nowhere, where Odysseus has been hidden away for seven years. Having started the homecoming of Penelope, and hence the reconstruction of his home, Athene, mastermind of the whole, can now give her full attention to Odysseus.

Penelope is never again indifferent to her fate. Recognizing the urgency of her need, she now plots and calculates her every move, even before she settles on a complete strategy. She shows herself to her suitors. She publicly rebukes them, confronting them with their own criminal behavior (xvi.431). She prays for the death of the suitors (xxvii.494). She listens attentively to the stories announcing Odysseus's return (xvii.150-61; 512-27). Indeed, she seems to turn the very homecoming of Telemachos into an inquisition about Odysseus. And from the moment the stranger, Odysseus disguised as a beggar, enters her halls, her attention is riveted upon him. We are brought to the threshold of Book xix, and the second stage in Penelope's homecoming.

It is evening. The halls of the palace have been emptied of the suitors and miraculously illuminated by a god-made light. Eager to question the beggar, Penelope orders her servant to set up a chair. Penelope and Odysseus sit beside the fireside, alone together for the first time in twenty years. As they begin to speak, each is guided by his own concern: Odysseus must discover whether Penelope can and will accept him back; Penelope must find a way out of her predicament, which will preserve her own future and the future of Telemachos. Both purposes depend, as Odysseus seems quickly to perceive, on Penelope's self-understanding. Though she has recovered the will to act, she still lacks self-knowledge. To know what she can or should do, she must first recall who she was and what she has become. She must, in short, reweave her past into her present. This is the main burden of Book xix, the central and decisive episode in the homecoming of Penelope. It is accomplished by the artful weaving of stories.

Penelope is the first to speak. She asks the stranger: "What man are you and whence? Where is your city? Your parents?" Odysseus responds with the utmost craft and cunning:

> Lady, no mortal man on the endless earth could have cause/ to find fault with you; your fame goes up into the wide heaven,/ as of some king who, as a blameless man and god-fearing,/ and ruling as lord over many powerful people,/ upholds the way of good government, and the black earth yields him/ barley and wheat, his trees are heavy with fruit, his sheepflocks/ continue to bear young, the sea gives

> him fish, because of/ his good leadership, and his people prosper under him./ Question me now here in your house about all other/ matters, but do not ask who I am, the name of my country,/ for fear you may increase in my heart its burden of sorrow/ as I think back; I am very full of grief (*polystonos*), and I should not/ sit in the house of somebody else with my lamentation/ and wailing. It is not good to go on mourning forever. (xix.106-120)

Mindful of the delicate task before him, Odysseus attempts to bring Penelope back into the past. Before he identifies himself as Odysseus twenty years older, he tries to bring the young Odysseus to mind. He does so by describing Penelope now as if she were Odysseus then, comparing her to a good king—faultless, famous, blameless, god-fearing, justly ruling a fruitful and powerful people. He identifies himself beguilingly as *polystonos* (one "very full of grief"), an epithet especially fitting Penelope. And, in the guise of explaining his reluctance to answer her questions, he offers Penelope advice: "It is not good to go on mourning forever." Odysseus has attempted to turn Penelope's attention away from the stranger before her; he has invited her to see how things stand with herself. In effect, he returns her question: "Who are you?" Penelope takes the bait:

> Stranger, all of my excellence, my beauty and figure,/ were ruined by the immortals at that time when the Argives took ship/ for Ilion, and with them went my husband, Odysseus./ If he were to come back to me and take care of my life, then/ my reputation would be more great and splendid. As it is/ now, I grieve: such evils the god has let loose upon me./ For all the greatest men who have power in the islands,/ . . . and all who in rocky Ithaka are holders of lordships,/ all these are my suitors against my will, and they wear my house out./ Therefore, I pay no attention to strangers, nor to suppliants,/ nor yet to heralds, who are in the public service, but always/ I waste away at the inward heart, longing for Odysseus. (xix.124-36)

Instead of the manly excellence, fame, and widespread power of which Odysseus had spoken, Penelope speaks of her ruined beauty and figure, her neediness and insufficiency. Instead of the good order and flourishing of Ithaka, she notes her own enslavement and the wearing away of her house. And, instead of respect for the gods, she gives evidence of her neglect—her long indifference to strangers, suppliants, and public servants.

Without further prompting, Penelope is now moved to tell her own story, the story of her web, from the moment the idea was put into her head until the moment it was detected and she was forced to finish it. Only this once do we learn about the web from the spinner herself. In concluding, she remarks:

> Now I cannot escape from this marriage; I can no longer/ think of another plan; my parents are urgent with me/ to marry; my son is vexed as they eat away our livelihood;/ he sees it all; he is a grown man now, most able/ to care for the house, and it is to him Zeus grants this honor. (xix.157-61)

Penelope's tale is indeed revelatory to the stranger before her but no doubt to herself as well. For in pulling together the threads of the story that can answer Odysseus's tacit question—"Who are you?"—Penelope must scrutinize her life and show its meaning also to herself. *She* articulates how, despite her good intentions, she neglected everything—her parents, her son, her house, her gods. No wonder she now sees only one alternative before her: to marry and to leave this house.

Once again, Penelope turns to Odysseus and asks, "Who are you?" Odysseus responds with care and tact, patience and respect, and with a story. He addresses the distraught Penelope for the first time as the "respected" (or "honored") wife of Odysseus, son of Laertes. He identifies his beggared self as a man of noble birth, the son of great-hearted Deukalion, the grandson of Minos, a King who conversed with Zeus, and tells of the time, twenty years ago, when he first met Odysseus and entertained him in his house. Odysseus thus artfully provides Penelope an opportunity to begin to overcome her neglect of strangers and her many years of estrangement. For in calling her "respected" wife of Odysseus, he invites her to think of herself as such. By producing noble credentials, he urges her to try to penetrate his ragged appearance. In reporting his own hospitality, he beckons her to reciprocate. Just at this point Homer remarks: "He knew how to say many false things that were like true sayings" (xix.203).

Odysseus's strategy hits its mark:

> As she listened her tears ran and her body was melted,/ as the snow melts along the high places of the mountains/ when the West Wind has piled it there, but the South Wind melts it,/ and as it melts the rivers run full flood. (xix.204-207)

The tears here prompted by the story, unlike the tears she had shed so often alone, melt her body and restore her to life. Penelope, like the mountain, frozen within for so very long, begins to melt. In the sequel, her words and deeds reveal the change.

In their subsequent conversation, Penelope moves ever closer in speech to the stranger, calling Odysseus first "pitiable stranger," then "stranger and guest," and then "guest dearer than any others." She recognizes the stranger as a contemporary of Odysseus's and, for the first time, she offers him hospitality. She asks Eurykleia,

Odysseus's own trusted nursemaid since birth, to wash "the feet of one who is the same age as your master," who "must by this time have just such hands and feet" (xix.358-59), but she does not yet penetrate Odysseus's disguise. At the moment Eurykleia makes her discovery of Odysseus's identifiable scar and precipitously drops his foot into the basin of water, Penelope's glance is averted, her mind is elsewhere.

After the foot bath, Penelope and Odysseus resume their conversation though it is by now quite late. Though still undecided about what to do, the alternatives Penelope contemplates are now somewhat different. She recalls the story of Pandareos's daughter, the greenwood nightingale. Grieftorn, like the legendary nightingale to whom she now compares herself, who killed her own son when "the madness was on her" (xix.523), Penelope wonders whether to stay beside her son *or* to marry the best of the Achaians. She no longer insists that she must go away.

Continuing, she asks Odysseus to listen to a dream she had and to interpret it for her. The dream is about numerous geese in her house, whom she "loved to watch" (xix.537). Suddenly, a great eagle swoops down and kills them all. She laments their death, crying out in sorrow as they are slain. But the eagle reappears, revealing himself to be Odysseus. The Odysseus before her readily agrees with the interpretation of the Odysseus in her dream, namely, that the dream portends the impending death of the suitors.

Though Penelope now insists that her dream was merely a vain wish, almost immediately after hearing the stranger's response, she knows exactly what she will do: she will select her new husband through the contest of the bow. Odysseus applauds her decision. Penelope abruptly ends their conversation, claiming now the need for sleep, the sleep she had moments before claimed never to be hers. What has happened?

Though one cannot be certain, we suspect that in trying to explain her situation to the stranger, Penelope brought *herself* to self-knowledge. In telling these tales, in comparing herself to Pandareos's daughter who unintentionally killed her own son and in her dream of the geese in her house whom "she loved to watch," Penelope recognized her own complicity. What the departure of Telemachos had begun seems here to have been brought to completion. Through telling her story, and with the aid of stories woven into it, Penelope has penetrated her own self-deception. She now sees herself clearly, and her self-recognition enables her, too, to penetrate the disguise of the man before her. Now that she knows herself, she also recognizes Odysseus, and immediately knows what to do. Consider her plan.

Both the bow and the contest Penelope proposes had belonged to Odysseus. They were his peculiar marks. He carried his bow and only he could string it.

The bow linked him to the generations of the heroes; it originally belonged to the hero Iphitos. The contest, in which he excelled, enabled him to display his manly excellence. The bow had been stored for the past twenty years in the "inmost recess" of the house (xxi.8). To retrieve it, and hence, to set up the contest, Penelope is in fact re-asserting and declaring her ties to the past, to her husband, and to the house of Odysseus.

That Penelope surely knows what she is doing is affirmed by the fact that she argues for letting the stranger participate in the contest and does not leave until he is given the polished bow. And, though *they* do not yet recognize the stranger, the suitors too recognize that they are being asked to compete against Odysseus.

As everyone knows, Odysseus strings the bow, wins the contest, and rids the house of the suitors. Penelope will not go to another house; her husband has reclaimed his home. And yet Penelope's homecoming is not yet complete. Though she has again committed herself to her home and revived her ties to the past, she now must wonder whether these are sufficient to secure the future. As she now too-well knows, time, wanderings, and hardships do strange things to the spirit; she must wonder about what they have done to Odysseus. No question, the stranger with the scar on his foot is none other than Odysseus. No question, in manly display with the bow he is the same Odysseus. But such signs do not reveal the heart. Penelope, perhaps all the more because of Odysseus's bloody slaughter of the suitors, wonders what twenty years of war and trouble have done to the best of the Achaians. She watches and waits, again holding herself aloof and steady, wondering just *who* it is, who has come home.

The answer comes in Book xxiii. His patience exhausted by her aloofness, Odysseus complains to Penelope:

> You are so strange. . . . / No other woman, with spirit as stubborn as yours, would keep back/ as you are doing from her husband who, after much suffering,/ came at last in the twentieth year back to his own country./ Come then, nurse, make me up a bed, so that I can use it/ here; for this woman has a heart of iron within her. (xxiii.166-72)

Penelope seizes the occasion to find out what she most needs to know, putting Odysseus to the test:

> You are so strange. I am not proud, nor indifferent,/ nor puzzled beyond need, but I know very well what you looked like/ when you went in the ship with the sweeping oars, from Ithaka./ Come then, Eurykleia, and make up a firm bed for him/ outside the well-fashioned chamber: that very bed that he himself/ built. Put the firm bed

> here outside for him, and cover it/ over with fleeces and blankets, and with shining coverlets. (xxiii.174-80)

Odysseus is enraged: "What you have said, dear lady, has hurt my heart deeply. What man/ has put my bed in another place?" (xxiii.183-84) And he proceeds to rehearse, in great detail, the construction, the look, the place, the adornment, and the character of the bed *he* had made so long ago.

It is Odysseus's reaction to her suggestion that their marriage bed, a bed fashioned out of a still-living olive tree rooted in the center of their home, had been cut and moved that finally shows Penelope what she needs to know. It is his memorable burst of anger that is so revelatory. For it shows that, despite his wanderings, Odysseus, like the marriage bed he built for himself and Penelope, still has living and deep roots in the home. Now, at last, Penelope "burst into tears and ran straight to him, throwing her arms around the neck of Odysseus, and kissed his head" (xxiii.207-208). Penelope embraces him, as swimmers embrace the shore after Poseidon has smacked their strong-built ship on the open water. Odysseus's affirmation of his own rootedness thus completes the homecoming of Penelope.

THE HOMECOMING OF HOMER

Penelope is home and so is Odysseus, yet Homer detains us a little longer. As Odysseus is reunited with his father, Laertes, and defending his home against the relatives of the suitors, the suitors descend into Hades and deposit there the story of Penelope's web and Odysseus's return. As in the two previous accounts of the web—by Antinoos (in Book ii) and Penelope (in Book xix)—the suitors say, "So against her will and by force, she had to finish it," but they *now* tell for the first time about the *completed* web itself: "She displayed the great piece of weaving that she had woven. She had washed it, and it shone like the sun or the moon. At that time an evil spirit, coming from somewhere, brought back Odysseus" (xxiv.146-49). The completed web, like the well-ordered home whose restoration it both images and makes possible, is the theme—and also the image—of the completed story, now deposited in Hades, the bank of memory and source of stories. Weaving, marriage, and story-telling, but especially stories of weaving, marriage, and story-telling, bring light like the very sun or moon to a world in which all that lives must die. Now, thanks to Homer, even in Hades, the repository of memory, not all is darkness. For stories that remind us of the best brighten our present and illuminate a way into the future.

2

The World through Ben's Bifocals

Ralph Lerner

Any author contributing to a celebratory volume has first to pose this question to himself: Is my theme or subject appropriate for the one being honored? On the face of it, one must confess, the fit between Benjamin Franklin and the interests, concerns, and character of Leon Kass goes only so far. To be sure, each savors a good story, both in the telling and the receiving. Each has channeled his great ambition to alleviating the misery, discomfort, and ignorance of a broad public. Each has probed long and hard into the operations of our moral understanding. Had they been contemporaries, Leon would (I believe) have enjoyed Ben's company. Indeed, who apart from John Adams could have failed to be charmed by the old magician? Yet for all that, Leon's admiration for Ben would have been tepid at best.

Ben's relations with his family lack warmth; they are cool and attenuated rather than intense. Ben's face gives few clues of his thoughts and feelings; his many masks are not merely literary creations. Ben's is not only a curious, searching mind but most probably also a deeply irreverent one. He was, in short, cut from a very different cloth than Leon, notwithstanding a certain degree of congruence. Which brings us back to the initial question: Is this a fitting gift for Leon Kass? Only to a point. But since our standards for enjoyment are laxer than our standards for admiration, this gift is offered in the hope that it may at least be enjoyed.

* * *

Typical autobiographers see no need to explain or excuse offering up their life-stories to the world at large. Having a tale to tell, they plunge in. Not so the author of one of the most widely read of all autobiographies. Benjamin Franklin finds it fitting to open his unfinished account of his life with the reasons or "inducements" impelling him to undertake such a project. They are several, a fact that might prompt the reader to be alert for redundancy; Franklin may be overdoing it. To begin with, he says he has always enjoyed hearing little anecdotes of his ancestors and imagines that his son (to whom this narrative is addressed) would enjoy hearing of his father as well. Beyond such idle sharing of enjoyment, however, is the thought that Franklin's descendants might find some utility in applying to their own situations the means he used in raising himself from poverty and obscurity to wealth and fame. Accordingly he promises to show them how he did it. Furthermore, Franklin is so pleased with his present happy condition that he says he is ready to relive his life, even without the opportunity of correcting some of its "errata." But that kind of repetition being out of the question, he settles for mere recollection; and to make that recollection "as durable as possible," he will commit it to writing. The final reason given in this catalogue of inducements is Franklin's admission that writing about himself will "a good deal gratify my own *Vanity*"—a gratification for which he is very grateful indeed (43-44).[1]

This opening paragraph, occupying a scant page and a half, is a tour de force, opening as it does a window into the mind of one of the subtlest and most charming observers of humankind. Looking in, we see that Franklin's most powerful inducement has been left at mere insinuation. Rather than sermonize, rather than state explicitly his largest lesson on how to look at the world and how to view our place in it, Franklin enacts a series of scenes in which we observe the drama and draw *his* conclusions on our own. With finesse and wit he accustoms us to borrow his bifocals and to observe and interpret the story he tells through his eyes. Consider again how this opening paragraph works.

The first inducement rests on the assumption that I'm like you and you're like me. I have always enjoyed hearing about my forebears and so might you. This, dear son, is less a matter of your being a chip off the old block than of our sharing a common human curiosity about our origins. The next inducement, however, rests on the assumption that I'm not like you and you're not like me. I am the noteworthy instance of a man who lifted himself quite a bit above the common dust of humanity. This ability is rare and not simply to be presumed in one's offspring. You, my posterity, might nonetheless wonder how I did it and whether the like might work for you. Franklin acknowledges that he must have had the blessing of God, but emphasizes how much is owing to his own efforts. For though a kind providence may have supplied "the conducing Means" for the autobiographer, it was "I [who] made use of [them]" (43). In the very course of announcing that he is now prepared to teach what every generation needs to learn, Franklin nudges us to realize that he is an autodidact, having found out this teaching on his own.

1. Page references are to *The Autobiography of Benjamin Franklin*, ed. Leonard W. Labaree, Ralph L. Ketcham, Helen C. Boatfield, and Helene H. Fineman (New Haven: Yale University Press, 1964).

On the whole, his has been a good life, not without its "sinister Accidents and Events" to be sure, but with what he calls "a considerable share of Felicity" (43). He sees no point in dwelling on what might have been; he has little taste or time for regrets and brooding. What's done is done, and one is better advised to get on with life. Yet, being an old man (he is 65 when writing these lines, though his brilliant diplomatic career still lies before him), he affects to be ready to indulge himself in recollections. Lest you imagine that this is an old codger in an assisted-living facility prattling away, note that Franklin is concerned that his recollection be made as durable as possible and spread as far as feasible. What we have here is not an aide-memoire of an old man with a short memory, but rather an ambitious production by a man very much possessed of his faculties and avid for ambitious readers. His audience extends far beyond his son, his immediate descendants, or even future generations of his countrymen. (It turns out that the full reach of this author's ambition for an audience doesn't emerge until later in the account.) Finally, there is this matter of vanity. There is no point in denying that it comes into play when I decide to tell you at length all about myself, nor is there any point in my apologizing for displaying this all-too-human trait. Franklin takes what earlier theologians and moralists had deemed a sin or a vice or at least a failing and adroitly transforms it into a socially and privately beneficial trait. In many cases, Franklin asserts cautiously, "it would not be quite absurd if a Man were to thank God for his Vanity among the other Comforts of Life" (44). With this amiable nod, the circle of inducements is closed with a blending of private and public concerns.

Franklin has suggested he will not hold back telling about some incidents that do him no credit, incidents where he would have behaved otherwise were he able to relive his life. In these pages, he leads us to believe, we shall see him portrayed warts and all. As he puts it later when refusing to excuse his decision to stop attending church services, "My present purpose [is] to relate Facts, and not to make Apologies for them" (198). He creates expectations that his story will be marked by candor, even if you the reader are put off by his open self-satisfaction and self-absorption. For now we need only to be reminded that we are not obliged by politeness to hear him out. The reader can close the covers of this book whenever he pleases. Ben's plain message is, Take me as I am. But that plain message is wrapped in such diffident language and delivered in so charming a manner that we are left with a general sense of warm geniality. Who can remain out of sorts with someone who confesses to having waged a losing war against pride and then wiggles out of this self-condemnation with this graceful flourish? "You will see it perhaps often in this History. For even if I could conceive that I had compleatly overcome it, I should probably be proud of my Humility" (160). Ben, tell us more! Please!

Nowhere is Franklin's mastery of artful speech more evident than in his discussions of religious belief. His tone of voice when alluding to divine providence suggests that he is on easy terms with the deity. His god is not that of his Presbyterian parents or of John Calvin, to say nothing of the Lord of Hosts who spoke to Moses out of a burning bush. Having planted in our minds the almost reasonable notion of thanking God for one's vanity, Franklin goes on immediately to acknowledge (as he puts it) "with all Humility" how much he owes to God for the happiness he has enjoyed up to this time. This expression of humble thanks is not without its own little twist. Ben speaks of "his kind Providence, which led me to the Means I us'd and gave them success" (45). It is not quite clear from this acknowledgment where the credit belongs: whether to the providence that pointed young Ben to the right means for attaining happiness, or to the "I" who used those means so effectively. However one understands it, Franklin is ready to hope, though not to presume, that his unknowable future fortune will be for the best. His is not a faith tortured by misgivings. He is ever-ready to enlist all of his *human* providence in support of whatever divine providence shines in his direction.

Immediately after this pious interlude, Ben sets out to satisfy the first-mentioned reason for writing the memoir. He presents a portrait gallery of some of his ancestors. Theirs is an old family of freeborn Englishmen, plain people with calluses on their hands, but by no means ordinary. From surviving genealogical records Ben discovers—and makes sure we register this fact as well—that he is "the youngest Son of the youngest Son for 5 Generations back" (46). In a world where being first-born carried distinct social, legal, and economic privileges, Ben's disadvantageous start in life seems all the greater. But in the context of his whole life's trajectory, this curious fact may strike us as neither a complaint nor an expression of regret, but as a boast. Consider the odds I have overcome; consider how far I have risen.

The individual ancestors Ben sketches are remarkably vivid. They come across as genuine characters. What is more, they are described in terms that invite the reader to see them as bearers of traits that one might observe in the author himself. His maternal grandfather, Peter Folger, labored for the repeal of Massachusetts Bay Colony laws that constrained the liberty of conscience of Baptists, Quakers, and others. His appeal to authorities was cast in a rustic poetry that Benjamin Franklin finds redeemed by what he characterizes as "a good deal of Decent Plainness and manly Freedom" (52). On his father's side, he singles out two uncles in particular. Uncle Thomas was a smith, but no ordinary laborer, as we can tell from his nephew's account: "being ingenious, and encourag'd in Learning . . . he qualify'd for the Business of Scrivener, became a considerable Man in the County Affairs, [and] was a chief Mover of all publick Spirited Undertakings." Ben draws attention to the "extraordinary" similarity of this forebear and himself, a resemblance that might suggest the one is a prefiguration of the other, or that the soul of Thomas Franklin has migrated to the body of his nephew (47-48). Uncle Benjamin elicits a comparison, even a silent contrast. Like his namesake, he was an "ingenious" man and lived to a great age. He was also pious and an avid "Attender of Sermons of the best Preachers" (48-49). His literary legacy consisted of two manuscript volumes of poetry of a rather moralistic sort that he had composed, along with many volumes of others' sermons that he had transcribed in a shorthand of his own invention. The latter he had proposed to offer to his young nephew should Ben become a clergyman. ("I suppose," Ben says, "as a Stock to set up with" [53].) But this was not to be, thanks in part to the decisiveness of the most influential ancestor, Ben's father.

Josiah Franklin, chafing under the Stuart laws aimed at suppressing religious practices at variance with prescribed Anglican rituals, had emigrated to New England with a wife and the first few children of what was to become a very large family. Ben describes this former dyer, who made himself into a tallow chandler and soap boiler, as a man of parts, able to draw and sing and play music and possessed of "a mechanical Genius." "But his great Excellence," he says, "lay in a sound Understanding, and solid Judgment in prudential Matters, both in private and public Affairs" (54-55). Here was a tradesman whose opinion was frequently consulted by others who recognized and respected his judiciousness. Josiah casts a long shadow in the autobiography, even after the teenager runs away from Boston and from the whole web of obligations that tie him to his parents and his apprenticeship. We note in passing that Ben is the third of Josiah's ten sons who rebels and escapes from paternal control.

Ben's account of his forebears is full of curious details but lacks warmth. More to the point, his depiction of his father's management of his education contains muted but unmistakable criticism. He writes, "My Father's little Library consisted chiefly of Books in polemic Divinity, most of which I read, and have since often regretted, that at a time when I had such a Thirst for Knowledge, more proper Books had not fallen in my Way, since it was now resolv'd I should not be a Clergyman" (58). The original resolve that Ben be trained as a clergyman was Josiah's; he had intended "to devote [Ben] as the Tithe of his Sons to the Service of the Church" (52). In keeping with this intention, Number 10 boy was sent to the grammar school where he flourished and shone for the bare year in which he was enrolled. But Josiah's second thoughts, prompted by considerations of the expense of a college education and the "mean living" that graduates might expect, led to his second resolve (53). After a further year in a school for writing and arithmetic, young Ben would learn a trade. At age ten he is back among the tallow pots making candles. Ravenous for books, he settles for what is at hand, works of polemical divinity that are, strictly speaking, good for nothing and good for none save other polemical divines. What a waste! Even worse, he insists, such works instill a disputatious turn of mind that all too soon turns into a nasty habit. A love of contradiction sours and spoils conversation. It is a sure way how *not* to win friends and influence people. Viewed in retrospect, Ben sees his youthful enthusiasm for confrontational argument as a disease: "I had caught it by reading my Father's Books of Dispute about Religion" (60).

Ben's account of his forefathers leaves us with a strong impression of a world suffused with religious doctrine and religious controversy, in which individuals with more or less practical wisdom try to wend their way. Prudence, above all, is needed, and any level-headed individual possessing it has in his hands an important instrument for making his mark. As though to reinforce that point by way of contrast, Franklin fills the rest of his autobiography with sketches of characters in high places and low who are very sure of themselves even while showing they lack good sense. Take Sir William Keith, governor of Pennsylvania. He proposes to help set up eighteen-year-old Ben in business as a printer, even while knowing he has no means for bringing that about. On the strength of Keith's vain assurances of a promised letter of credit, Ben sets sail for England to buy the necessary equipment only to be left high and dry and to discover this damning truth about the governor: that "He wish'd to please everybody; and having little to give, he gave Expectations" (80-82, 86-87, 92-95). Or consider the ill-fated British Major General Edward Braddock. Confident of himself and of his redcoats, and dismissive of both the colonists and the Indians whom he has been sent to pacify, he rejects and loses the advantage of local knowledge and experience. When warned by Franklin of the danger of ambushes awaiting his army's extended line of march through the wilderness, "He smil'd at my Ignorance" and proceeded into the disaster he could not envision (216-17, 223-25). On a more amusing and triumphant note, listen to Ben's account of the Abbé Jean-Antoine Nollet, preceptor in natural philosophy to the French royal family and an early experimenter in electricity. When first encountering Franklin's scientific pamphlet, *Experiments and Observations on Electricity*, Nollet refuses to believe that such a work could emerge from America (of all places) and is persuaded that his enemies in Paris have concocted this fraud the better to attack his reputation. Even after being satisfied that the alleged author is not a hoax, Nollet proceeds to contest Franklin's experiments and deductions. Ben reports that he thought better of responding:

either his experiments could be replicated or not, and he was not under any obligation to defend observations which had been offered only as conjectures, not delivered dogmatically. In the end, he says, "I concluded to let my Papers shift for themselves"; other scholars came to the defense of Franklin's theories; while the poor Abbé, fallen from favor, now lives to see himself barely a footnote in the annals of science (243-44).

Overweening people provide endless opportunities for a careful observer to draw a lesson and make his move. Perhaps the most engaging and rewarding parts of Ben's narrative are those describing how Ben observes and learns from others' folly and where we too are able to observe and learn from his education in life. But we are not yet done with his vignettes of character. Here is another sketch, a splendid instance of chicanery and misplaced confidence offering much matter for reflection:

After stealing out of Boston, incognito as it were, the young apprentice seeks work in New York City, but with no success. The local printer there, William Bradford, tells him that his son Andrew, a printer in Philadelphia, may well have need for an extra hand. On the strength of this intelligence, Ben continues southward and after many misadventures finally makes his memorable entry into town. Presenting himself at Andrew Bradford's shop, whom should he meet there but the elder Bradford, on a visit from New York. Andrew can offer no immediate employment, but in a spirit of helpfulness suggests that his competitor, Samuel Keimer, might. And even more helpfully, the senior Bradford volunteers to accompany Ben to the interview. Now the comedy begins. Before it is over, a fool shows his true colors, and readers who reflect upon these scenes may be the wiser for it. This is how Ben picks up the story:

> And when we found him, Neighbour, says Bradford, I have brought to see you a young man of your Business, perhaps you may want such a One. He ask'd me a few Questions, put a Composing Stick in my Hand to see how I work'd, and then said he would employ me soon, tho' he had just then nothing for me to do. And taking old Bradford whom he had never seen before, to be one of the Towns People that had a Good Will for him, enter'd into a Conversation on his present Undertaking and Prospects; while Bradford not discovering [i.e., not disclosing] that he was the other Printer's Father, on Keimer's saying he expected soon to get the greatest Part of the Business in his own Hands, drew him on by artful Questions and starting little Doubts, to explain all his Views, what Interest he rely'd on, and in what manner he intended to proceed. I who stood by and heard all, saw immediately that one of them was a crafty old Sophister, and the other a mere Novice. Bradford left me with Keimer, who was greatly surpris'd when I told him who the old Man was. (77-78)

The sixty-five-year-old man who tells this story clearly relishes exposing Keimer's profound ignorance of the world. Presuming that someone who addresses him as "Neighbour" is indeed such leaves this naïf naked and exposed. Getting the better of such a dunderhead is child's play, and the seventeen-year-old who witnesses the encounter understands "immediately" what the man twice his age does not. The humorless Keimer is in for it once he hires Ben. This boy with more than a touch of spite knows how to deal with his future employer so as to secure his own interests and at the same time provide a steady source of amusement.

How ought one to understand the unthinking readiness of Keimer to spill the beans? He was clearly an eccentric and perhaps mentally unstable. Though a rotten printer, he was no illiterate and even had some scholarly pretensions. But he was a congenital believer. In Franklin's words, "He had been one of the French Prophets and could act their enthusiastic Agitations. At this time he did not profess any particular Religion, but something of all on occasion" (79). Franklin's reference to French Prophets is to a sect of "French Protestant refugees [Camisards] in England in 1706, given to trances and revelations, proclaiming a Messianic kingdom soon to come" (79 n. 7). Keimer's yearning for some kind of religion-inspired transcendence led him to try on different ones for size, but finding none suited him for long, he was prepared to make his own. It is tempting to say much the same about young Ben. He abandons his parents' Presbyterianism, goes on to "become a thorough Deist," fabricates his own private credo and liturgy, and ultimately envisions forming a world-wide secret "sect" in which the "Virtuous and good Men of all Nations" would unite around a single creed, a creed stripped of anything "that might shock the Professors of any Religion" and hence acceptable to all (113-14, 147, 161-62). This demands a much closer look, but we cannot turn to what Ben calls his "*great and extensive Project*" until we have finished our business with the inimitable Keimer (158, 163).

Ben is now working full-time at Keimer's print shop. They are on good terms, the employer having no wind of the fact that his pressman, backed by the promised patronage of the provincial governor, is aiming to set himself up as a competitor. Keimer's skewed preoccupations keep him from appreciating that this skilled, hyperenergetic young man will not long settle for being an underling. Further, he finds Ben good company, a perfect complement (as he sees it) to his own strengths: namely, his indulgence in old religious enthusiasms and his love of argumentation. As Ben reports, "We therefore had many Disputations" (88). Only gradually does Keimer come to realize that they are not fighting on a level field. A few years earlier Ben had learned from a book (as you the reader might learn from *his* book), that there are better ways of dealing with the world's stupidity than by what he calls "abrupt Contradiction, and positive Argumentation." A lesson he took away from Xenophon's *Memorabilia*, recollections of the life of Socrates, was the utility of the method whereby Socrates affected a profoundly ironical humility. Ben reports, "I was charmed with it, adopted it . . . and put on the humble Enquirer and Doubter" (64). (For more on Franklin's promotion of this noncombative stance and his insistence on the value of keeping a low profile, see 65, 117, 143, 159, 193.) Ben was drawn to this method for a deeper reason than that it would permit him to win arguments on the cheap, though that undeniably had its own attraction. He had a very strong inducement for becoming a master practitioner of a strategy of humility: "being then . . . become a real Doubter in many Points of our Religious Doctrine, I found this Method safest for my self and very embarassing to those against whom I used it" (64). Given this background, it was a near-certainty that Keimer would soon find himself flummoxed, even paralyzed, by the artful snares that Ben laid for him. "I us'd to work him so with my Socratic Method, and had trapann'd him so often by Questions apparently so distant from any Point we had in hand, and yet by degrees led to the Point, and brought him into Difficulties and Contradictions that at last he grew ridiculously cautious, and would hardly answer me the most common Question, without asking first, *What do you intend to infer from that*?" (88)

You might think that Keimer suffers from a lack of self-esteem, but you would be off the mark. He is too dull-witted for that. Instead he sees a new opportunity, with Ben as his sidekick, "in a Project he had of setting up a new Sect." Ben explains that Keimer "was to preach the Doctrine, and I was to confound all Opponents" (88). From each according to his abilities! The comedy now begins in earnest as master and apostle negotiate over the content of the doctrines to be preached. Keimer, inspired by the Law of Moses, insists on his essentials: wearing one's beard untrimmed and keeping the seventh day as the Sabbath. Ben reluctantly concedes, provided he can have his way too: let there be strict vegetarianism. Keimer objects: "I doubt, says he, my Constitution will not bear that. I assur'd him it would, and that he would be the better for it. He was usually a great Glutton, and I promis'd my self some Diversion in half-starving him. He agreed to try the practice if I would keep him Company. I did so and we held it for three months" (88-89).

Again, one ought to view this episode in the spirit in which it is offered. Although he had once been a vegetarian on principle, Ben no longer is, having been seduced from his higher commitment by the delicious smell of cod coming hot out of the frying pan. His covenant with Keimer is prompted, rather, by "the Cheapness of it"—that is, by the economies in keeping to a vegetarian diet—and by the prospect of the fun he will have in tormenting this intemperate carnivore. "I went on pleasantly, but poor Keimer suffer'd grievously, tir'd of the Project, long'd for the Flesh Pots of Egypt, and order'd a roast Pig. He invited me and two Women

Friends to dine with him, but it being brought too soon upon table, he could not resist the Temptation, and ate it all up before we came" (89).

Here is a vaudeville version of how yet another high-minded movement for the elevation of humankind bites the dust. There are more than a few laughs in this episode, but not only that. We are entitled to ask, what kind of religion are master and apostle preaching to the gentiles? The doctrines, insofar as we are informed about them, make no pretense of explaining how the believers would be better men and women by virtue of their adherence. The hollow core of this would-be sect anticipates a criticism Franklin would later make of a preacher whose sermons he described as "very dry, uninteresting and unedifying, since not a single moral Principle was inculcated or enforc'd, their Aim seeming to be rather to make us Presbyterians than good Citizens" (147). Disgusted with that preacher's missed opportunity, Franklin finds better use for his Sunday's leisure and thereupon, if we are to believe him, resumes use of his private liturgy as laid down in his *Articles of Belief and Acts of Religion* of 1728. It seems to him that there has to be a better way than the inanities of a Keimer and the self-satisfaction of the Presbyterian sermonizer. And indeed, now something grander and more challenging heaves into sight: "It was about this time," he says, "that I conceiv'd the bold and arduous Project of arriving at moral Perfection" (148).

Ben is famous not only for the book he began but never finished—the story of his life—but also for the book he intended to publish but never wrote—*The Art of Virtue* (157). He explains in the autobiography that his long-cherished design was frustrated by the press of his private business when he was still young and by the press of his public involvements during his mature years. Those preoccupations have effectively barred his ever bringing his book to light. He adds these words, pregnant with meaning: this book, *The Art of Virtue*, "being connected in my Mind with a *great and extensive Project* that required the whole Man to execute" (158). These few words offer a glimpse into his far-reaching design. Nothing less than the "whole Man" will suffice. We are teased into wondering why that should be so.

Clearly, if it were simply a matter of bringing together the sundry "short Hints" he has been composing over the years, arranging and amplifying those notes, developing his commentaries on the various virtues he means to promote, or even refining "the Utility and Excellency of my Method" by showing "the *Means* and *Manner* of obtaining Virtue" (157)—all these could have been accomplished over the years, bit by bit, by even a very busy man if he steals odd interludes from his schedule. Indeed, this is a fairly adequate description of how Franklin manages to compose as much of his memoir as he does. One might also dismiss his excuse as being superfluous, for he has in fact folded into his autobiography what amounts to a twelve-page executive summary of the whole *Art of Virtue* (148-60). A more likely account of what is afoot here would focus less on the little book itself and more on the "*great and extensive Project*" to which it is connected in Ben's mind. It is that "Project" which requires the whole man.

Recall that Franklin's point of departure is "the bold and arduous Project of arriving at moral Perfection. I wish'd to live without committing any Fault at any time; I would conquer all that either Natural Inclination, Custom, or Company might lead me into" (148). This is a tall order indeed, and even in merely trying to reshape himself into something better than he is, Ben falters and stumbles. The path toward individual perfection is steep and rocky. Ben readily confesses that. But thanks to his excellent method of habituating himself to better words and deeds, he does inch closer to his goal. Now enlarge the field of vision and multiply the number of those who are to be enlisted in a "united Party for Virtue" (161). At age twenty-five Ben contemplates forming a world-wide party of believers, a secret society composed at first of young single men who will submit to the prescribed thirteen-week cycle of moral reform and reinforcement as prescribed in *The Art of Virtue*. Combining self-help with mutual promotion of "one another's Interest, Business, and Advancement in Life," Ben endows this support group with a nondenominational "Creed" at which no one would take offense, referring as it does to a creator, providence, prayer, the immortality of the soul, and reward and punishment "either here or hereafter." Critical to this new religion is the notion "that the most acceptable Service of God is doing Good to Man" (162). Plainly put, this "Sect" (Ben's own word) has a god whose message to men is that they ought to focus their thoughts on their own business here on earth and leave the deity (however understood) to take care of his. With a breathtaking blandness, Ben proposes calling this new sect "the Society of the *Free and Easy*; Free, as being by the general Practice and Habit of the Virtues, free from the Dominion of Vice, and particularly by the Practice of Industry and Frugality, free from Debt, which exposes a Man to Confinement and a Species of Slavery to his Creditors"—truly a sect given to works over faith (163). Note that Ben does not explain in what sense the adherents of this society will be "Easy," though the implication is left for us readers to draw after asking, "Easy—compared to what?"

The plainspoken answer to that question has to be sought, not in the pages of Franklin's memoirs, but in the preface he wrote in 1773 to a proposed revision of the Anglican *Book of Common Prayer*, an undertaking in which he collaborated with a fellow-deist. In that preface the anonymous editors, speaking in the singular, profess pious admiration for the work they are about to dismantle. Their book purports to be only an "Abridgement"; and they are motivated to make this effort out of regard for the suffering, or at least inconvenience, caused by the overlong liturgy of the Church of England. Think of the aged and infirm shivering away for hours in a wintry cold church. Think of the young who are put off by those endless, repetitive services. Think of busy, gainfully employed people who might be tempted to drop in for a weekday service if only the prayers were reduced to a much narrower compass. The language suggests that this editorial project is driven by compassion for parishioners and care for the renewed vigor of the established church. Yet the bland tone of the preface smacks rather of a time-motion engineer focused on his stopwatch, and it prefigures the heavy hand to be visited upon the liturgy: "this humble performance may serve to shew the practicability of shortening the service near one half, without the omission of what is essentially necessary."[2]

Judgments of what is "essentially necessary" must differ of course. But it was unlikely that orthodox Anglicans would have quietly suffered the virtual excision of references to the Holy Ghost, the mediating role of Jesus, and his real presence in the consecrated bread and wine—and they did not. Even modern commentators on Franklin feel compelled to view this revision less as an abridgement than as an evisceration of the *Book of Common Prayer*.[3] Still, it is undeniable that congregants using this trimmed-down version would have found their accustomed religion suddenly and markedly made more "Easy."

* * *

We might well wonder how far the Great Projector got in realizing his "*great and extensive Project*." Ben turns rather vague; it is, after all, hard to recall details fifty-seven years after the event. But he does remember sharing his project—"in part"—with two young men "who adopted it with some Enthusiasm" (163). Far from regarding such results as slim pickings, Ben is in no way dismayed. He couldn't spare time to do more then, but remains firmly convinced that his scheme is both practicable and useful. "And I was not discourag'd by the seeming Magnitude of the Undertaking, as I have always thought that one Man of tolerable Abilities may work great Changes, and accomplish great Affairs among Mankind, if he first forms a good Plan, and, cutting off all Amusements or other

2. The text of Franklin's "Preface" is printed in *The Papers of Benjamin Franklin*, ed. William B. Willcox, et al., vol. 20 (New Haven: Yale University Press, 1976), 345-51 (quotation at 349).

3. Ibid., 345 introductory note, and 349 n. 4. See also Alfred Owen Aldridge, *Benjamin Franklin and Nature's God* (Durham, North Carolina: Duke University Press, 1967), 172: "In tackling the liturgy, he slashed right and left. Gone completely were the Absolution and the Canticle—nearly all of the Exhortation, the Te Deum, the Venite exultemus—and a large section of the Confession. Over half of the Apostles' Creed went by the board." The ribald deist agenda behind this editorial project is nicely, if gently, developed by Aldridge at 166-79 as he traces the relationship between Sir Francis Dashwood (Baron Le Despencer), the principal "abridger," and Benjamin Franklin, his aider and admirer.

Employments that would divert his Attention, makes the Execution of that same Plan his sole Study and Business" (163). Here if anywhere, we find the credo of the authentic Benjamin Franklin.

Ben remains to the end an evangelist of a new kind. He is proselytizing for a "Scheme [that] was not wholly without Religion," or a "Method . . . that might be serviceable to People in all Religions" (157). The artful blurring of lines in this account suggests powerfully that Franklin's religion of the future aims, over time, to transform popular preoccupations and orientations. The change he has in mind is encapsulated in a little story he tells about his friend George Whitefield, who was so prominent in the first major religious revival in America—the "Great Awakening." Franklin had offered to have this famous evangelist as his house guest when he came to Philadelphia to preach. "He reply'd, that if I made that kind Offer for Christ's sake, I should not miss of a Reward. And I return'd, *Don't let me be mistaken; it was not for Christ's sake, but for your sake*. One of our common Acquaintance jocosely remark'd, that knowing it to be the Custom of the Saints, when they receiv'd any favour, to shift the Burthen of the Obligation from off their own Shoulders, and place it in Heaven, I had contriv'd to fix it on Earth" (178-79).

Benjamin Franklin lived a life full of accomplishments. He made his mark in technology, science, politics, diplomacy, music, and literature. His many acts of benefit to others still entitle his memory to be held in regard not only by his countrymen but by humankind at large. Yet there is no denying that he was motivated to perform these public-spirited deeds by considerations lying outside the moral and religious mainstream. Recall how in his memoir's opening paragraph he planted the notions that a mixture of many motives may lie behind a simple action, that the seemingly private may have important social consequences, that a useful public action may be driven by intensely private desires. He knew from first-hand experience that very many of his contemporaries would have been ill at ease with his unorthodox reasonings had they been stated baldly and decisively. He had, then, good cause to adopt the strategy he used in presenting his life-story. Close reflection upon his thoughts and words discloses that both his starting-point and his end-point were firmly lodged in *this* world, in *this* life. He would have us readers come to understand that it is *here* that we ought to focus our attention and care. His cautionary tales, told with so much understated wit and grace, are meant to work upon our understanding and then upon our will. He could not have expected that his readers would move as far from the preoccupations of their fathers as he had from his, but perhaps it is a measure of his long-term success that today his bold project hardly seems revolutionary at all.

3

Medicalizing Childhood

Gilbert Meilaender

When in August of 2001 President George W. Bush named Leon Kass as Chairman of the newly formed President's Council on Bioethics, his action inevitably forced a redirection of Kass's scholarly energies. But it was also a great gift to the discipline of bioethics.

A major player in bioethics since it had burst upon the scene in the 1960s, blessed with a distinctive and profound angle of vision, Kass had in more recent years turned to exploration and explication of biblical texts (the fruit of what he once called "a late onset rabbinic gene"). That work reached one terminus with the publication in 2003 of *The Beginning of Wisdom: Reading Genesis*. Had the presidential appointment not intervened, he would no doubt simply have moved on to Exodus—which would have been a very good thing.

Not as good, however—though how we make such judgments is hard to say—as the forced refocusing on bioethics. For his store of knowledge about the development of the discipline and his unique perspective on how it might best be done would, then, never have been given the kind of scope for development made possible in the work of the President's Council—and bioethics would have been the poorer.

The Council was, of course, a body of eighteen highly independent and diverse thinkers, and the reports it produced during Kass's tenure as chairman surely reflect that diversity and independence. The reports are the Council's, not Kass's. Nonetheless, there were moments when his distinctive perspective surely shaped the focus of the Council's work and the manner (a "richer" bioethics, as he liked to say) in which it approached that work. Perhaps nowhere is this more evident than in *Beyond Therapy*, a report released by the Council in October 2003.[1] While it surely has its weaknesses as well as strengths, *Beyond Therapy*

1. *Beyond Therapy: Biotechnology and the Pursuit of Happiness*. A Report by the President's Council on Bioethics (New York: Regan Books, 2003). Citations will be given by page number in parentheses within the body of the text.

is a striking example of how bioethical reflection is enriched when its subject matter is placed within reflection about abiding human desires and aspirations. By taking up just one topic—the danger of medicalizing childhood—I hope to continue here the exploration begun in *Beyond Therapy* and to honor some of the central concerns of the work of Leon Kass.

One of the ironies of our world is that, although we eagerly use technology to exercise a distinctively human mastery of will in the production of our children, in the rearing of them we now often seem to act as if human beings were little more than animals—"just body." This reduction of our full humanity is hardly better than that which, exalting will and choice, thinks of us as free spirits who transcend the body's meaning and limits. For if we turn childhood's problems only into occasions for seeking the right prescription, we may miss essential aspects of being human. But, in order to think about these matters, I begin very far from our contemporary concerns.

Augustine's Discontent

"You have made us for yourself, and our hearts are restless until they rest in you."[2] Thus St. Augustine, in one of the most well-known lines of one of the most influential books ever written. The *Confessions* is a story of discontent and longing, of a search to quiet that discontent, a search that—Augustine thinks—can succeed only when our hearts rest in the God for whom we are made.

The roots of his later discontent and of his impulsive and (even) self-destructive behavior were evident, Augustine believes, in the effort he made even as an infant to have his wants met and in the anger he displayed when they were not. As a young boy in school, his restless heart was evident. He preferred playing to studying and was disciplined harshly for that preference. He disliked some subjects that he was compelled to study—Greek, for example, which he never really mastered even as an adult. He was entranced by other subjects—Latin literature—and describes himself "weeping at the death of Dido" (1.13). He told lies to his teachers and parents, "all for love of play, eagerness to watch worthless shows, and a restless hankering to imitate them" (1.19).

Indeed, "in that youth of mine," he says, perhaps with the exaggerated seriousness of the convert, "I was on fire to take my fill of hell" (2.1). And, in an episode his recounting has made famous as a paradigm of youthful vandalism

2. St. Augustine, *Confessions* 1.1. Although I have modified it in this passage, I will generally quote from Rex Warner's translation, *The Confessions of St. Augustine* (New York: New American Library, 1963). Citations will be given by book and chapter number in parentheses within the body of the text.

and the mystery of evil in the human heart, he and some friends stole pears from a neighboring vineyard—not because they were hungry, but because "our real pleasure was simply in doing something that was not allowed" (2.4). Indeed, by the time he was well into adolescence, he had become to himself "a wasteland" (2.10)—as he writes, in words that provided a title for T. S. Eliot's most famous poem.

Then, "I came to Carthage, and all around me in my ears were the sizzling and frying of unholy loves" (3.1). His restlessness and discontent, having never really found any good that answered to them in his early years, were now full grown. "I was not yet in love, but I loved the idea of love. . . . I hated security and a path without snares" (3.1). Despite the lack of focus and the impulsive behavior that he describes, one could not say that the maturing young man's achievements fell short of those in his peer group. In fact, he advanced professionally and became a teacher of the liberal arts. If he fell short, it was in terms of his own potential and his own desires—a failing that is painful enough, of course.

Successful as he was in some senses, however, he was far from content—and still "panted for honors, for money, for marriage" (6.6). He was struck by the fact that a poor, drunk beggar on the street appeared to be happy and enjoying himself, having found without trying, it seems, the contentment Augustine lacked. And when he eventually resigned his position, it was partly because, as he writes, "my lungs had begun to give way as the result of overwork in teaching. I found it difficult to breathe deeply; pains in the chest were evidence of the injury and made it impossible for me to speak loudly or for a long time" (9.2). This ailment, which, so far as we know, never recurred later in his life, invites our speculation. "It is more than probable," Peter Brown, Augustine's biographer, suggests, "that . . . Augustine had come to develop the physical manifestations of a nervous breakdown"—the end point, perhaps, of problems that had been developing throughout his life.[3]

Out of this experience of his restless heart Augustine made a great story—and, indeed, something more than that. He constructed a narrative that—in his mind and the minds of many readers since—unfolds important truths about every human life, not just his own. Moreover, although Augustine believed that only the grace of God can bring healing and wholeness to the restless human heart, he by no means absolves us of responsibility for the sad state in which we find ourselves. The fetters that bound him, as he engaged in a seemingly endless pursuit of something that would end his discontent, were not "put on me by someone else, but by the iron bondage of my own will" (8.5). The self is divided—longing

3. Peter Brown, *Augustine of Hippo: A Biography*. A New Edition with an Epilogue (Berkeley, California: University of California Press, 2000), 102.

for a contentment that only God can give, but simultaneously grasping at one or another passing pleasure—and "I, no doubt, was on both sides" (8.5). That is to say, Augustine will not pretend that the discontent, the restlessness, the impulsivity, the lack of focus and readiness to be distracted are simply a misfortune he suffers—as if these characteristics were one thing and his character another. No, it is he himself who is discontented, impulsive, distractible—and to feel shame and guilt for the person he has become is a hopeful sign.

Thus, the discontent and restlessness that he experiences are not entirely bad, nor would he necessarily be better off were he completely content. For God uses this discontent to draw Augustine on toward his true happiness, which alone can offer the heart lasting peace. "You were always with me, . . . scattering the most bitter discontent over all my illicit pleasures, so that thus I might seek for pleasure in which there was no discontent and be unable to find such a thing except in you, Lord, except in you" (2.2). Or again: "My God and my mercy, how good you were to me in sprinkling so much bitterness over that sweetness" (3.1). And yet again: "Your graciousness to me was shown in the way you would not allow me to find anything sweet which was not you" (6.6). And even after his momentous conversion experience in the garden, Augustine knew himself to be only on the way—seeing in the distance the land of peace, but not yet there. Hence, the God who is our happiness may not make us happy here and now. Were a pill available that seemed to make us perfectly content, we should reject it, lest we lose that *eros* for the God who is truly our good. That is, we can have a false happiness, which cannot ultimately satisfy, or we can relinquish the desire for perfect contentment here and now, leaving open in our being a gaping wound that God must fill in his own good time. "Here I have the power but not the wish to stay; there I wish to be but cannot; both ways, miserable" (10.40).

We might ask ourselves whether we should regret the historical happenstance that Augustine came along too soon in history to have received the kind of medical treatment recommended by Dr. Joseph Biederman in a presentation to the President's Council on Bioethics about the use of psychopharmacology in treating children.[4] Had Augustine's symptoms—his inability to attend to what he found boring, his impulsive behavior, his restlessness—been diagnosed as Attention Deficit/Hyperactivity Disorder (ADHD) early enough, he might have been treated with Ritalin and spared years of anxiety and discontent, years of feeling that "myself to myself had become a place of misery, a place where I could not bear to be and from which I could not go" (4.7). He might have been spared

4. The transcript is available at: bioethics.georgetown.edu/pcbe/transcripts/feb06/session5.html.

the "horrendous inner sense of restlessness" that Dr. Biederman discerns even in many who are well past childhood. It is true, of course, that—compared to many of his peers—the young Augustine achieved a good bit; nevertheless, as Dr. Biederman noted, "dysfunction" is a relative term. Despite his achievements relative to those of others, Augustine may not have been able to use his "intellectual ability to the fullest." Given that, in Dr. Biederman's words, "academic progress is a fundamental passport for a good life," perhaps with treatment Augustine could have lived out his life in Rome as rhetorician for the well-known and powerful, rather than in Hippo, carrying out the thankless duties of a bishop in the struggling African church. But then, of course, we would not have his *Confessions*. How easily we forget that one may become a philosopher through loneliness or discontent.

I exaggerate—but in search of an important point that the work of the President's Council on Bioethics may help bring into focus. In *Beyond Therapy: Biotechnology and the Pursuit of Happiness* the Council noted that powerful stimulant drugs used, for example, to treat ADHD "have the capacity to enhance alertness and concentration in children without any symptoms whatsoever" (76). That is, the primary focus in *Beyond Therapy* is on "what it means *in general* [and not only in clear cases of over-treatment or under-treatment] to seek better or better-behaved children by pharmacological means" (75). A concern about medicalizing childhood is a concern about the means used to achieve an undeniably desirable end: happy, successful, and well-behaved children. And the use of drugs both to treat childhood disorders and to enhance children's accomplishments invites us to think more carefully about the meaning of childhood; for we cannot know what we should want for our children unless we reflect upon what it means that they are children.

THE MEANING OF CHILDHOOD

There are places where *Beyond Therapy* may take an insufficiently nuanced view of childhood—as when, for example, it suggests that "the sweetness, freshness, and spontaneity of life are available in their purest form only to the as-yet-unburdened young" (94).[5] Children have problems and anxieties aplenty, even

5. A few dissenting opinions: Wilson Carey McWilliams, *The Idea of Fraternity in America* (Berkeley, California: University of California Press, 1973), 36: "The impression that childhood is a dulcet time suggests how kind are the failures of memory." George Orwell, "Such, Such Were the Joys," in *A Collection of Essays* (New York: Harcourt Brace Jovanovich, 1953), 4-5: He writes of "a deeper grief which is peculiar to childhood and not easy to convey: a sense of desolate loneliness and helplessness, of being locked up not only in a hostile world but in a world of good and evil where the rules were such that it was actually not possible for me to keep them." To which I might

when their problems fall short of any diagnosable psychiatric disorder. They are often very far from feeling unburdened, as Augustine's story demonstrates so acutely. They already experience the longing of the restless heart, well before they can articulate it. They need, therefore, nurture and direction. But having recognized this, we in turn need to think about how best to help them deal with their problems and anxieties as they mature.

If childhood is not as "unburdened" as the sentence from *Beyond Therapy* quoted above suggests, it is nonetheless true that we could easily impose burdens on children if we think of childhood only as a step on the way toward adulthood. So, for example, as part of his case for the importance of medicating children diagnosed with ADHD—indeed, even for denying entirely that our society has any problem of over-diagnosis or over-medication—Dr. Biederman asserted more than once to the Council his belief that "there is a connection between what you accomplish in school and where you end up in life." If a distinguished clinician approaches his young patients in that spirit, perhaps the Council was not wrong to worry that adult expectations might unduly burden children.

Gareth Matthews is that rare philosopher who has actually given thought to the meaning of childhood, and he has argued quite persuasively that we make a mistake if we think of it simply as a stage on the way toward adulthood.[6] Matthews characterizes developmental models of that sort—whether ancient, as in Aristotle, or more modern, as in Piaget—as "deficit" models. They describe childhood primarily in terms of those aspects of adulthood which childhood lacks (but toward which it is oriented): "The nature of a child is to be a *potential* adult."[7] Thinking that way, we are likely, with Dr. Biederman, to assume that children should naturally be anxious when taking a test (on which a bit of their future depends), rather than to wonder whether we should alter their school environment and our expectations in order to create less anxiety. We are likely to emphasize, with Dr. Biederman, how important it is that children be attentive even to material that is boring (lest, I guess, they end up with deficits, like Augustine's in Greek, that plague them the rest of their lives and make it difficult for them to live up to their potential). If we envision childhood as "an essentially *prospective* state, what is good for a child can only be something that

add the wisdom of my mother who not only raised her own five children but cared at various times for a number of other children as well, and who often said: "Children have problems of their own."

6. Gareth B. Matthews, *The Philosophy of Childhood* (Cambridge, Massachusetts: Harvard University Press, 1994).

7. Gareth B. Matthews, "A Philosophy of Childhood." A monograph published by the Poynter Center for the Study of Ethics and American Institutions, Indiana University (January, 2006), 7.

will contribute to its good in adulthood."[8] So if we find ourselves thinking in the terms of such a "deficit" model, the point of childhood will be simply to become an adult. And the point of adulthood will be—well, what? To be satisfied?

I do not want to press the matter farther than we should. Although I would resist—for reasons I will come to in a moment—describing the child as a kind of "incomplete" human being, there is surely some sense in which it is right to think of the child as immature and in need of nurture. Because we are not simply animals, parents must help their children to develop, as best they can, the full range of human capacities. Hence, the Council noted in *Beyond Therapy* that parents rightly want their children to become attentive, well-behaved, and well-adjusted. If they want this in part for reasons of "parental pride," they also want it in part because they think—with Dr. Biederman, reasonably enough—that "children who possess these qualities are more likely to succeed and flourish later in life." We might even, as the Council notes, "find fault with parents who did not share" these aims, "at least to some considerable degree" (73).

It is very common to think of our lives in terms of a life cycle, for which the meaning of earlier stages lies partly in the way they prepare us for stages still to come. And thinking in terms of a life cycle might incline us, then, to picture the child as an incomplete human being—on the way toward full or complete humanity. But it is better, I think, to envision the child as (simply) "young" than as "incomplete." If we permit too much of the meaning of childhood to be gathered into its prospective and preparatory functions, we will see it relentlessly as a means to an end, and we are likely to try to take more control of its trajectory than is wise. Because we are not gods, parents are right to recognize limits to their work of shaping and forming their children.

Thinking in terms of the life cycle is not entirely mistaken, and it does point us toward a part of the truth about human life. It is not wrong to see childhood as, in part, oriented toward later stages of maturation still to come. That, of course, is why we are especially pained when someone dies in childhood; the full course of life's cycle has been cut short. Nevertheless, human beings do not "flourish" only in their adult state. A child can "flourish" precisely as a child; the meaning of its flourishing does not depend on future development or improvement. If the meaning of each stage of life were composed entirely of its prospective or preparatory functions, we would be hard pressed to see any point or worth to the last stages of life, when we have no further prospects.

For one image of life—that of the cycle—each stage of life has its meaning in terms of a trajectory of development that takes place over time. And this image does display a part of the truth about our lives. But equally true is the

8. Matthews, "A Philosophy of Childhood," 7.

quite different image of a "circle" rather than a "cycle" of life. For that image every moment and stage of life, each point along the circle, is equidistant from its center. It may be that the persuasiveness of this image relies upon some background religious beliefs. As all people, whatever their respective talents or accomplishments, are equal because equidistant from God, so each moment of life—whatever its stage of "development"—is equally meaningful and not just a step on the way toward some later stage. What, one might wonder, would heaven be like without children? The praise of God without the voices of children in the chorus? Each age, each moment of life, has its own distinct worth. Hence, we will miss certain truths about life if we think of our early years only as incomplete or as preparation for what is still to come.

In addition, when we think of childhood as only a prospective state, a means to the end of adulthood, we may try to take more control than is wise of the trajectory of a child's development. This is a constant temptation for both parents and teachers (and, dare we add, clinicians?). Paul Holmer taught for many years at Yale Divinity School. The story goes that at a banquet on the occasion of his retirement,

> after various faculty had spoken of him in glowing terms, the honoree was asked to respond. Holmer rose and read a short letter that he had received, saying that this was "my most treasured compliment to my teaching." The letter was from a young man who said that Holmer had changed his life, that his teaching had made a world of difference to his spiritual development.
>
> After reading the letter, Holmer sat down, saying only, "That young man is in jail serving a life sentence for murdering his father."[9]

Cutting still closer to the bone, John Ames, the 76-year-old preacher who is the narrator of Marilynne Robinson's *Gilead* and who is writing a long letter about life to his young son, recounts a sermon he had preached on Abraham and his sons Isaac and Ishmael. Abraham had been prepared to sacrifice Isaac at the Lord's command; Ishmael he sent off into the wilderness with his mother Hagar. Ames reflects that "any father, particularly any old father, must finally give his child up to the wilderness and trust to the providence of God. . . . Great faith is required to give the child up, trusting God to honor the parents' love for him by assuring that there will indeed be angels in that wilderness."[10] Perhaps, then, recognizing the limits of our ability to shape our children or to

9. William H. Willimon, "Hard truths: William H. Willimon on Paul Holmer," *The Christian Century*, 122 (Feb. 22, 2005), 27-28.

10. Marilynne Robinson, *Gilead* (New York: Farrar, Straus & Giroux, 2004), 129.

guarantee the course their development toward adulthood will take should lead us to discern our need not only for the image of the life cycle but also for the image of the life circle. Without it we cannot say all that needs to be said about the nature of a child.

Thus, while recognizing that some children have serious psychological disorders and badly need medical treatment, we must also be alert to deeper philosophical questions—such as what it means to be a child—that will shape our thinking on diagnosis and treatment. If we think of childhood solely as a prospective state, and the child only as a potential adult or incomplete being, we are likely to see distracted, discontented, and difficult children simply as problems to be solved through powerful behavior-modifying drugs now available. But if we listen both carefully and critically to the medical experts and reflect upon those moments when they themselves are puzzled, we may become hesitant to medicalize too quickly such characteristics of children.

BEHAVIORS, CAUSES, EXPERTISE

In preparing *Beyond Therapy* the President's Council heard from two physicians—Dr. Lawrence Diller and Dr. Steven Hyman—who discussed our attempts to improve the behavior of children through the use of psychotropic drugs.[11] At a later moment in its existence, studying more generally the problems of children in our society, the Council heard from Dr. Joseph Biederman and Drs. Fernette and Brock Eide.[12] To consider some of the disagreements about both diagnosis and treatment that grow out of these discussions is, surely, to be invited to puzzle a bit over complicated questions about childhood.

Both Dr. Hyman and Dr. Biederman seemed relatively content with an approach to psychiatric diagnosis based less on an understanding of causes than on observation of (possibly symptomatic) behaviors. (Perhaps I should not describe Dr. Hyman as entirely "content" with this, for he emphasized that the science is for now "very early" and that observation of behavioral symptoms gives, at best, "reliability," not "validity.") While a disorder such as ADHD may have multiple causes—genetic, neurological, environmental—much about its origins remains uncertain. Nonetheless, so long as trained clinical observers, using standard behavioral criteria, agree in their diagnoses, we can—or so the hypothesis goes—regard their diagnosis as reliable, even if, in a sense, this

11. The transcripts are at: bioethics.georgetown.edu/pcbe/transcripts/dec02/session3.html (for Diller) and bioethics.georgetown.edu/pcbe/transcripts/march03/session1.html (for Hyman).

12. For Biederman see note 4 above. For the Eides: bioethics.georgetown.edu/pcbe/transcripts/feb06/session4.html.

tells us very little about what is actually happening to cause the behavior that concerns us. I pass over here, though we should not ignore, the fact that an initial "diagnosis" often comes not from a trained clinician but from parents or teachers. If, as may often happen, a child then behaves more or less appropriately in the doctor's office, the doctor may rely on these reports of symptoms manifested elsewhere. Even Dr. Biederman, who is not inclined to grant the possibility that over-treatment is occurring, admits that the symptoms are variable, that they may occur in some contexts and not in others, and that a clinician may therefore simply rely on reports from others.

Dr. Fernette Eide and Dr. Brock Eide were, by contrast, far from satisfied with this approach. In their view, many of the learning or behavioral problems that can result in a diagnosis of ADHD are caused by neurologically based disorders of cognition and learning (such as visual problems, partial hearing loss, dyslexia, language disorders) or by instruction that is not suited to the ways in which a given child may learn best or most efficiently. In their view, "many children who struggle in school do not have cognitive "impairments" or "abnormalities" in any absolute sense, but simply differences in learning-style—many of which actually render them well-suited for various adult occupations" (a viewpoint that is engagingly flexible when contrasted with the Biederman vision of academic progress as the passport to a good life). Yet, whatever the causes may be of such children's behavioral problems, the odds are increasingly good that they will be diagnosed with ADHD (and additional psychiatric disorders)—and then medicated to control their behavior. But medicating is not quite the same as "rearing," and in turning too quickly to a pharmacological fix we may treat the child as "just body," failing thereby to recognize the child's full dignity. Some of these children surely are genuinely disturbed; they need, and may benefit from, medication. But, at least in the clinical judgment of the Eides, it is less certain that others are really helped. They may be enabled to conform better to the schedules they are given, but it is not clear that they make measurable gains in learning.

Another factor complicating diagnosis came out especially clearly in the presentation to the Council made by Dr. Diller: namely, complexities buried in the concept of "impairment." Dr. Biederman, as I noted earlier, was concerned to argue that impairment or dysfunction are relative terms. One's achievements may be quite respectable and may even surpass those of many of one's peers (as, in my extended example, was true of Augustine) while, nonetheless, one is never really able, in Dr. Biederman's words, to use one's "intellectual ability to the fullest." Whereas Dr. Biederman seemed to have relatively little hesitation about the good of medicating such persons, Dr. Diller raised doubts and questions.

He recounted, for example, an instance of medical students who had failed the national credentialing exam and had then sued the National Board of Medical Examiners—claiming that, because of an ADHD disorder, they needed unlimited time to take the exam. The court ruled against them, noting—reasonably enough, it might seem to the lay observer—that, though they may be impaired in terms of their potential, as persons capable of completing medical school education they could hardly be said to be impaired when compared to the population in general. Any of us, even if our talents are many, may set the bar of our aspirations so high that we will almost inevitably experience anxiety; yet, it is hard to think that we are then best described as impaired. If such comparatively talented and capable people are afflicted with a disorder, it may have to do at least as much with their (or their parents') desires and aspirations, their sense of what could count as a good life, than with any medical disorder—more, that is, to do with morality than with medicine.[13] Perhaps a clinician could medicate them and they might feel they had been "helped," but we should not be entirely indifferent to the distinction between help that works "with" them as they struggle to become persons of a certain sort and help that merely works "on" them, making adjustments of biochemistry.

These disputes are seldom, if ever, merely about facts. Deeper issues—which, for lack of a better term, we may simply call philosophical—are generally buried in the discussion, needing to be uncovered. Thus, for example, at least in my judgment, the Eides have a considerably richer and more nuanced understanding of the meaning of childhood than Dr. Biederman's rather monochromatic sense of childhood as an essentially prospective state, a stage on the way toward adulthood. No amount of medical expertise alone can tell us how best to think about childhood. Even a psychiatric clinician is not an expert on the meaning of the good life or how to live well.

In raising children, educating them, and shaping their behavior, we hope for certain results, and we look for means to achieve those results. But that is not all we should hope for. We should want something more than just a certain *result* (a disciplined, thoughtful, and cooperative child). If that were all we wanted, there would be little reason not to turn almost at once to medication. But our aim is not just to produce certain behavior, desirable as it, of course, is. We want a child who has begun to become a person of a certain sort—whose character is such that he or she is increasingly disposed to be disciplined, cooperative, kind. In search of such results, however, we cannot simply want

13. Cf. Peter Conrad, *The Medicalization of Society* (Baltimore: Johns Hopkins University Press, 2007), 64: "What is interesting about adult ADHD is that many of those who are given the diagnosis are by some measures successful individuals."

to make a young Augustine less restless; for that discontented *eros* draws him, finally, toward God. Simply medicating to achieve a desired result would be to substitute "the language and methods of medicine for the language and methods of moral education" (91). What we want is an Augustine whose restless desire has been directed toward the goods of life in loves that are—to revert to the language he himself used—ordinate rather than inordinate.

From some perspectives, of course, such a position may seem out-of-date. Thus, for example, Dr. Biederman noted that in the past many would have described the case of a child who plays Nintendo for hours while seeming unable to do homework for two minutes as a "volitional" problem. But in Dr. Biederman's view, to characterize it as a problem of the will calling for moral discipline would be mistaken. Perhaps it sometimes is mistaken. But is that determination the province of any single group of experts? It raises deep questions about the nature of the self, the meaning of the self's involvement and agency in human activity, and the difference between achieving a certain result and becoming a person of a certain sort. As Council member Francis Fukuyama noted in the discussion that followed Dr. Diller's presentation, approaching these diagnostic issues too narrowly "reduces our understanding of moral agency" and "medicalizes a whole range of behaviors that traditionally were thought of as moral behavior," which had to be "socialized and taught." Of course, physicians must attend to such matters, but these are not questions for them alone to ponder.

In his presentation to and conversation with the President's Council, Dr. Steven Hyman leaned in the direction of a view like Dr. Biederman's, but the puzzling complexity of the phenomena eventually compelled him to draw back somewhat. There is, he said, no fundamental difference between using psychotropic drugs to affect the brain and using our disciplined experience to do so. Both are probably ways of accomplishing the same mechanistic aim: remodeling synapses within the brain. If that is really true, of course, it should make no difference to us which means we choose to reach the desired end when behavior needs to be altered.

Nevertheless, Dr. Hyman could not bring himself to be entirely indifferent, and he drew back somewhat from the implications of his own assertion. He preferred treatment approaches that do not immediately turn to drugs, fearing that doing so would send a message that this was the best way to deal with life's problems. The message to children would be something like: "Behavioral control comes from a bottle." Dr. Hyman added, "We have the problem of anabolic steroids for the soul." If, however, there were really no significant difference between moral education and prescription drugs as means for reshaping behavior, it would be hard to know why Dr. Hyman should draw back from medicalizing behavioral problems (assuming the drugs being used are safe). Thus, his scientific/philosophical view of mind and brain stands in some tension with his reluctance to turn at once to medication as a solution to misbehavior and its accompanying discontents.

I do not say this with any intent to criticize him. On the contrary, honest puzzlement here is a sign of humane insight. It recognizes the peculiar character of human beings, those organisms whose mediated relation to the world gives rise to the capacity for reflection and the ability to act purposively. The action of such agents, unlike simple behavior, integrates body, mind, and spirit in ways that express the peculiar character of being human.

Because Ritalin functions as a kind of universal stimulant—enhancing alertness and attentiveness not only in those children with a true disability but also in all who take it—we are tempted to reduce a wide and complex range of behaviors (and behavior problems) to just one thing: chemistry of the brain, to be fixed with a pill. Surely, however, this is no better than obstinately insisting that the cure for all a child's behavioral problems lies in disciplining the will.

The philosopher John Wisdom told the story of a keeper at a Dublin zoo, who had a record of great success at breeding lions. When asked the secret of his success, he replied, "Understanding lions." Asked, then, what understanding lions entailed, he answered, "Every lion is different."[14] We should say no less of children—at least if we remind ourselves to think of them as human beings, those in-between creatures who can be reduced neither to will alone nor to brain chemistry alone.

14. John Wisdom, *Paradox and Discovery* (Oxford: Basil Blackwell, 1965), 138.

4

Washington Square

Harvey C. Mansfield

Henry James's short novel *Washington Square* is about Dr. Austin Sloper, a resident of that Square in New York City, who cannot persuade his daughter Catherine not to marry Morris Townshend, whom he correctly regards as an idle mercenary. Although he is a successful doctor, he fails as a father. Besides being a doctor, he is several times called a philosopher, as having an aura above practical science, and in confirmation is said to have "an idea of the beauty of reason" (2:32).[1] But he cannot rule his daughter with the authority of his reason and ends up losing her respect. The novel is a story of loss: Dr. Sloper loses his daughter, and she loses both him and her lover Morris Townshend, who also loses her. In the end, Catherine is vindicated as the heroine of the novel because only she is able to come to terms with her loss.

To say that the novel "is about" this or something else betrays my amateur status as literary critic, for I cannot read a book without wondering whether the author has a point to convey, and about the conventions of criticism apart from that point I am ill-informed. I came to this book to honor my friend Leon Kass, also a doctor and a philosopher (a more serious one) but, though he has a daughter—indeed, two daughters—he does not otherwise resemble Dr. Sloper. Kass has, however, been concerned with the problem of authority as it appears in *Washington Square.* I believe that James has something valuable to say about authority, in America or anywhere, at the time of "republican simplicity" of his novel or at any time, and in particular about the authority of science and the resistance to it that continues today.

Let us begin as does Henry James with the character of Dr. Sloper, very definitively set down at the beginning of the novel. Dr. Sloper was a distinguished physician, a member of a profession known in America more than elsewhere as liberal. James is writing, or the narrator is telling, of the recent past, "the first half

1. References are to chapter and page in the Penguin Classics edition: Henry James, *Washington Square*, ed. Brian Lee (London: Penguin Books, 1984). The novel was first published in 1880.

of the present century," in early nineteenth-century America when things were different. Yet it is constant in America that, to "play a social part," one must earn or appear to earn one's income, thus be practical, while at the same time to be "touched by the light of science," like the physician, is also accounted a merit. Americans have a "love of knowledge . . . not always . . . accompanied by leisure and opportunity"—James's typically indirect way of saying that Americans are not quite satisfied with the practical but not willing to devote themselves to an impractical love of knowledge for its own sake (1:27).

This was a "scholarly doctor" who always gave his patients a prescription, a remedy as well as an explanation, neither theoretical without a remedy nor vulgar without an explanation. He was popular and had a first-rate reputation, which are equivalents in the American democracy. His public character easily survived two grievous blows, the death of his first-born child, a son, followed by the death of his wife in giving birth to his second-born, a daughter. For these failures he was pitied rather than blamed by others, but he blamed himself for the rest of his days. He was and was known to be a "clever man," but he suffered disappointment in his own life, in the application of his cleverness to his own affairs. His disappointment fell most heavily on his surviving daughter, Catherine, who was both plain and dull, yet so robust and healthy that the doctor could have no fear of losing her as he had lost his wife and son.

James also says that Dr. Sloper was "an observer, even a philosopher," as if the science of medicine were touched by the light of something higher than science (1:28). The word "philosopher" occurs eight times in the novel in different forms, loosely as befits a democracy that sees value in science but not in the love of knowledge undirected toward practice. Most frequently James uses it in the loose and popular sense of being able to accept disappointment, like a Stoic (though to be sure without mentioning "Stoic"). He later says that Dr. Sloper was a philosopher in this sense (2:36), but in the novel he proves to be very far from reconciled to the disappointment of his daughter's rejection of his advice—which becomes a command—not to marry Morris Townshend. Morris Townshend for his part seems much more philosophical in this sense than Dr. Sloper, yet his last word in the novel, as he is sent away by the daughter, is "Damnation!" (35:210) The only one who calmly accepts disappointment is Catherine Sloper, who, having lost her father and her beloved, ends the last scene by sitting down to her embroidery "for life, as it were."

Philosophy in this loose sense means acceptance of the reality that for certain human ills there is no remedy—the very contrary of science, which tirelessly seeks a remedy for everything. James insistently calls Catherine his "heroine" in order to indicate by his choice that he has something to tell to Americans (and to others like them) about the necessity of acceptance. That Americans use "philosophy" in this sense as praise shows some appreciation for the resistance of reality to our wishes, but suggests too that they have no considered understanding of it. In *Washington Square* James sets himself as the narrator above his characters, to whom he condescends, I think because he wants his readers to feel disappointment in a novel with no obvious hero or heroine—he has to identify Catherine as the heroine for us six times[2]—that is lacking in drama and that does not have a happy ending. He takes pride in producing a novel that makes us feel disappointed in order to understand better the nature of disappointment, particularly as it comes to a country that in its young history, and with its belief in progress, does not suffer it well. "Philosophy" is so far from being an accidental expression in *Washington Square* as to be the name for the wisdom, in its loose sense of intelligent resignation, that James actually teaches his readers. As an intellectual virtue it includes science while opposing the false optimism of science, and as a moral virtue it is democratically available to non-philosophers such as Catherine and very useful to democracy while opposing the false optimism that is characteristic of democracy as well as of science.

Morris Townshend is Catherine's beloved, the lover whom Dr. Sloper rejects as a son-in-law. The novel is a contest between the two for Catherine's mind, won by neither.[3] Townshend is introduced very differently from Dr. Sloper, for whom James wanted to be seen as "describing a clever man," with all his virtues and accomplishment set forth in the first few pages of the book. We see Townshend only by stages, first through the eyes of Catherine as she meets him, but with the narrator looking over her shoulder and correcting her. Townshend speaks to her with easy charm, dances with her, amusing and beguiling her, so that she has to learn his first name from her aunt Mrs. Almond. As soon as she learns it she seems to hear it repeated in her ear, but as she leaves the party she pretends to her other aunt Mrs. Penniman and to her father that she does not know it. Catherine is quite taken with Townshend and wants to keep him to herself, a first sign of the rebellion to come.

By contrast to Dr. Sloper, Townshend is never described either definitely or completely, but is left in vagueness throughout. His doings are mostly a matter of rumor, also of his own unspecific confession that he had been "wild" (12:91). He had been "knocking about the world, and living in queer corners" (4:44). He has spent the small amount of money he inherited, led a "life of

2. James, *Washington Square*, 2:34, 3:40, 4:46; 10:78, 79 (this time in the mind of Mrs. Penniman); 25:158. In *Portrait of a Lady* Isabel Archer is also so identified several times.

3. Cf. William Veeder, *Henry James, the Lessons of the Master* (Chicago: University of Chicago Press, 1975), 188, who emphasizes "the sinister bond" between Dr. Sloper and Morris Townshend.

dissipation," but he was amusing himself and he doesn't owe a penny (11:86, 12:91). He has "never concealed" his "great follies," but they are never revealed either (12:91). Disputing with her father, Catherine says, "you know a part of him—what he has chosen to show you. You don't know the rest." When her father asks her what is the rest, Catherine does not know but merely says, "there is sure to be plenty of it." At the end, when Townshend comes back to see Catherine years later, the narrator says, "he had made himself comfortable, and he had never been caught" (35:217). Caught doing what? And by the police or by public opinion? It is not said. Having said early on that he was looking for a "position," Townshend later gets one—but as what? He is in "partnership with a commission merchant," Mrs. Penniman tells Catherine—perhaps the vaguest possible employment, trading rather than earning (25:159). Earlier his sister, the widowed Mrs. Montgomery, admitted to Dr. Sloper that Townshend had not actually brought up her children for her but had assisted in their education by teaching them Spanish (14:102). "That must take a great deal off your hands!" the doctor laughed, and then went on to ask directly whether Townshend was not sponging off her, an impecunious widow with five children.

With this question, which Dr. Sloper admits is crude, we come to the opposition between Dr. Sloper and Morris Townshend. The reason why Dr. Sloper rejects Townshend as a son-in-law is that he regards him as an idle mercenary who wants to marry Catherine for her money, the money she will inherit from him. James gives us reason to suppose that Dr. Sloper may be right, when Mrs. Penniman relates to Townshend that Dr. Sloper pretends he likes the money he would get from marrying Catherine. "I *do* like the money!" replies Townshend (16:113). Then, while Dr. Sloper takes Catherine on a trip to Europe to distract her from the idea of this disastrous marriage, Mrs. Penniman lives in his house and invites Townshend frequently to tea. Townshend makes himself at home there. He spends time "turning over the curious collections of its absent proprietor," whatever they were. He "found the house a perfect castle of indolence," and it became for him "a club with a single member" (23:151). Earlier he had said that this is "a devilish comfortable house," rueful but still relishing the prospect of living there with Catherine after her inheritance upon the doctor's death (16:116).

All this is clear evidence that Morris Townshend was indeed an idle mercenary, if "idle" means not twiddling one's thumbs but having no position, and if "mercenary" means not greedy but living without earning an income. But what is wrong with that? Henry James does not quite pose this question, though in some ways, we shall see, he invites it. It may seem strange to ask why "sponging" is wrong, still stranger to try to find a defense for it. For we today still commonly have contempt for that sort of dependency, and apart from that fact, one, and only one, definite answer to the question is given in the novel, and that is by Dr. Sloper as he condemns it. Dr. Sloper is suspicious of Townshend from the start, as soon as he sees him take an interest in Catherine. His view was pre-determined; he thought his daughter as plain and dull as Henry James describes her, "neither pretty nor lively," so that any attraction to her could only be for her fortune (6:60). After Morris had called on his daughter once, he jokingly asks her, "did he propose to you today?" She returns, with humor that surprised him: "Perhaps he will do it the next time" (6:58).

After this retort, Dr. Sloper moves quickly to establish "what sort of gentleman" is Morris Townshend. Dr. Sloper's intelligent sister Mrs. Almond sends him to Morris's sister, Mrs. Montgomery, who confirms his impression that Townshend sponges off her, as we have seen. He observes Morris carefully at a dinner party, from which he sees that Morris "has a very good head if he chooses to use it," and Morris concludes, correctly, that Dr. Sloper does not like him. At an evening at Mrs. Almond's, the Doctor tries Morris again, from which Morris escapes, impudently the Doctor thinks, with his claim that he is "amateur tutor" to his sister's children (9:74). After Catherine tells her father that she is engaged to be married, he tells her directly that he does not like Morris and on the following day confronts him as he arrives to ask him to approve the engagement. In this meeting the Doctor comes out on top. He explains to Morris why he disapproves of him as a son-in-law in a critical scene in which Morris argues that he is not an idle mercenary and the Doctor asserts to his face, "I don't want to believe in you" (12:90). Catherine would be miserable as Townshend's wife, the doctor believes, and yet he does not care if she were miserable even for a lifetime as a result of following his strong recommendation.

But to defend his disapproval, Dr. Sloper does not say that he knows Morris's character for sure. He merely says he belongs to the wrong category, the category of those whose absence of means or profession or resources or prospects would make it imprudent for him to "select" Morris as a husband for his daughter, "who is a weak young woman with a large fortune" (12:89). He will not forbid the marriage, he says, for "I am not a father in an old-fashioned novel" (12:93). In an old-fashioned novel the father would simply forbid, but in this one he reasons, using a category based on his medical trade in which, he tells Mrs. Almond, he is right in estimating people nineteen times out of twenty (13:94). Later he refers to the "philosophic trick" of induction that resembles his use of a category here (14:101-102, cf. 27:168). New-fashioned he may claim to be, but still he wants to "select" his daughter's husband. His "category," his habit of "dividing people into classes, into types," enables him to avoid the task of judging Morris Townshend as an individual and as a husband, and it assumes that earning one's living is the only respectable life.[4]

Two difficulties in this premise appear in *Washington Square*, the first having to do with Dr. Sloper, the second with Catherine. Dr. Sloper himself started with an income he did not earn, the result of marrying a rich wife. True, he would have been a doctor without this "accident," and he had not become a doctor merely to make money but "to learn something and to do something" (1:29). Nonetheless, this good start enabled him to be a doctor "in the best possible conditions," which meant having patients among "the best people." Then, in addition, he earned enough because of his merit and the good start to make a fortune of his own, which was improving at a rate of $10,000 a year; this was not an accident (3:37). Merit was Dr. Sloper's guiding principle—the idea that "you are good for nothing unless you are clever"—but his merit has received an assist at the beginning of his life and will leave a "fortune" for his heirs that they have not made on their own. His own fortune, which Catherine stood to inherit, is the very thing, the topic of the novel, over which he and Morris Townshend dispute. He does not object to the acquisition by marriage of a large sum: "It's right to get all one can" in that case (14:100). In Dr. Sloper's own case, however, merit begins and ends with unearned income, with one inheritance that is received from his wife and another that is left to his heirs without any but an accidental relation to merit.

Dr. Sloper makes a great point of Morris's "living *upon*" his sister (6:61), or, he also says, "living with her and doing nothing for himself" (8:71). He does not want such a person for a son-in-law and he refuses to give Catherine a penny of his fortune if she marries him. Now, how does this judgment affect Catherine, his daughter, who lives with him and does nothing for herself to earn her income? After she learns from him of his refusal and still insists on marrying Morris, she says to him: "If I live with you, I ought to obey you." Here "living with" requires obedience, as opposed to "living off," which perhaps has no requirements. Dr. Sloper agrees with this theory, to which she replies to his surprise: "But if I don't obey you, I ought not to live with you" (22:146). To live with and not obey is sponging. Dr. Sloper's principle makes a slave of his daughter and in general does not apply to women; it applies only to those men who take advantage of women. "You women are all the same!" the doctor declaims. Women tolerate and make excuses for men who are weak, who accept nothing of life but its pleasures, and who secure pleasures mainly from the "complaisant sex" (14:101). In sum, the doctor has no place for women in the merit

4. Veeder, op. cit., 192-94, applies this inadequacy to the doctor's judgment of Catherine, but it also applies to his judgment of Morris.

principle, the standard by which he denounces Morris Townshend. Catherine sees this and—in her "striking argument" to her father, not Townshend's but "my own," she says—she discovers the independence that makes her the heroine of *Washington Square*.

The merit principle has a political aspect, which we must now begin to unfold. It is enshrined in the "temple of Republican simplicity" to which Dr. Sloper pays his devotions by his distrust of luxury. Early on he worries that Catherine dresses too richly, on the occasion of the party at which she meets Morris, in a red satin gown trimmed with a gold fringe that is described as "royal raiment." It is all right to make money, but vulgar to show it. Yet just as merit leads to a fortune, so also it brings on the desire for luxury, and the novel expressly chronicles the rising "tide of fashion" that accompanies the growth of trade in New York City from "murmur" to "uproar" (3:38). The trend shows in the movement of the most fashionable real estate from Canal Street and the Battery on the lower tip of Manhattan to Washington Square and then uptown beyond that.[5] When Dr. Sloper married his wife Catherine in 1820, she was one of the pretty girls of the "small but promising capital" at the Battery, referring perhaps to the fact that New York was the first Capital of the United States in 1789-1790 (though not, of course, in 1820); it was the place where George Washington was sworn in as first President (1:28). Dr. Sloper then built, in 1835, a handsome house described as "modern" in Washington Square, uptown at Fourth Street, today a park in Greenwich Village. At the close of the novel the same house is called "old" and considered unfashionable in comparison with the brownstones further uptown (34:210). The Washington of the Square is George Washington, and the title of the novel marks a stage in the progress of the American republic in which wealthy, earned fortunes make their troublesome appearance and republican simplicity comes to be doubted and evaded.

There is worse to come for republican simplicity, but after this account of Dr. Sloper's merit principle, let us first see what might be said in behalf of Morris Townshend or the life of the idle mercenary. As little is said to describe Morris's life or to define his character, so he himself says little to defend either of them. Certainly he does not have a principle strong and clear enough to oppose effectively Dr. Sloper's powerful rejection of him. We have seen that he makes a weak defense of himself as an amateur tutor of Spanish to his nephews, that later he claims to have a job as partner of a commission merchant, out of which nothing solid ever emerges, and that when he returns to see Catherine at

5. New York is "a great city in which everyone is both literally and metaphorically moving uptown." Richard Poirier, "*The American* and *Washington Square*: The Comic Sense," in Harold Bloom, ed., *Modern Critical Views: Henry James* (New York: Chelsea House, 1987), 68.

the end, years later, it is said of him that he had made himself comfortable and "had never been caught," hardly a recommendation. What does Catherine see to have fallen in love with him? She sees charm and intelligence, an entertaining husband, but then after Morris refuses to marry her without the inheritance her father has denied her, she turns against him for good.

One person in the novel intercedes for Morris, defends him in every situation and regards him as a "hero," the only one to do so, and that is Mrs. Lavinia Penniman, Dr. Sloper's sister (10:79). Mrs. Penniman is the widow of a preacher (with whom Dr. Sloper had once had an angry exchange) who, having no money, comes to live with the doctor after her husband died. But Mrs. Penniman, we are told, was a "goose" (2:35). Morris had originally used her as an intermediary to recommend him to Catherine, who "was not wise enough to discover" her aunt's stupidity. Later, she does discover it when she learns that Mrs. Penniman has met privately with Morris and is taking his part against her father. To Catherine Mrs. Penniman conveys greater assurance of Morris's desire to marry her than is the fact and in doing so helps to increase her disappointment when she finds that Morris will not marry her disinherited from her father's fortune. Catherine has great respect for her father and felt that to displease him would be like "an act of profanity in a great temple" (18:121). When she does then deliberately displease him, it is not because her aunt had with her usual levity suggested it. Later, she finds that her aunt had encouraged Morris to leave her or justified his leaving, as if she had agreed to it (30:192). And at the end of the book, after the doctor's death and years have passed while aunt and niece live together in the house in Washington Square, it is the aunt, always seeking drama and now providing the climax of Henry James's novel, who tells Catherine that she has seen Townshend and who then "takes the liberty" of inviting him, despite Catherine's discouragement, to see her again, as it turns out, one last time. In sum, the case for Morris, and the management of what Mrs. Penniman regards as "the real romance of his life" (words attributed by her to him), are in the charge of a goose (34:212).

Yet there is a case for Townshend that one might begin to state from a summary of him by Mrs. Almond, Dr. Sloper's younger and wiser sister. By no means wishing to compliment Morris, she says that if he marries Catherine, and gets the doctor's money, "he will be an idle, amiable, selfish, and . . . tolerably good-natured fellow" (23:151). She goes on to say that if she does not get the money, he will take revenge and be "pitiless and cruel" as a husband. This last is a judgment not borne out in the novel, because Morris has the sense not to marry her. He is indeed looking for someone to live upon, and under that condition he would be a perfectly good husband for Catherine, a better one, perhaps, than a man Dr.

Sloper would respect.[6] We do not know what Morris really does with his life, besides not earning a living and seeking an unearned income for himself. There are people wrapped up in themselves—philosophers come to mind—who could be considered selfish, idle, sponging mercenaries, perhaps even cruel if distracted from their preoccupation, without being worthless.

I do not suppose that Henry James's repeated references to philosophy in *Washington Square* are casual or distant or unserious; there was, after all, a philosopher in his family. But there is an appearance of casualness arising from the fact that philosophy is seen from underneath in his book, for its upshot and not as a philosopher would see it.[7] As it appears there, "philosophy" means reasoning strictly, as by inference or induction, and it also describes a moral attitude of equanimity, especially the latter. Looking at Dr. Sloper and Morris Townshend, we see that the former is called a philosopher and the latter is not. Summing them up, we may judge that Dr. Sloper is knowing (or "clever"), is a gentleman, accomplished, has a sterling reputation, and has his own means—whereas Townshend is looking (always looking around without finding anything, 5:52), is not a gentleman (so Dr. Sloper, though Morris claims to be one), a ne'er-do-well, held to be "wild," and lives upon others. Each has one aspect of the philosopher—Dr. Sloper the knowledge and belief in the beauty of reason, the scientific part of philosophy, and Morris Townshend the life of seeking rather than finding—but each also falls short. Neither has equanimity of mind, the most prominent characteristic of the philosopher as given by James, apparently casually but I would say with purpose, in this book. Each of them curses Catherine, the heroine. Dr. Sloper gives her a father's curse in disinheriting her, even insulting her in his will; Morris Townshend, though coolly facing his opponent and cautious in considering his prospects, ends by calling out "Damnation."

I was going to say that each of them curses *poor* Catherine, but she is the one who shows equanimity. After her father's death she lives contentedly with one-fifth of his inheritance, not contesting his will but only remarking that she "wish[ed] it had been expressed a little differently!" (33:208) Her response to Morris Townshend, if she heard him as he left the house, was to go back to her embroidery.

What is wrong with the two men? To Morris, when at the end after many years he comes back to ask for her friendship, she says: "You treated me badly"

6. See S. Gorley Putt, *Henry James: a Reader's Guide* (Ithaca, New York: Cornell University Press, 1987), 51.

7. Richard Poirier, a fine critic of *Washington Square*, disparages any "mole-like search for buried philosophic treasure" in it. I begin from the surface fact that James uses the word and proceed to wonder why. See Poirier, op. cit., 59.

(35:218). He had won her love, promising to stay with her regardless of the inheritance though urging her to do her best to persuade her father not to deny it. When the denial comes, they have a confrontation that Catherine, James's undramatic heroine, refuses to accept as a "scene" (29:181). Morris, trying to make a quarrel that would ease his abandonment of her, says he is too proud to owe her anything (agreeing with Dr. Sloper that earning is the only way to live). She replies that she will take him as he is. He departs New York, refusing to see her as she begs him, forcing her into the shame of going to his home to ask for him, and then sends her a letter in which he deplores the necessity of this abandonment, claiming that the two of them are "innocent but philosophic victims of a great social law" (31:196). The great social law is that they cannot marry each other because she is rich and he is poor; he would necessarily have to live upon her, thus making him dependent on her, hurting his pride and violating the freedom and equality of republican simplicity. In this statement Morris translates earning one's income as "rich," and failing to do so as "poor." His wanting an unearned income to live upon made him poor, and he could not find a way to justify himself to Catherine.

Mrs. Penniman suggests to Catherine, as if in his name, that Morris's "scruples" keep him from agreeing to the marriage that would bring down her father's curse on her and cost her an inheritance (30:194). This argument has the effect of justifying Dr. Sloper's conduct rather than Catherine's: he was right to think Morris was an idle mercenary and she was wrong to think he loved her. Her love for him was unrequited and she thought it just that he return it. He would have made a good husband under his terms but, as Mrs. Almond said, he could not meet hers. He was cruel to her as lovers feel and understand cruelty—the injustice of loving another and not being loved in return. Republican simplicity requires that love be requited—mutuality for the sake of equality—as opposed to marriage between unequals based on mutual advantage. Republican simplicity renders spenders like Morris unequal to earners like Dr. Sloper, thus unfit to marry the daughter of an earner. Morris was too republican to defend himself, and Henry James does not suggest a republican defense he might have used. All he does is to make his readers wish for such a defense so that Morris could marry Catherine and the novel have a happy ending.

If Morris Townshend had too little justice to offer, Dr. Sloper had too much. It is time to return to the question of authority raised earlier. James shows by stages the breakdown of reason to authority, from the doctor who has an idea of the beauty of reason, to the father who becomes a tyrant as the idea of reason is carried into practice. We have seen Dr. Sloper suspicious of Morris Townshend from the beginning. He has a natural father's concern for the happiness of his daughter, but it is narrowed and framed by the principle that merit is shown in the earning of one's own income by contrast to the idle selfishness of living upon others, a principle that ignores possible merit in not earning one's income. By chapter six, the doctor is moving to apply this principle to Morris, and he tosses aside Mrs. Penniman's rosy view that Morris is a "young man of great force of character, and of remarkable powers of satire" (5:56). He determines (as seen above) from his other sister, Mrs. Almond, that Morris lives with his widowed sister and considers that this means living upon her. In the next chapter he decides, based on a quick view of Morris and his long experience as a doctor, that Morris is not a gentleman, is in fact a "plausible coxcomb" (6:65). His daughter, he decides too, is a "grievous simpleton" whose view of Morris can be dismissed if not ignored, and he turns on Mrs. Penniman, who tells him correctly that his daughter is not a "weak-minded woman" (8:71).

The next chapter, the ninth, in which Dr. Sloper foils Morris Townshend but loses his daughter, is the crux of the novel. Dr. Sloper admits that Morris is intelligent and keen, but believes that this makes him more dangerous to his weak-minded daughter, and he sees that Morris is calm and affable, with no sign of evasiveness, but puts this down to his amazing conceit. Catherine agrees to meet him, not at a tryst as Morris proposes but in the parlor of the Doctor's home rather than behind his back, in his face one could say, declaring her independence.

Not being an old-fashioned father, Dr. Sloper will not forbid his daughter's marriage but he will disinherit her if she goes ahead with it. This move sets a love test for the couple and has the effect of exposing the mercenary motive of Townshend by separating it from his good will and decency as well as love. To the extent that he treats Catherine badly it is because he was compelled to give up his interest, necessarily "selfish," in order to have her. Dr. Sloper makes Morris behave worse than he wants; this is not the voice of reason being reasonable. Though "determined to be very mild" with his daughter (11:83), he proceeds to Morris's sister, Mrs. Montgomery, and gets her, with promises of financial help, to say to him "Don't let him [Morris] marry her!" (14:104). He also wanted her to say that Morris is "abominably selfish," though Mrs. Montgomery denies him this "moral satisfaction" (14:103). He states that the function of a son-in-law is to be a protector and care-taker of "my child," who cannot take care of herself. His premise is that Catherine remains his child, not that, being his daughter, she might be grateful for his advice.

Catherine tells Mrs. Penniman that she has not seen Morris "because my father has forbidden it" (17:117). But her will is now her own if not her behavior. In a subtle passage James shows her father demanding that she make him happy by giving up Morris: "It all depends on your will" (18:123). But he means that her will is to depend on his, as Catherine sees in asking, "Is it to give him up?" "It" means *his* will, and he answers, "yes." Have you no "faith in my wisdom . . . ?" he inquires. Catherine believes, we have noticed, that to displease him would be like "an act of profanity in a great temple" (18:121). Her father was sorry for her but was "so sure he was right" (18:126). In the next chapter Dr. Sloper demands of Mrs. Penniman that she cease giving encouragement to Catherine, who is "in deliberate opposition to my wishes." To give her aid and comfort would be "distinctly treasonable" (19:127). You talk like a "great autocrat," says Mrs. Penniman, and Dr. Sloper replies that he talks like his daughter's father. His reason has become his will, and his will is stated by Mrs. Penniman in political terms. Mrs. Penniman does not think that Dr. Sloper is an Orthodox Christian, but Catherine begins to think that she has broken a "sacred law" in opposing him (21:140, 22:144).

With this phrase the question of the relevance of divinity makes a slight but significant intrusion into the novel. For it is obvious that the difference between making one's own living and living upon someone else is affected by man's relation to God. If Dr. Sloper depends for his existence and prosperity on the providence of God, then he can be said to earn his own living only in a limited sense. His earning would be consequent to a gift, for which he would have to be grateful rather than proud as if it were entirely his own doing. Thus it is no accident that he represents the modern science that brings benefit to human beings because it doubts God's beneficence and believes that progress will occur only from adopting that doubt as its premise. Nor is it a surprise that the belief in one's own self-sufficiency, which is both cause and effect of earning one's own living, should excite a certain phantom sense of divinity in one's own authority, such as happened to Dr. Sloper.

The doctor takes his daughter on a trip to Europe in the hope that she will be distracted from her love, and Catherine consents in the hope that he will be mollified in his will. Europe seems to stand for the beauties of life as they soften its willfulness, but it doesn't work this time. Catherine accompanies her father dutifully, but at last, in a desolate scene high in the Alps, he challenges her to say whether she has given up Morris, and she answers no. To which he replies that he is very angry, he is "not a good man," and he can be "very hard"—as indeed he proves to be (24:154). The doctor is "exasperated" (27:170). Morris justly observes that he "combines the properties of a lump of ice and a red-hot coal," so far is he from equanimity. In an exchange with his wiser sister Mrs. Almond, Dr. Sloper refuses sympathy to Catherine and insists that there was nothing cruel in saving her from an abominable marriage (32:101).

As Dr. Sloper descends from the temple of republican simplicity to the autocracy of a patriarch enshrined by sacred law, Catherine ascends in the other direction from plain and dull to her own "authoritative speech" (25:163). When telling her father of her engagement, she obliges him to give his reasons for opposing it but only succeeds in hardening his authority (11:86). She does give herself authority, however. Soon she finds herself "thinking over her situation" and considering how to be a good daughter (15:105-106). While doing so she sees herself as another person "who was both herself and not herself." She was making up her mind, a phrase we use both for reflecting on something and for settling on a solution, both reason and authority.

James gives a picture of self-knowledge at work in the one character in the novel who learns something, who "grows," as we say now. "I am braver than I was," she says to Mrs. Penniman (25:161). She never does anything drastic, and *Washington Square* is a rather dull romance. Catherine has to be identified as its heroine because she does nothing dramatic to demand our interest in her. She lives in a republic that is not as simple as it thinks itself to be, for it is devoted to making money—Dr. Sloper himself, we recall, says that "it's right to get all one can"—but morally contemptuous of one who appears to be mercenary (14:100). James invites us to foresee trouble arising from this two-faced attitude. The honesty that distinguishes earning from non-earning can transform itself into high-minded contempt for those who do not earn, above all women, of whom Dr. Sloper has little good to say. For this he receives a deserved reproof from the author, who makes a woman the heroine. Hardly a siren, no sort of queen, she is a woman who says to her supposed lover: "I disappoint every one" (20:135).

The most notable point that could have been made in Morris Townshend's defense can be glimpsed in Dr. Sloper's strongest attack on him. While Dr. Sloper is away in Europe, Morris, as noted above, was "making free" with his house by invitation of Mrs. Penniman. The doctor calls this "inconceivable bad taste" and says of Morris, who passes through the novel undefined, as we saw, "if that doesn't describe him, he is indescribable" (27:170). What Morris does is to spend Dr. Sloper's money in his absence, just as he might have done as his son-in-law after he died.[8] Morris is a spender as opposed to an earner. Now, what does one earn money for if not to spend it at some point? If so, what good is it to earn money if one doesn't know how to spend it? One could even say, and the classical philosophers said it, that money, and indeed all things, belong truly, as opposed to legally, to those who know how to use them best.

8. "A club with a single member," as Dr. Sloper's house became for Morris Townshend, would be a nice description of philosophical reflection (23:151). But one does not know whether it took place.

What most infuriates Dr. Sloper about Townshend should impress him the most—"why, here is a man who can spend my money better than I! I should let him go to it." Dr. Sloper does not appreciate that his true objection to Morris is not that he does not earn but that he will not spend well. Earning one's own money does not guarantee that one will use it well, as is obvious in Dr. Sloper's case. Although claiming, and wishing, to act in his daughter's interest he did his best to make her life miserable.

One can see why the American republic respects earners rather than spenders, for most everyone can earn and very few can spend well. Earning is more democratic than spending as the test of merit, and the honest earner does not take from other earners, whereas the spender uses another's money. But if we relax the requirement that one be a philosopher in order to spend well, a more political, even more republican view emerges. The multitude of those who earn does not, at this time, include women; so half the citizens are left without the republican respect due to merit. But if women are not allowed to earn, they can at least spend well; they can excel at home economics. This possibility does not occur to Dr. Sloper, and if it had, he would probably not have extended the principle to include Morris. Catherine, however, spent her money well in charitable activities and "became an admirable old maid . . . with an even and noiseless step," an unspoken example to all (32:203). After Catherine had been jilted, she refused at least two offers of marriage, one from a young man who was "seriously in love" with her (32:202). She was not going to learn and move on from her experience, for her love was serious because it had made her free. Because she knew how to live in leisure, she was in fact freer than her father.

The men in the American republic are unerotic earners, doubtful of love and suspicious of lovers, and they do not offer material for drama. At their best they are mostly like Dr. Sloper, too hard and too sure. After all, Dr. Sloper was a type of the kind he was fond of conceiving: it was his virtue mixed with his concern, and not his evil, that made him cruel. A few men are like Morris Townshend, reflective but too pliable, and unable to find a principle by which to sustain a leisured way of life with time for love as well as wine and cigars. The two men represent philosophy in the two loose senses of too rational and too unworldly. Henry James's heroine is philosophical in the loose sense, featured in *Washington Square,* of the ability to live with disappointment. This popular sense of "philosophy," no doubt connected to the stricter, more demanding notion that philosophy is learning to die, is perhaps needed most in a country devoted to progress like America. A commercial country, always on the rise, always moving "uptown," needs a source of equanimity for the times when its optimism proves false. James assigns it to women with the inner strength of soul that Catherine develops and displays.[9] In two novels following *Washington Square*, James follows the advancing course of the emancipation of women. *The Portrait of a Lady* (1881) has for its heroine Isabel Archer, a young American "very fond of my liberty," whose father has died and who receives a fortune to spend from her uncle. In *The Bostonians* (1886), Verena Tarrant is the object of a contest for her soul between a retrograde conservative man and a feminist woman. In both cases the modest "philosophy" of Catherine is left behind if not rejected, and in neither is the result a woman's happiness.

There is another woman in the novel whom I have mentioned throughout—Mrs. Penniman, the sister of Dr. Sloper who is labeled a goose by the narrator almost as soon as she appears. I have an idea that Mrs. Penniman, the mediator between the three main characters, who always fails because she tries to add drama to every occasion, is James's alter ego—as opposed to his heroine.[10] She brings the characters together and, by overdoing it, keeps them apart. She in her "innocent falsity" prides herself on "always saying the right thing"—even though she speaks twice of the "ruins of the Pantheon," mixing it up with the Parthenon (7:65, 25:159, 23:147-48). She flatters herself that she is "philosophic" (28:175). James's hallmark as a novelist is irony, and the word is used twice in the novel by Dr. Sloper,[11] who praises it and then lays it aside (27:169). Mrs. Pennington represents false drama, setting off by contrast to herself the sober good sense of Catherine, who needs no drama to see her way to independence. Yet readers need the contrast in order to see the point. James the novelist supplies the need of his readers for drama. All drama is false drama, as it is life dramatized, and yet true when the drama brings out a truth otherwise hidden. James amuses himself by appearing as a goose, and with his literary art he outdoes philosophy in the spirit of philosophy.[12]

9. It is sad that a feminist critic speaks only of "the dreadful confinement of Catherine." She does not blame Henry James: "It is not the plot imposed by the writer that is at fault but the plot that real-life social conditions impose on all women." She overlooks the strength of women that the supposedly patriarchal James makes manifest, for which she should have praised him (and modified her opposition to patriarchy). Mary Doyle Springer, "Closure in James: A Formalist Feminist View," in Daniel Mark Fogel, ed., *A Companion to Henry James Studies* (Westport, Connecticut: Greenwood Press, 1993), 275. Cf. Poirer, op. cit., 64, on the "hidden depths of [Catherine's] character," and Veeder, op. cit., 204-205, for a fine tribute to Catherine.

10. No critic has been found who shares this idea. Springer states the difficulty well as "the problem of the extra character," *extra* meaning one who has no necessary place in the story; see Mary Doyle Springer, *A Rhetoric of Literary Character: Some Women of Henry James* (Chicago: University of Chicago Press, 1978), 76-89. Springer underestimates both Henry James and his character Catherine Sloper, for Mrs. Penniman gives definition to Catherine's virtue, which without her would be too inconspicuous. Mrs. Penniman allows James to make fun of himself as the analyst who dramatizes the sober, undramatic American democracy.

11. The word appears eight times altogether.

12. See Machiavelli, *Discourses on Livy* III 2.

As a novelist James shows himself more accurate than Dr. Sloper, the character in his novel whom he ironically calls "philosopher." Dr. Sloper understands human beings scientifically and professionally according to "types" that may work in the practice of medicine (though not unfailingly) but that do not disclose the whole human being when it comes to judging a possible son-in-law.[13] James's refusal to describe Morris Townshend, leaving it unclear whether Catherine's love or her father's science supplies the truer judgment of him, is his way of showing the incompetence of science in the business of life. In the scene where Dr. Sloper declares definitely that he knows the character of Morris Townshend "well enough," he says to Catherine that she can wait to marry until he dies. "Your engagement," he says, "will make you extremely impatient for that event." The doctor enjoys making this point, as Catherine recoils in "natural horror." She regarded it as like a "logical axiom," not "in her province to controvert," yet a "scientific truth" she felt wholly unable to accept. Resistance to science, i.e., resistance to *his* science (for science in practice is always some human being's science), was the basis for her equanimity and her freedom. Science cannot understand resistance to science, hence cannot understand either the need for equanimity when science brings disappointment or the value of freedom from the sort of "scientific truth" that Catherine's father tried, unsuccessfully, to impose on her.

One could also consider whether Henry does not cast a doubting glance in the direction of his brother William's optimistic philosophy of pragmatism. In a way he is below philosophy, because one could reflect on the principle of earning one's own living without the aid of his characters and the action of his plot, brushing them aside to find more directly what the novel "is about." But in giving one to think with the help of the qualities of a novel, he keeps philosophy all the more alive because in his treatment it does not reek of answers and conclusions—and when it does overreach, in the person of Dr. Sloper, it can bring on the grand disappointments against which it should have armed us. Yet again, if one wants to be given to think, one must be in a receptive mood, not just looking curiously but looking for what the author, in the slightest details as well as in obvious features, shows the novel is about.

13. On this see Poirier, op. cit., 70.

5

The Silence of the Spartan: City, Soul, and Study of the Stars in the Epilogue to Plato's Last and Longest Dialogue

Harvey Flaumenhaft

The following was delivered as a lecture on August 27, 2004, at St. John's College in Annapolis. Surrounding its central part, "The Nocturnal Council in the *Laws*," are a part on "The *Laws*" and a part on "The Epilogue to the *Laws*," which in turn are surrounded by a prologue and an epilogue. Attached to the lecture as delivered is an epilogue to the epilogue.

Prologue

Two old men set the tone of the St. John's College community when I arrived, almost forty years ago, as a young man. They were Jacob Klein and Simon Kaplan, who had found refuge here in their flight from Bolshevik Russia and Nazi Germany. These old friends were men of very different sorts.

Mr. Klein had been Dean of the College, and achieved distinction by showing how the proper study of Plato could be the beginning of a truly liberating education. Mr. Kaplan had paid special attention to German philosophy, especially Kant, but for many years put his heart into leading an extracurricular study group on the Hebrew Bible. Mr. Kaplan once suggested the following college curriculum: first year, the Bible—with beatings; second year, Kant—to show the limits of reason; third year, Hegel—to show reason gone astray; fourth year, the Bible—without beatings.

Wisdom is often conveyed in jest. Consider a few noteworthy features of the curriculum put forward in Mr. Kaplan's curriculum: it begins and ends with the study of the Bible; beatings accompany the study at the beginning, but not at the end; in between, equal time is given to the study of a pair of authors who deal with reason; and that time is given to them with a view to what reason cannot do and what reason does do when it does what it shouldn't do; there is no study of an author to show simply what reason can do or what reason does do when it does what it should do. Mr. Kaplan's curriculum has no place for the pre-eminent author of the St. John's Program: there is no place for Plato. Why not?

For many lovers of Greek wisdom, Plato is the peak. But just what is the worth of Greek wisdom? In the writings of the medieval Jewish poet and dialogue-writer Yehudah Ha-Levi, there appears the remark that Greek wisdom bears flowers, not fruit. If the Plato that appears in the St. John's program were the *whole* of Plato, rather than being the flashy *part* of Plato that's devoted to the seductive and possibly corrupting celebration of that questionable character his questioning teacher Socrates, then the study of Plato might very well seem questionable to a serious, sober, and respectable adult responsible for raising the young to live their lives as serious, sober, and respectable grownups in the community. To give a solid reply to such a charge might take some doing. If, quickly recovering from surprise at such a critique, one replied without hesitation that Plato, far from being a seducer and corrupter, is rather a teacher of spirituality, one might then be taken aback by some wielder of the Nietzschean critique which says that Plato himself is boring, and that Platonism vulgarized is the calamity that is Christianity.

But there is another part of Plato—one that might seem more commendable to a serious, sober, and respectable adult responsible for raising the young to live their lives as serious, sober, and respectable grownups in the community—namely, Plato's longest book, his *Laws*. This book, however, is widely held to be the long-winded even tedious product of the failing powers of Plato's old age. This opinion might be less widely held if the *Laws* were more widely read in the way that Mr. Klein, among others, showed that Plato's writings should be read—not as mere quarries from which to extract arguments for analysis, but as action-packed dramas, in which the interplay of the speeches is inseparable from the interaction of the souls of a variety of characters. Properly read, the *Laws* might be called Plato for adults. This is not to deny that it is also for the serious youths, the youths who are to become serious adults; after all, in the regime that's depicted in the *Laws*, the great instrument of education is to be the reading of this dialogue the *Laws*.

In reading the *Laws*, and not only the *Laws*, one might do well to keep in mind a shrewd remark by President Lyndon Johnson, who said that he hired young people to generate new ideas and old people to tell him if the ideas were any good. Much of human life is constituted by a variety of things that we cannot do without but also cannot easily fit together. We want to get the good new things and also to keep the good old things. At the root of this desire to combine progress and preservation is an interplay of daring and of prudence.

Some ancient authors were much more daring in their thinking than might at first glance appear in the very prudent expression of that thinking in their writings. One such author was Plato. Beyond what is manifestly daring in Plato lies even greater daring than is readily apparent. That is not so widely recognized as it might be, because Plato was read by generations of Europeans through lenses fashioned by the heirs of the preaching of St. Paul and the confessions of St. Augustine. What often escapes the attention of those readers in Christendom is more likely to be noticed by those who read Plato through lenses fashioned by al-Farabi, a Turkic Central Asian who wrote in Arabic a few centuries after Mohammed. The Plato of the Christians, who have been preoccupied with faith, has looked different from the Plato of the Muslims and the Jews, who have been preoccupied with law, specifically with divine law. The Plato of the *Laws* goes on and on and on about law, taking as his starting-point the asking of the question whether the sources of the Spartan and the Cretan laws were divine or merely human.

The *Laws* might be called Plato's most serious book: it has been called his most pious book, and also his most political book. Philosophy was made political by Socrates in its subject-matter; in its manner, though, it was made political by Plato—and it is in the *Laws* that Plato is at his most politic. In the *Laws*, he presents the best polity for a real city, one constituted of city fathers, in contradistinction to the best polity presented in the *Republic* for an impossible made-up city constituted of makers or craftsmen.

The chief interlocutor in the *Republic* makes a city in speech which has features, borrowed from the comic dramatist Aristophanes, that he says he expects to be laughed at; the chief interlocutor in the *Laws* calls the theme of the *Laws*—which is identified as a whole polity constructed as an imitation of the most beautiful and best way of life—the truest tragedy. The *Republic* might be called Plato's comedy; the *Laws*, his tragedy.

In the *Republic*, the polity constructed in speech culminates in a proposal that philosophers be kings and kings philosophers—a ridiculous proposal from the viewpoint of ordinary citizens, for whom philosophers appear to be either impractical loquacious fools or impious subversive knaves. In the *Laws*, despite its length, philosophizing does not get mentioned as such until very late, and then it is mentioned only twice, both times very briefly. (The first mention, in Book Nine, when laws are said to need not only to compel but also to persuade, reports that when physicians who are free men treat patients who are free men, they almost philosophize, carrying on a dialogue that grasps the disease from its source and goes back to the whole nature of bodies—which causes them to be laughed at for being not physicians but rather educators of physicians. The other mention, in Book Twelve, when writings on physical science are said to be a cause of atheism, reports that the poets have compared those who philosophize to howling bitches.)

The *Republic* presents a polity that is manifestly unable to satisfy humanity's yearnings; the *Laws*, a polity that seems able to. But even though the *Laws* does not seem to be as glaringly wild and inconclusive a dialogue as the *Republic*, it is a strange book.

Right now, however, my concern is not so much with Plato's dialogue the *Laws* as it is with the relation of that dialogue to the Platonic dialogue that is its even stranger epilogue, the *Epinomis*. The conversational journey of the *Laws*, after going through a surprising institutionalization of dialectical theology as the highest and the most extensive stretch of its traversing of the penal law, reaches its peak, at the end, in the claim that what's most needful is wisdom and the recognition that this need has not been met in the dialogue; its epilogue, the *Epinomis*, presents the astonishing teaching that wisdom, which is the highest need of a sound political community, is provided by mathematical study of the stars, and that this is the pinnacle of piety too.

In the seven lectures that I've given as Dean to open the school year of this college, my themes have been largely either political or mathematical. This lecture now will bring those two sorts of themes together—by treating a certain aspect of the relation between, on the one hand, laws, founding, and the ancient city and, on the other hand, wisdom, divinity, and the mathematical study of the stars. To do that, I'll be considering a part of the Platonic writings that is not a part of the St. John's curriculum, even though it helps to illuminate writings, both Platonic and non-Platonic, that are. The freshman year at this college is devoted to a quest for wisdom with writings of ancient Greeks, Plato most prominently. The sophomore year begins with what is, within our great tradition, the great radical alternative: the study of the Hebrew sacred scriptures. The Hebrew scriptures teach (at Proverbs 1:7) that "the fear of the Lord is the beginning of wisdom"; the very beginning of the first book of instruction in this opens with the phrase (at Genesis 1:1) "in the beginning," and goes on to give an account that demotes the heavens and what's in them—so that, far from being divine, they are mere creatures, whose business is only telling time for the Adamite earthlings. Later, it is written (at Deuteronomy 4:19) that the worship of the stars has been allotted to the nations who have not received the instruction of the Hebrew scriptures, and (at Psalms 19:1) that the heavens recount the glory of the divinity who created them. This last statement is the first line of a psalm that, after saying more about that divine glory displayed in the sky, goes on to glorify the divine instruction given in the Hebrew scriptures. What law is to rule human life and what is the proper view to take of the lights that shine on high are closely linked questions in Biblical wisdom. They are closely linked questions in Greek wisdom too. We can get some glimpse of how, by considering the part which Plato suggested that the mathematical study of the stars might play in prudently dealing with a most serious difficulty that was a prime concern for him. The difficulty is this—that sound civic life needs wisdom, and the quest for wisdom requires radical and comprehensive questioning, but radical and comprehensive questioning endangers sound civic life.

Let us therefore consider what is said, and what is being done by what is said, in Plato's *Laws* and in its epilogue.

THE LAWS

The *Laws* is Plato's longest dialogue. It seems also to have been his very last. At least it had not appeared in finished form when the old man died at the age of eighty-one, less than ten years before the Macedonian victory at Chaeronia ended the era of the independent Greek city as a political form.

The situation that the dialogue depicts is this: three old men are conversing as they walk from the ancient city Knossos to the Cave of Zeus, an ancient place of pilgrimage on Mt. Ida in central Crete. Crete at that time was populated by the Greek tribal group called Dorians, which included the Spartans—but not the Athenians, who belonged to the group called Ionians. The Dorians were old-fashioned folk, whose laws and customs went back centuries. The Cave of Zeus was said to be the place where Zeus had met with his son Minos, who, instructed by his father, gave the Cretans their laws. The Spartans in many of their ways resembled their fellow-Dorians, though the Spartans' laws were adapted to their own peculiar circumstances. The Spartans, few in number, lived among more numerous peoples whom they had reduced to serfdom, even to slavery; and to keep their subjects industrious and submissive, they themselves took part in no activities but those that would make and keep them invincible warriors firmly in command of those whom they had subjugated. From cradle to grave, by abstemiousness, discipline, fortitude, and valor, their life was an unrelenting exercise in service to their city. In the dialogue, one of the old men is a Spartan named Megillos; another, old but not as old as he, is a Cretan named Kleinias; the youngest of the three old men is an Athenian, but, strangely, his name is not given—he is called merely "stranger."

Since the battles of Salamis and Plataea are mentioned, the conversation must be set in the time after the Athenians and the Spartans together had defeated the Persians who were attempting to conquer Greece; but, since there is no mention of any of the momentous events or the prominent personages of the subsequent decades of war between the one-time allies Athens and

Sparta—things which one might expect such men to mention in so long a conversation about the matters they discuss—one may reasonably presume (as Catherine Zuckert has pointed out) that the conversation is set no later than the time between the Persian and Peloponnesian Wars. The time of conversation, then, is pre-Socratic.

So much for the who, the where, and the when of the conversation depicted by Plato in his *Laws*. Now let's turn to the content of the conversation—and, first, to a brief overview of the whole and its chief parts.

The *Laws* consists of twelve books, the first three of which display the inadequacy of the Dorian laws and regime, Cretan and Spartan. When, at the conclusion of this display, the Athenian innocuously says that the whole conversation thus far serves to clarify how a city or an individual human being could live best, but asks how they could tell whether what they've said is at all useful, the Cretan Kleinias replies by disclosing his membership on a ten-man commission that's preparing to send out a colony composed of persons recruited from much of Crete. In framing the colony's laws, the commission need not restrict itself to Cretan legislation if foreign modifications will result in improvement. To help with that, the Cretan asks the others to join him in founding a city in speech, making a selection from what they have said. The Athenian agrees to join in doing so unless the Spartan finds it irksome. The Spartan declares his willingness to join the Athenian, and the three of them go on to found a city in speech.

Let's look a little closer at what happens in the first three books and then go on to consider the founding of a city in the final nine. The reader of the *Laws* encounters what seems to be a sprawling mass of detail, treating all manner of things—dances and funerals, prisons and schools, children's toys and the municipal water supply. One's grasp on all of that will be firmer if one sees how much of it is set in order by means of the device which Eva Brann has shown that Plato uses heavily in the *Republic*—namely, the placing of items in concentric rings around a center.

The *Laws* opens with a question. This opening question concerns the source of the Dorian laws, which Dorian legend claims originate in divinity. The Athenian stranger opens the dialogue by asking: "a divine or a human being—which is responsible for laying down your laws?" The ensuing conversation quickly moves from the allegedly divine source of the peculiar Dorian laws to the human purpose that they serve. Victory in war is given as the dominating purpose. Difficulties arise in making sense of this, and thus the subject of discussion becomes the virtues that make human beings excellent, which are characterized as the divine goods in human life.

The Dorian arrangements attend to the virtue that deals with pains and fears, namely, courage; but what about the one that deals with pleasures and desires, namely, sobriety? The Dorians' dining together in public mess-halls and their working out together in public gyms may foster warlike spirit and camaraderie, but don't they also foster shameful sexual practices among the men and make the women loose? The angry Dorian response is that the Athenians are dissolute drunks because of the parties that they hold for riotous drinking together. The Athenian response to this is that any collection of human beings goes astray if not properly led, and the same is true of drinking-parties, which have an important use in testing and in forming character. The central book of these first three then moves smoothly on, from treating wine as an instrument for education in sobriety, to treating song and dance, along the way considering wine and music as instruments for rejuvenation of the old. Having discussed the musical half of the choral art, the interlocutors then agree, at the end of the second book, to go on to the other, the gymnastic half—but instead, at the instigation of the Athenian, who says that the proper viewpoint for their conversation is civic development toward virtue and vice, they spend the third book doing political archaeology: first they trace the development of civil life from original primitive conditions up to the beginnings of the Dorian regime (which is where they were, says the Athenian, when they "digressed" to talk about music and drinking) and then they examine what went wrong with the Dorian regime.

Not until then is the Cretan colonizing mission at last disclosed, and the third book ends with the Spartan Megillos and the Athenian stranger agreeing to help the Cretan Kleinias with his task. Selecting from what has come up in their conversation so far, they will help him found a city in deed by joining him now in founding a city in speech.

This founding occupies the dialogue's remaining nine books, and may be divided into three parts.

Books Four and Five make up the first part, which is a preliminary to the presentation of the polity itself. Book Four begins with the nature of the city's territory, and Book Five ends by returning to that. After that first discussion (in Book Four) of the nature of the city's territory, comes discussion of the origins of its population; and before that final discussion (in Book Five) of the nature of the city's territory, comes discussion of the property relations of its population. In between those brackets, a brief consideration of the role of chance leads to a long central discussion of the art of laying down a city's laws. This involves considering the role of tyranny as well as piety. The core of this central discussion is the treatment of the need to add persuasion to compulsion. The harsh commands of law, it is emphasized, need to be accompanied by what are called "preludes," playing upon the fact that the word for law in Greek also refers to a song of a certain sort. An example is given: the legal requirement that citizens marry will not suffice as bare command. The prelude to the laws as a whole reaches its completion in the first half of Book Five, which lays out the proper way of honoring one's soul, namely, by displaying virtue. The discussion of preludes to the laws nears its end earlier, in Book Four, with the Athenian stranger remarking that it is now high noon, and they have been walking and talking since dawn, but the whole conversation has been a prelude to the laws. The mention of high noon might remind us that earlier, in Book Three, when the Athenian stranger pointed out that the conversation had returned from its digression, the Spartan Megillos had remarked that they were near the day when "the god" turns from summer toward winter. That was his way of saying what we might say more naturally this way: they were near that day of the year when the sun's position in the sky at noon no longer keeps getting higher-and-higher day-by-day, and instead keeps getting lower-and-lower day-by-day afterward. That day of the god's turning, when Crete gets sunlight for fourteen hours, is the longest day of the year.

The central part of the presentation of the city's founding consists of Books Six, Seven, and Eight. The first half of Book Six presents those laws which designate what officials will lead the city and what procedures will be used to select the persons to serve as those officials. The rest of Book Six begins the presentation of the laws proper; first come laws that have to do with what is highest, that is, the sacred things; and then Book Six concludes with laws concerning marriage, the household, married life before children, and the generating of children. Book Eight concludes with laws which have to do with what is most basic, that is, with the supply of food and other necessities; and, before that, come laws that have to do with festivals, which, while held in honor of the gods, are largely a means of training for war, and which, since they provide opportunities for licentious sexual activity, require legislative attention not only to enabling the citizens to make war but also to restraining them from making illicit love. In between those brackets, Book Seven, which is the most extensive book, and is the central book of this central part of the nine-book treatment of the city's founding, presents laws that have to do with child-rearing and education. Education was also the subject in the central book of the three-book preparation for the presentation of the city's founding.

The final part of the presentation of the city's founding, which consists of Books Nine through Twelve, comes when afternoon is over. It deals, for the most part, with crime and punishment. But while going on at length about matters that are very low and vile, it deals as well with matters that are beautiful and lofty. We must look at this more closely.

Back in Book One, when the Athenian criticized that exegesis of the Dorian laws which gives victory in war as their dominating purpose, he sketched the items that would need to be covered in an adequate presentation of a system of laws. For the most part, the items in that list match up with the items that would constitute a table of contents for the *Laws*. The glaring exception is the unexpected discussion that occupies Book Ten. Instead of merely laying down punishments for impious behavior, including blaspheming speech—which is what would have satisfied the Dorian interlocutors, and would have resembled the practice of the somewhat liberal city of Athens—the Athenian stranger goes on at great length: first, he presents arguments from writings on physical science that say there are no gods but only chance motions of material bodies which eventually give rise to human beings who fabricate the gods; then, he presents arguments, which bring in the priority of soul over material bodies, for persuading unbelievers that the gods exist, that they care about human beings, and that they can't be bribed through offerings of sacrifice and prayer by wicked human beings; and, after that, he offers a myth about a divine maker of the whole cosmos and about a life after death in which better souls go to better places. The Athenian's suggestion that the theology be a prelude leads the Cretan to say that the argument for the existence and goodness of the gods would be the most beautiful and best prelude for all the laws.

THE NOCTURNAL COUNCIL IN THE LAWS

The need for all that theological bother is news to the Dorians. Kleinias mentioned, back in Book Three, that the Cretans weren't even familiar with Homer, and here in Book Ten the Athenian is informing him and Megillos that among the Greeks there are now available books about nature, books so outrageous as to promulgate atheism. The remedy suggested by the Athenian is a prison of a peculiar sort. He calls it the "sobriety place" (coining the Greek word *sôphronisterion*, which is a reference to the *phrontisterion* or "sagacity place," a coinage of Aristophanes, in his comedy the *Clouds*, to name the place where Socrates dwelled with his disciples and supposedly pursued natural science that promoted atheism as well as promoting rhetoric that defended injustice). Those who make a display of impiety in the city that's depicted in the *Laws* are to be punished by doing time in isolation in a jail meant to sober them up. Impiety in this city is a capital crime only upon a second conviction. The five years of confinement after the first conviction, if the violation stemmed from intellectual failings rather than from such moral failings as angry passion or despicable greed, are to be spent in theological conversation with the members of a certain council that meets before morning.

About this Nocturnal Council nothing more is said until the last book of the *Laws*. Here, in Book Ten, it comes up twice. As Leo Strauss has pointed out, Book Twelve begins with seven items that deal with various public matters, including crimes against the city, and it ends with seven items that deal with various other public matters; in between are five items that deal with private law or crimes against individuals. In the seventh item of Book Twelve's first part, and also in the seventh item of its final part, the Nocturnal Council comes up again. All that we've heard of it previously is that its members, in order to rescue the souls of fellow-citizens who have been foolish but not wicked, risk danger to their own souls by exposure to discussion of pernicious doctrines about the gods. What more do we learn about it now? Back in Book Nine, when discussing responsibility and the punishment of crime, the Athenian suggested that just as proper treatment by free men of disease in free men is a kind of educating, so going through laws in the way that they were doing might be called educating the citizens rather than laying down the law. Now we learn how far that thought leads.

The end of the first part of Book Twelve treats intercourse with foreigners, either by citizens going abroad or by foreigners being admitted to the city. Since this city is designed to be as good as possible, corrupting innovations may be expected from indiscriminate travel to other cities. Travel is therefore restricted. Indeed, it is forbidden, except that very good men above the age of forty are to be allowed to go as heralds, ambassadors, and official visitors to sacred games or sacred places located elsewhere in Greece. And there is another exception: some men of good repute are to be allowed, between the ages of fifty and sixty, to visit other cities in order to view their laws and ways of education, and also to learn from any individuals of divine good nature, who do spring up even in cities without good laws; only thus can the ways of the well-designed city be placed on a firmer footing and be improved if they are somehow lacking. For this purpose, these viewers, on their return, must immediately report to the Nocturnal Council. In this connection, the Athenian says more about the Nocturnal Council. It is required to meet every day from dawn until the sun has fully risen. Half of its members are older men—namely, the priests who have won prizes for excellence, the ten oldest of the officials called Law-Guardians, and the present Minister of Education along with all former holders of that office; the other half are younger men, between the ages of thirty and forty, each of whom is picked for membership by one of the older members.

Later, when the Nocturnal Council comes up again in Book Twelve, the membership mentioned in characterizing it is slightly altered: there is no mention of those who are members for being or for having been in charge of the administration of education—and those who are members for having won prizes for excellence are characterized as "all" who have done so, not as "priests" who have done so; that item at the end of the final part of Book Twelve comes immediately after the item treating the inevitable end of the life of the individual citizen, namely, the laws about burial of the dead. The final item treats the need for something that will save the city and its laws from decay and destruction. This savior is the Nocturnal Council. It meets before the day has started—a time when all its members have the most leisure from their other activities, both private and communal. The Athenian says that if the city lacked such a council it would be like a human being without a head: the older members of the council are the brains of the city; the younger are its eyes and ears. The work of the Nocturnal Council, it turns out, is not just to talk theology with atheists who are of good character and therefore might be saved: we learn now that its members are to be always talking about the city and its laws—and about whatever learning may contribute to a clarification of those matters.

The complete and lasting safeguard that the city needs is the presence in the city of some who understand what the city and its laws are for. This presence is to be supplied by the Nocturnal Council. The Council supplies this presence by engaging in conversations through which it gives itself a higher education, a more "precise" education, than the rest of the citizenry can be expected to acquire. The content of this higher education has to do with inquiries of the following sorts.

In the first place, what one thing makes courage, sobriety, justice, and sagacity each a virtue—or is virtue not a unity but a whole of differentiated parts that are the various virtues—or is virtue both a unity and a whole—or what?

Secondly, what about what's beautiful and good—how is each of these things one as well as many? (That recurring phrase "beautiful and good," which in the Greek is *kalos kai agathos*, often fused into a single word *kalokagathos*, originally referred to someone "nice-to-look-at and good-for-battle," since it was by dazzling beauty and daunting brawn that a first-rate man in archaic times stood out from the human herd. The term later came to be applied in ways that went beyond the cruder senses that relate to love and war. The classical Greek *kalokagathos* had some resemblance to what was later called a "gentleman.")

And finally, isn't one of the most beautiful things what pertains to the gods—knowing, insofar as humans have power to know, about their existence and power (and didn't we see, earlier in the conversation, that this follows from considering the priority of soul—that is, how it is the eldest of things that come into being and is deathless and rules over all bodies) and also considering the intellect that's the leader of what is in the stars? Having viewed what's common to these things and the things belonging to the Muse, all together, one needs to fit them together with a view to arrangements of character and custom, having an articulate account to give of whatever can be given an articulate account. Whoever can't acquire those things in addition to the virtues of ordinary people can't be an official sufficient for leading the whole city but can be merely a subordinate to other officials who do lead it.

Without abolishing political life, as does the city in the *Republic*, the city in the *Laws* looks as if it has been made safe for philosophy—even, indeed, has been made a source of philosophy. Without suffering the deprivations of the *Republic*'s philosopher-kings, the Nocturnal Councilmen in the *Laws* have as their work the quest for wisdom.

Plato's profound presentation of alternative ways of life receives its most comprehensive treatment in his two dialogues the *Republic* and the *Laws*. Perhaps the film director Howard Hawks was on to something when he remarked, "The only difference between comedy and tragedy is the point of view." In the *Republic*, political life is viewed from the standpoint of philosophic life; in the *Laws*, philosophic life is viewed from the standpoint of political life. In the *Republic*, philosophy is Spartanized; in the *Laws*, politics is Athenianized. Reading the *Republic* but not the *Laws* is like reading Homer's *Odyssey* but not his *Iliad*; it's like taking Odysseus as the only heroic possibility and ignoring Achilles.

Not that the Athenian stranger is an Achilles. The Athenian stranger moves the Dorians beyond the ethos of a warrior society where exuberance of strength is tantamount to valor and accumulation of experience is tantamount to sagacity—beyond an ethos, that is to say, where youth is identified with courage, and age with wisdom.

The fundamental question of the *Laws* is the Nocturnal Council's prime question: what is the oneness or wholeness of virtue. The *Laws* moves from valor to sagacity; it begins by singling out courage from the quartet of cardinal virtues, and it ends by singling out prudence or wisdom. The conversation it depicts takes place in a time when philosophy, albeit pre-Socratic philosophy, has been let loose upon the world, but hasn't yet quite reached the hicks in the sticks. For all practical purposes, nonetheless, the question of the unity or the wholeness of virtue comes down to the question of the relation of the warrior and the philosopher, or of the life of action and the life of thought—that is to say, of the highest thing in Sparta and the highest thing in Athens. The question amounts to asking whether the city need be hostile to philosophy, and philosophy need be subversive of the city. The city in speech that emerges in the *Laws* contains the best of Sparta and the best of Athens. The distorted form of political life that is Dorian and the distorted form of philosophic life that is Athenian both seem to be avoided in the Cretan city in speech. This city, resisting ambition and avarice, superstition and scoffing, brings together valor and sagacity, cautious old-fashioned social solidarity and innovative intellectual daring. The promotion of radical and comprehensive inquiry need no longer be opposed to the promotion of civic health. From below, this city is supported by a Dorian foundation, but at its peak it has an Athenian direction.

Not that the Cretan city in speech is an Athens. The lid, as it were, is still on the city. In the *Laws*, the love of wisdom almost dares not speak its name. The dialogue, as we noted earlier, barely mentions philosophizing as such. If we consider the two prime aspects of human life—that is, seeing things as they are, and acting nobly and justly as a member of a community (let's call them "viewing" and "doing")—we might say this: whatever justice the *Republic* does to "viewing," it does at the price of neglecting "doing," except to show how "doing" can only be kept from conflict with "viewing" by being kept from coming into its own—whereas the *Laws* sees "doing" as what it is only at the price of not showing "viewing" in its fullness. This limitation of the *Laws* results from the need to promote a new kind of piety that restrains both ignorant zeal and heedless scoffing, so that awe can curb insolence and activate mutual aid.

At the very end of Book Twelve, and therefore of the entire dialogue, after the Athenian has revealed the magnitude of the Nocturnal Council's need for wisdom and of what would be required for its members to meet the need, Kleinias wants to talk about how to do what it will take to meet the need. The Athenian replies that laws for such men can't be laid down in advance—that men who haven't already learned what they will need to learn couldn't understand it if it were written down beforehand—but he is willing to continue the conversation. Megillos now re-enters the conversation. He has not said a single word since, way back in Book Ten, he uttered a few words to register his agreement that, since private prose-writers and poets have started spreading around atheism, counter-arguments should be put in writing by lawgivers. Now the Spartan says to the Cretan that either the city's founding must be abandoned or the stranger must by entreaties and by all contrivances be made to stay and share in the city's founding. The Cretan replies to the Spartan that what he's said is true, and that he (the Cretan) will do just those things—and that the Spartan must help. The Spartan then says that he will help. There the dialogue ends—with no further word from the Athenian in the *Laws*.

THE EPILOGUE TO THE LAWS

Laws in Greek is *Nomoi*. An epi-logue to that Platonic dialogue called *Nomoi* is the Platonic dialogue called *Epi-nomis*. Among the Platonic dialogues, the *Epinomis* stands alone: it is the only one whose name makes it a mere appendage of another one. But then it doesn't stand alone after all; indeed, it stands alone least. There is another Platonic dialogue whose title connects it to the *Nomoi*—by its alliterative sound and by the person whom it names; this is the *Minos*, which somehow serves the *Nomoi* as a preface. But the *Laws* is not a continuation of the conversation in the *Minos*, whereas the *Epinomis* is a continuation of the conversation in the *Laws*. The *Laws* and the *Epinomis* also stand together as the only Platonic dialogues in which Socrates doesn't appear. The persons who do appear in the *Epinomis* are the same trio who appeared in the *Laws*, and the *Epinomis* begins with a reference to a previous agreement to meet to continue the conversation of the *Laws*. Doubts have been raised about whether Plato is indeed the author of the *Epinomis*; but it would, in any case, be worthwhile to try the experiment of seeing what turns up if the text is studied very hard on the assumption that it is authentic. If the *Epinomis* is authentically by the author of the *Laws*, then a question to be answered is what is appropriate about its being a separate dialogue rather than a thirteenth book of the *Laws*.

Although the *Laws* is the longest of the dialogues, the *Epinomis* is one of the shortest. The Athenian stranger is the person who initiates the conversation in the *Laws*, where the last words belong to Kleinias followed by Megillos, each of whom utters only a very brief sentence in closing—which is not surprising since Kleinias does not say very much in the course of the conversation and Megillos says much less. In the *Epinomis*, by contrast, Kleinias is the person who initiates the conversation, where the last word is a very long speech by the Athenian, and in the entire course of the conversation not a single word is uttered by Megillos. The silence of the Spartan is obtrusive. After all, right at the beginning Kleinias mentions him by name as one of the three who have agreed to meet again, and not very long after that the Athenian addresses by name the two Dorians, Megillos and Kleinias. So, another question to be answered is just what the Spartan is doing here.

The questions pile up. The form of the dialogue is, in a way, easy to grasp. Kleinias speaks first, then the Athenian does, then Kleinias again, and then the Athenian—back and forth in alternation, with a total of fourteen speeches by Kleinias and fourteen by the Athenian. The conversation is a series of statements by the Athenian in response to what Kleinias says. But what Kleinias says is also a response to what the Athenian says; and, while some of what Kleinias says in response is a cue to which the Athenian responds, some of it is deliberately provoked by the Athenian so that he can then go on to follow through on what he himself has begun. So, another question to be answered is just what the Athenian is doing.

That must be related to the dialogue's three-part structure. In the first part, the Athenian holds forth; in the final part also, the Athenian holds forth; in the central part, however, there's give-and-take between the Athenian and Kleinias. There is, to be sure, some give-and-take in the first and in the final parts, but nonetheless there's not as much of it there as in the middle; and while in the middle there's some holding-forth, there's not as much of it there as in the opening and closing. What's central to the dialogue is the interaction between the Athenian stranger and the Cretan, in the silent presence of the Spartan. The turning-point in that interaction consists of the two central speeches in the dialogue. One of those central speeches is the Athenian's seventh speech, which—beginning by asking the Cretan what they've meant and ending by asking the Cretan what he means—piously suggests that they offer the most beautiful and best speeches to the gods. The other central speech is the speech of response by the Cretan, who enthusiastically exclaims that that's "wondrously" so and addresses the stranger by calling him *daimonie*, that is, an uncanny semi-divine being.

The reader of the *Epinomis* needs to ask why Kleinias just then uses that special word *daimonie* to address the Athenian—and why, at another point in the dialogue, the Athenian addresses by name the two others, naming the silent Megillos first and then the interlocutor Kleinias. With respect to terms of address, perhaps the most obtrusive unintrusive detail is the following: Kleinias in his opening speech addresses the Athenian as "stranger," but the Athenian responds, in his very first words in the dialogue, by addressing the Cretan as "friend Kleinias." The drama is in many respects very understated, and what is overstated can easily distract the reader from small details that are most significant, like this: the only question that the Cretan asks is a very little one that is his last speech, but questions are asked by the Athenian at the ends of the following speeches: his first and his seventh (which are, in the first half of the totality of his speeches, the opening and the closing speeches) as well as his tenth, eleventh, and twelfth (which are, in the second half of the totality of his speeches, the three middle speeches). Thus do the details accumulate as clues to answering our questions.

There isn't time now to describe the subtlety of the Athenian stranger's handling of these Dorians—which is to say, the subtlety of the Athenian author who deftly depicts the Athenian stranger's seemingly heavy-handed heavy-lifting of the Dorian heavies. For now it must suffice to make a few suggestions that may induce you to consider it worth your while to study these dialogues that are so foolishly neglected by so many of those who look to reading Plato as a source of wisdom.

To do that, I first must briefly sketch the doctrines that the Dorians hear from the mouth of the Athenian stranger whom they have urged to help them on the way to wisdom. What he tells them is something like the following. Life for human beings is very harsh, and the harsh fact is that only a few can become truly happy and blessed in this life. Wisdom is essential. Wisdom is not the possession of the mental capabilities useful for producing necessities, or for playing with representations, or for protecting against dangers natural or human—nor is it merely the mental ability to take things into the mind quickly and keep them there long. The source of the distinctively human mental capabilities, it turns out, is the ability to number, and the source of the ability to deal with number at a high level is Heaven, a divinity which, although not worshiped in the cities of the Greeks, is, according to the poetic theogeny, older than the pre-Olympian male divinities and older than all of the Olympian divinities. Human beings developed their mathematical ability by keeping count of the motions of the lights in Heaven. Between those lively fiery bodies high up there (belonging to the visible gods) and the lively earthy bodies deep down here (belonging to us the mortals), there are intermediate lively bodies—ethereal ones, and (lower down) airy ones, and (lower still) watery ones—uncanny, or omen-bearing, or spritely. We find that the lit-up heavenly bodies that move around across the star-bespangled Heaven seem to wander, seem not to move uniformly—but since they are, like Heaven, divinities, to think them to be in any way disorderly is impious and ignorant. Indeed, it is the deepest piety and the highest wisdom to be able to give a mathematical account of the heavenly divinities, showing the beautiful cosmic order that prevails up there and relating it to harmonies of number that are not restricted to what moves up there.

That's the gist of the argument in the *Epinomis*. What about the action? Plato shows us what the Athenian tells the Dorians; what else does Plato show us—and what does this indicate?

Consider the opening few speeches of the *Epinomis*. The conversation depicted in the *Laws* was initiated by the Athenian stranger, but it is not he who initiates the sequel to it in the *Epinomis*. In suggesting a departure from the Dorian theologico-political position, the Athenian will only go so far. He will go further only after having sufficiently provoked the Dorians to beg for help in going after wisdom. The *Laws* came to its end with the Dorians begging for help and the Athenian not responding. The *Laws*, that is to say, ended in the silence of the hitherto loquacious Athenian. The conversation depicted in the *Epinomis* is initiated by the Dorian Cretan Kleinias. But although he has come to see that the city cannot be preserved unless wisdom resides in the city, he nonetheless has some unease about the stranger's views: after all, the stranger has said some very uncivil things—about human things not being truly serious, about lawgiving being perhaps impossible because it seems that laws originate not through human choice but rather by chance and through the harsh necessities of war and poverty and disease. Kleinias in the course of his first speech keeps some distance from the Athenian, whom he still addresses as "stranger," while the Athenian in the very first word of his reply addresses the Cretan as "friend," and in course of his speech calls the two Dorians by name. But the Athenian's reply seems harsh, putting down human life again, grimly confining the prospects for happiness in this life to a blessed few. The reply ends with his including in our misery the difficulty of saying what wisdom is. This difficulty derives from his denial that wisdom can have anything to do with what is useful. It is then that he goes on to exhibit the root of the matter in the human ability to number, attributing the development of this ability to our looking up to what is literally the highest god, the one that is said by the poet to be older than all the divinities except for those pre-Olympian females called Darkness, Daylight, Attraction, and Earth. After he attributes that development of our numbering ability to our looking up to Heaven and counting the motions of the heavenly bodies in their courses, the response of Kleinias is noncommittal: that's a big discussion of big things, the Cretan says.

In the ensuing conversation, Megillos continues to be completely silent: in a way, it's all beyond the simple old jock from Sparta. But (as we noted earlier) the Athenian manages to leverage the interest of the Cretan and elicit his enthusiasm: Kleinias is delighted when he sees how nicely the Athenian's wisdom can enter the city of the *Laws* with a bow to what the city bows to. Kleinias glimpses something of how the sober city can be open to the daring quest for wisdom. How reassuring it must be for him, that the most solid sobriety doesn't have to clip the wings of those who can fly the highest, and that the highest daring need not be reckless.

These old men form an interesting trio: the stranger is a man who can see for himself and can, with his insight, guide the thinking of those who lack it; Kleinias is a man who can take a leading part in action that is guided by hearing what's said by someone who can see for himself; and Megillos is a man who can't himself do much more than go along with that. The youngest of them, the Athenian, would be able to take a place among the philosophers; the older Dorian, the Cretan, would be able to take a place among the princes; the oldest of them all, the Spartan, would have to take a place as just one of the people.

Megillos is incapable of any quest for wisdom. Kleinias may be inferior to the stranger in this respect, but still he's much superior to Megillos—and he is aware that he's superior to him. The stranger and Kleinias speak with a view to the limitations of Megillos. Kleinias may go along with what he takes to be the stranger's adaptation of his speech to the limitations of Megillos, but it's likely that Kleinias is unaware of how the stranger adapts his speech to the limitations of Kleinias. Since the limitations of Kleinias are not the same as those of Megillos, the stranger must speak on three levels: for Megillos, for Kleinias, and for whatever reader may be akin to the stranger himself.

The interlocutors in the *Laws* are founders of a city in speech that, while normal and healthy, is somehow open to and even nurturing of philosophy. The *Epinomis* presents the most delicate part of that enterprise: enlisting the full support of the non-philosophical gentleman who is open to philosophy, while overcoming any possible resistance from the non-philosophical gentleman who is not. The most politic part of the highest political act is the progressive and preservative double act of stimulating the quest for wisdom while at the same time reforming piety.

Megillos may not have a clue about what the stranger is concerned for, but Kleinias is not so dumb. He is aware that wisdom beyond the ordinary is needed for ruling, let alone for laying down the laws that will rule over the rulers. He is also aware that the stranger's notion of wisdom is better than his own: he has learned that the stranger can provide much that he himself lacks. The *Laws* ended with the silence of the stranger; before the reader can see what the *Epinomis* depicts, it had to be made clear that it is not in the stranger's nature eagerly to rush to take part in the founding of a city. The stranger will be at most a willing teacher of founders. But does his natural reluctance to be one of the founders indicate that he is somehow lacking the qualifications to be a teacher of founders? The action of the *Laws* was partly the stranger's testing of Kleinias: the stranger sought to find out how teachable this founder is. The action of the *Epinomis* is perhaps partly Kleinias's testing of the stranger—and is even perhaps partly his teaching of the stranger. If the stranger's concern for wisdom transcends the city, how can that concern fit the city? Kleinias needs to know what the stranger's concern for wisdom will look like to the city. The stranger has come bearing the strange foreign gift philosophy. Can the stranger's philosophy be politic? The dialogue shows the stranger presenting an image of wisdom not as atheistic talk about what's natural (what those Greeks called *physiologia*) but as cosmic talk about what's divine (*theologia*). He can make philosophy safe for the city as he makes the city open to an image of philosophy that will open a part of the city to philosophy. Kleinias is sufficiently reassured by the image not to worry about what he doesn't understand. The stranger may be strange, he may say some strange things, but he is not a menace. Indeed, the founder may take him as a teacher.

Epilogue

To students of the *Laws* and its epilogue the *Epinomis*, the Platonic enterprise looks much more interesting—both more daring and more prudent—than it looks to those who confine themselves to studying the *Republic* alone. Plato's work culminates in what might be called a cosmologico-theologico-political discourse. Through this politic treatment of the highest things that there are to see, piety, which raises human beings above the beasts and brings them together under what's divine, is preserved but made more thoughtful, while radical and comprehensive thoughtfulness is made less threatening to the citizenry of a healthy city. We are taught to deal seriously with human life as it ordinarily appears, while relentlessly pursuing the implications of the insight that there's more than meets the eye.

Now it is surely pleasant to have a reassuring happy ending. Happy endings, however, happen in comedies—and the *Laws*, in the *Laws*, is called a tragedy. Perhaps we're missing something. Perhaps the *Laws*, even with its epilogue, is not the end of the story. Perhaps the story doesn't have an end. This lecture, however, must come to an end. Unlike the *Laws*, which begins with an opening question, this lecture will end with a closing question. To ask it will require some prefatory words. Plato's most manifestly daring dialogue, his grim comedy the *Republic*, closes with Socrates telling a tall tale, in the course of which it is suggested that when extraordinary intellect and courage have liberated a man from the restraints that communal brainwashing had previously led him to accept, a relentless quest for wisdom is the only alternative to a resolute quest for tyrannical power. That may be a shocking thing to say—but what if it's true? A thought like that led one of Plato's greatest readers—the medieval codifier of Jewish law, Maimonides—to write, in a book about the perplexities of interpreting the divine instruction, that the outward looks of human beings obscure how few are inwardly very human, the rest being rather more like beasts of prey or beasts of burden. My closing question, then, is this: what does that Socratic suggestion about tyranny and philosophy say, in particular, about the work of college education?

EPILOGUE TO THE EPILOGUE

With that last question, this lecture as it was delivered came to an end. Nonetheless I now continue, in a kind of second epilogue, addressing some questions elicited by delivery of the lecture.

What the lecture treats may seem to be an antiquarian or merely academic affair, of concern only to those with a somewhat precious taste for books from long ago. But consider the following passage from a novel written in the midst of the long nightmare that constituted much of the century concluded very recently. That novel, entitled *Darkness at Noon*,[1] appeared a few years after Stalin sought to consolidate his tyranny through show-trials to purge the leadership of Communist Russia in the run-up to a struggle for the mastery of the world. In

1. Arthur Koestler, *Darkness at Noon* (London: Jonathan Cape, 1940).

the novel, Arthur Koestler tells the story of Rubashov, a fictional old Bolshevik who is broken down under ruthless interrogation and is thus prevailed upon to make a false confession of acts betraying the revolution to which he has devoted his life. Each of the novel's first three parts depicts a hearing in which Rubashov is interrogated, at the end of the third of which he agrees to confess—as his final duty to a party whose dictatorship is necessary for leading the proletariat, and therewith all mankind, into the promised land of the classless, finally free society. The last part of the novel is called "The Grammatical Fiction"—a reference to the first person singular pronoun "I", use of which was frowned upon by those who sought to construct a totally collectivist reality. Before the novel ends, with Rubashov's execution, there is this:

"So now it was over. . . . He had paid, his account was settled. . . . The hours which remained to him belonged to that silent partner. . . . He had christened it the 'grammatical fiction' with that shamefacedness about the first person singular which the Party had inculcated in its disciples. . . .

"He continued pacing through his cell. . . . He was puzzling over certain questions to which he would have liked to find an answer before it was too late. They were rather naïve questions; they concerned the meaning of suffering, or, more exactly, the difference between suffering which made sense and senseless suffering. Obviously only such suffering made sense as was inevitable; that is, as was rooted in biological fatality. On the other hand, all suffering with a social origin was accidental, hence pointless and senseless. The sole object of revolution was the abolition of senseless suffering. But it turned out that the removal of this second kind of suffering was only possible at the price of a temporary enormous increase in the sum total of the first. So the question now ran: Was such an operation justified? Obviously it was, if one spoke in the abstract of 'mankind'; but applied to 'man' in the singular, to the cipher 2-4 [i.e. the prisoners' tapping code for the letter "I"], the real human being of bone and flesh and blood and skin, the principle led to absurdity. As a boy, he had believed that in working for the Party he would find an answer to all questions of this sort. The work had lasted forty years, and right at the start he had forgotten the question for whose sake he had embarked on it. Now the forty years were over, and he returned to the boy's original perplexity. The Party had taken all he had to give and never supplied him with an answer. And neither did the silent partner, whose magic name [that is, "I"] he had tapped on the wall of the empty cell. He was deaf to direct questions, however urgent and desperate they might be.

"And yet there were ways of approach to him. Sometimes he would respond unexpectedly to a tune, or even the memory of a tune, or of the folded hands of the *Pietà*, or of certain scenes of his childhood. As if a tuning-fork had been struck, there would be answering vibrations, and once this has started a state would be produced . . . the 'oceanic sense.' . . . One's personality dissolved as a grain of salt in the sea; but at the same time the infinite sea seemed to be contained in the grain of salt. The grain could no longer be localized in time and space. . . .

"Rubashov wandered through his cell. In the old days he would have shamefacedly denied himself this sort of childish musing. Now he was not ashamed. In death the metaphysical became real. He stopped at the window and leaned his forehead against the pane. Over the machine-gun tower one could see a patch of blue. It was pale, and reminded him of that particular blue which he had seen overhead when as a boy he lay on the grass. . . . Apparently even a patch of blue sky was enough to cause the 'oceanic state.' He had read that, according to the latest discoveries of astrophysics, the volume of the world was finite—though space had no boundaries, it was self-contained, like the surface of a sphere. He had never been able to understand that; but now he felt an urgent desire to understand. He now also remembered where he had read about it: during his first arrest in Germany, comrades had smuggled a sheet of the illegally printed Party organ into his cell; at the top were three columns about a strike in a spinning-mill; at the bottom of a column, as a stop-gap, was printed in tiny letters the discovery that the universe was finite, and half-way through it the page was torn off. He had never found out what had been in the torn-off part. . . .

"When he had read that newspaper notice, then also alone in his cell, with joints still sore from the last bout of torturing, he had fallen into a queer state of exaltation—the 'oceanic sense' had swept him away. Afterwards he had been ashamed of himself. The Party disapproved of such states. It called them *petit-bourgeois* mysticism, refuge in the ivory tower. It called them 'escape from the task', 'desertion of the class struggle'. The 'oceanic sense' was counter-revolutionary.

"For in a struggle one must have both legs firmly planted on the earth. The Party taught one how to do it. The infinite was a politically suspect quantity, the 'I' a suspect quality. The Party did not recognize its existence. The definition of the individual was: a multitude of one million divided by one million."

Darkness at Noon so deeply impressed me when I read it in my youth, that many incidents and even phrases from the novel stayed with me through what is now some fifty years. Something from that passage which I have just quoted sprang to my mind as I was writing this lecture. What I have already quoted supplies the context that is needed to understand what I have saved for last—namely, the following paragraph from the middle of the passage: "Rubashov stood by the window. . . . As a boy he had really meant to study astronomy, and now for forty years he had been doing something else. Why had not the Public Prosecutor asked him: 'Defendant Rubashov, what about the infinite?' He would not have been able to answer—and there, there lay the real source of his guilt. . . . Could there be a greater?"

That remarkable concluding question does make it hard to avoid seriously entertaining the possibility that astronomy is, after all, profoundly relevant to politics and psychology—to city and to soul. And perhaps even more so now, when, with the collapse of the Soviet Union and the discrediting of the doctrine for which it stood, humanity nonetheless faces, not an easy road to the lasting prevalence of the liberal state and the free market, bringing security and prosperity to a global society of equal individuals living as they please, but rather age-old minefields strewn with questions about the relation between polity and divinity—about what divinity is, and about how to interpret laws for which multitudes of human beings believe divinity is responsible. A scholar of my acquaintance who joined a Washington public policy institute a few years ago later said that he had been expecting to feel like a marginal figure there—someone who would have to try hard to justify his presence among colleagues who were experts on matters like trade agreements and military spending—only to discover, in the wake of 9/11, that his specialties—medieval Islamic political philosophy, and the role of religion in public life—were at the center of world politics and national crisis. Reading al-Farabi on Plato's *Laws*, or al-Farabi's successor Maimonides on the perplexities that astronomy poses for those obedient to a divine law, no longer seems to be a merely academic affair. Views of what is loftiest now seem once again obtrusively to shape the down-to-earth actions of men entangled in life-and-death political struggles.

Not that the Platonic Athenian stranger should be called an impious manipulator of opinion for such narrowly political purposes as controlling mobs or preventing tyrannies. The Athenian stranger knows that we do not know that we can get answers to all our questions by thinking in terms of the pushes of necessity, and he therefore knows that soul for all we know may well be older than body. He has reason to believe that our view of things should include attraction as well as mere pressure—the attraction, in particular, which is love of what is higher than blind and dumb material necessity. The Athenian stranger knows that viewing the cosmic spectacle can lead our souls to be lifted up and moved by what somehow lurks unmoved behind the circling heavenly lights. The Athenian stranger is after something that resembles what Maimonides was after. Both men are aware that imagery adapts the presentation of divinity to the capacities of the audience to which it is presented. Both of them seek less anthropomorphic thought about divinity and more theomorphic thought about humanity. Consider Maimonides more closely for a moment. Although he teaches that calling the human being an image of the divine being does not mean that the divine being has a body or even passions, he also teaches that the sacrificial law remains binding in perpetuity, despite its low occasion and its inferiority to what develops in prayer. Prayer, however, though superior to sacrifice, is still a kind of action, and Maimonides teaches that truly divine instruction concerns itself not only with action but also with opinion. As Chesterton remarked, men who don't believe in God will believe in anything. Divine instruction liberates human beings from the blindness, the burdens, the distractions, and the terrors of superstition, however much it is compelled to do its good work by means of speech in the tongue of the human-all-too-human Adamite earthlings—speaking, that is to say, neither perfectly reasonably nor altogether unreasonably in order to make those who listen to it as reasonable as it would be reasonable to expect them to become. The reasonableness of limited expectations of reasonableness is the reason for Maimonides's adherence to limitations on the teaching of what the sages called "the affair of the beginning" and "the affair of the chariot," although he does say that these correspond to physics and metaphysics, and he does refer to the heavenly bodies as "the holy bodies." Maimonides follows Farabi who follows the Platonic Athenian stranger in thinking it good for the citizens to have a better albeit inadequate image of divinity not only because it is useful but also because it is uplifting.

Since the *Laws* does not seem tethered to the context that passed away a mere few years after its author passed away, a question arises about the contemporary relevance of the Nocturnal Council. In a liberal modern state, of course there cannot be a complete counterpart of the virtuous classical city's Nocturnal Council. The liberal modern state arises, after all, by rejecting the establishment of a single religion—it is essentially committed to the liberty promoted by the existence of a multiplicity of sects within the state. (The very principle of the extended republic set out by James Madison in the 10th *Federalist* paper is a generalization of David Hume's adaptation of the commitment to a multiplicity of religious sects found in Spinoza's defense of liberal democracy, which made possible Spinoza's novel philosophical defense of democracy.) But the non-establishment of a single religion does not as such mean the establishment of non-religion: the modern liberal state combines non-establishment of religion with the free exercise of religion. This combination does, however, generate a tension. That tension's persistence requires a rationale for religious pluralism. True pluralism cannot be the product of atheism or of religious indifference. It must derive from an appreciation of how images of divinity adapt the presentation of divinity to the capacities of a multitude of human beings—an appreciation of how what is taught about the very highest things is like a radio emission that passes through different sorts of devices for transmission and ultimately reaches devices of varying capabilities, with the result that none of the many messages received fully corresponds to the one originally emitted. According to such a pluralism, the variety of inadequate finite views of what is infinite should not be homogenized and then imposed, but at best be merely refined when circumstances are propitious. The propitious circumstances are unlikely to arise from non-official rule de facto by a disciplined avant-garde party, or from an enthusiastic movement dedicated to mobilizing multitudes, or from clustered devotees of contemplative friendship who wish only to be left alone in their walled gardens. Only institutions devoted to promoting thoughtfulness can do the job. It would be unreasonable to think that such institutions can be official bodies in a modern liberal state. It does seem, however, that the liberal modern state cannot flourish without institutions which, while independent of governmental authority, are prudently mindful of the need for such authority and of what such authority itself needs, as well as being ardently devoted to a feasible public enlightenment. The liberal modern state needs to be informed by true thoughtfulness as much as by liberal modern principles. Plato's *Laws* and its epilogue need not provide a constitutional blueprint in order to constitute excellent means of becoming informed by true thoughtfulness.

6

Torah Transformed

Michael Fishbane

It is a great pleasure to honor my dear friend and colleague Leon Kass on the occasion of his seventieth birthday. According to an ancient rabbinic tradition, this age marks the entrance into *seivah*, or elderhood—a time of ever-deepening reflection and counsel.[1] It is a time for the cultivation of a wisdom that is not for one's self alone, but for future generations as well. Such an onset of maturity is not a natural happenstance, but must itself be nurtured; and it is just such a cultivated thoughtfulness, wholly grounded in the concreteness of mortality and the human condition, that has marked Leon Kass's life and life-work. A personal memory is apropos, and carries my mind back to one of our first of innumerable meetings in his office, when the conversations entered the depths of dialogue. On that occasion, I vividly recall my friend invoking the great scriptural phrase found at Psalm 90:12, "[God] has enjoined us to number our days, (so as) to cultivate a heart of wisdom." In doing so, he cited and produced a manuscript in his possession from his own mentor, Hans Jonas, for whom this passage was a by-word. As indeed it must be for all who might convert the thoughts of one's lifetime into a gift for the future, that ensuing generations might benefit from those experiences transmitted with due regard for their well-being. Such is the life task: a cultivated responsibility for one's personal integrity and for the fate of one's children (in the fullest sense). It has been Leon Kass's task to exemplify such a commitment, with ever-new ethical regard for the nature and meaning of life itself, and for the ethical discourses that may ensue through devoted pedagogy and the study of texts.

In Kass's devotion to the fundamental literary sources of culture, the Hebrew Bible has emerged in the last decade as a personal paradigm, captivating his heart and mind. In this sense, 'Torah' has become for him a fundamental axis for cultural reflection—since it reveals a vigorous model of family and society grounded in

1. *Mishnah Avot* V.21. In his sixteenth-century commentary *Midrash Shemuel*, R. Shemuel Uzeida notes the precious quality of temporality, and emphasizes that *seivah* not only marks a fullness of years, but also an ideal time for the fulfillment of piety and learning.

value, respectful of tradition, and devoted to a responsible future. Accordingly, in my present contribution in his honor, I would like to trace a trajectory of this very term 'Torah' from biblical to rabbinic antiquity and toward something of its contemporary meaning. Over this span, the term has undergone numerous fundamental transformations, in response to new values and circumstances. At the outset the term 'torah' simply referred to specific ritual instructions. But as its scope widened, new modes of inquiry into its meaning were initiated, and as torah became a term of larger and more comprehensive instruction ('Torah') it too was subject to ethical and spiritual extensions, until it even became a focus of devotion and piety as well—as the study of the instructions for ritual practices came to take the place of the practices themselves, which became impractical after the fall of the second Temple. In this way study became the preeminent center of Jewish religious praxis—virtually absorbing and transcending all other activities.

For those like Leon Kass, whose life is devoted to the explication of classical and sacred sources, this process, whereby texts become the all-inclusive frame of existence and their study becomes an exercise in piety, can only be a matter of marvel.

Torah as Teaching and Scripture

In order to put the subject of 'Torah' in biblical antiquity into context, it behooves us first to review several contours of its nature and occurrences. In the course of time, these elements come together in significant ways. So we may first ask: What is Torah and its instruction(s) in the major genres of Scripture?

We begin with the Priestly literature and its traditions. In this corpus, the noun *torah* refers to specific ritual or cultic instructions, or better, to a specific domain of priestly concern and activity. *Torah* is thus literally an 'instruction' bearing on the priestly ritual practices and concerns. It may therefore mark the instructions for various sacrificial procedures, as in Leviticus 6:2, 7, 18; 7:1 and 11 where we find the phrase, "This is the *torah* of the *olah* (holocaust)," "the *minhah* (meal)," "the *hata'at* (sin)," "the *asham* (guilt)," and "the *shelamim* (peace or vow-redemption)" offerings respectively. Or, as this catalogue is re-specified seriatim in a related summary colophon (7:37): "This is the *torah* for the *olah, minhah, hata'at, asham* ... [and] *shelamim*" offerings. In addition to such sacrificial practices, there were also specially marked instructions for matters of purity and holiness, and for the ritual separation of the holy and profane, as we are told in a comprehensive way in Leviticus 10. In this passage, Moses informs Aaron that both he and his lineage are duty bound "to make a separation between the holy and the profane, and between the impure and the pure, and to instruct (*le-horot*) the Israelite people in all the statutes which the Lord their God spoke via Moses." These matters are taken up in considerable detail in Leviticus 11-15, which delineates the *torah* of permitted and forbidden foods and their separations (ch. 11; with a colophon beginning at verse 26); the *torah* pertaining to a childbearing woman and the regulations of her impurity and purification (ch. 12; and its colophon at vv. 7-8); the *torah* pertaining to the diagnosis, containment, and purification of skin lesions, scabs, and discolorations, and also to some types of related infections and 'plagues' affecting clothing and building of various materials (chaps. 13-14, and the summary colophons at 13:59 and 14:54-57); and the *torah* dealing with male and female fluxes and emissions (ch. 15, and its colophon starting at verse 32). In other sources, the priestly texts delineate a "*torah* statute" dealing with the purification of persons defiled by corpses (Numbers 19:2 and 3-13), and enunciate the *torah* dealing with a person who dies in a tent, specifying various potential miasma and purification rites pertaining thereto (vv. 14-22).[2]

Such instructions are provided to the priests in significant detail. Presumably such rules and more were the types of technical matters referred to by Moses when, in an old poetic designation, he states that Levi (and his priestly descendants) "shall instruct (*yoreh*) Jacob with laws and Israel with Your (God's) *torah*" (Deuteronomy 33:10). However, it is not possible to determine from this passage if the *torah* referred to has a comprehensive sense (including judicial matters), or whether it refers only to those specific ritual matters which the priests might themselves adjudicate or diagnose. The later designation found in Jeremiah 18:18 is similarly ambiguous in its warning that through their disobedience the people are subject to the loss of leadership and instruction—stating trenchantly that the sinful people will suffer an absence of "*torah* from the priest, *davar* (oracular word) from the prophet, and *etzah* (counsel) from the wise." Certainly such an old tripartite division of teachings (one that anticipates in fact the tripartite division of the later Jewish canon) is most striking both with regard to the forms of instruction and to the kinds of instructors highlighted. Whatever the scope of these terms, the context suggests that the priests deal with matters already revealed as divine *torah*, as against new prophetic oracles or teachings of natural wisdom. According to a probably contemporaneous tradition recorded in the book of Deuteronomy, we learn that *shoftim ve-shotrim* (judges and magistrates) were to be set up in the various locales to "judge (*ve-shafetu*) the people with due justice (*mishpat*)" (Deuteronomy 16:18); whereas in baffling or difficult cases, bearing on capital or civil rulings, as well as torts and injuries, one should go to a

2. For these and other colophons, and their text-critical implications, see my discussion, "On Colophons, Textual Criticism and Legal Analogies," in *Catholic Biblical Quarterly* 42 (1980), 438-49.

higher authority—namely to "the levitical priests or the judge" (or magistrate) of that time, and "seek out" (*ve-darashta*) a legal ruling from them (17:8-9); and that one should then carry out the verdict delivered, enacting all in which the judges "instruct you" (*yorukha*), "in accordance with the *torah*-instruction in which they instruct you and the ruling (*mishpat*) handed down" (vv. 10 f). In these complex cases, the priests or magistrates administer public rulings and their provisions, designated as *torah* instructions of a specific type.[3]

It would seem from the context that there is an expansion of the term *torah* here, in order to cover the administration or technical execution of the judicial rulings; though it is certainly possible that the double designation of *torah* and *mishpat* may distinguish priestly rituals from other adjudications. In any event, the decisions of *torah* (by priests or others) are reached through some ratiocinative or customary procedure. There is no reason to assume otherwise from these texts, even if the *mishpat* announced by the Levites is oracular in some other cases (as we may deduce from Exodus 29:30). By contrast, in the late post-exilic prophecy of Malachi, we are clearly told that the people "seek out (*yivaqshu*) *torah*" from the mouth of the priestly Levite, "because he is a messenger (angel) of the Lord of hosts" (Malachi 2:6-7). Clearly, in this setting the 'seeking out' referred to is oracular in nature (as also in Ezekiel 7:28). This mantic dimension of priestly *torah*-instruction is thus linked to the medium-like personal status of the Levites. Other post-exilic sources will similarly introduce an oracular dimension to *torah* learning but will locate this elsewhere.

As we have seen, the verb *darash*, with the sense of an application or searching for a decision, is used to describe the action taken in puzzling cases, when the people (or local administrators) were to go to higher courts and 'seek out' a remedy or ruling. In this setting the verb has a human, deliberative quality. Similar usages occur also in Deuteronomy 16:4, in cases dealing with the examination of evidence dealing with persons accused of false worship. And the formulation is given in a more expansive way in 13:15, in connection with persons inciting others to false worship, and there is no doubt that it involves a careful scrutiny of and 'inquiry' into evidence and details. Such a ratiocinative process reflects the larger emphasis in Deuteronomy on wisdom and rational procedures. And thus it is instructive to compare this material with the earlier traditions of legal remedies found in the book of Exodus—specifically the change in procedure indicated in chapter 18. In that setting we are told that Moses sat "from morning to night" administering justice. He explains his actions to Jethro his Midianite father-in-law,

3. For a consideration of the text, and the possibility of diverse judicial elements integrated herein, see Moshe Weinfeld, *Deuteronomy and the Deuteronomic School* (Oxford: Clarendon Press, 1972).

telling him that when the nation comes "to seek out (*lidrosh*) God," they come to him and he "judges" their cases and informs them of "the statutes of God and his *torahs*" (Exodus 18:15-16). Certainly, the sense of the text is that Moses functions as a legal medium of sorts, administering divine justice through his own person. Upon hearing this, Jethro suggests a more viable plan and proposes upright and God-fearing persons to serve as magistrates who will deal with the easier cases, and only the difficult ones would come before Moses. This hierarchical structure of adjudication is again articulated in Deuteronomy 1:9-18—where, however, the judicial innovation is presented without reference to any foreign suggestion or source, the appointees are specified as "wise, sage, and knowledgeable," and there is no reference to people seeking out God or to Moses functioning as a judicial medium (rather, Moses 'hears' the cases and commands the verdicts to be complied with). Surely the same 'rational' spirit pervades this revision as occurs in Deuteronomy 17, which now appears as an instantiation in the settlement period of the hierarchical judiciary founded in the desert and pre-settlement periods.

This focus on deliberative, investigative clarification affects the nature of Torah itself. In the book of Deuteronomy, the great bulk of priestly *torah*-instructions are deleted (with the exception of the rules of permitted foods, truncated and slightly revised in chapter 14), and it is now *only* the entire corpus of divine instructions that is called a 'Torah'. Indeed, at the very outset, we are informed that at the end of the desert sojourn Moses said to the people "all that the Lord had commanded" (Deuteronomy 1:4), and that he then began "to explain (*be'er*) all this Torah" to the people (verse 5). The deictic reference ('this') is prospective of course, and points to the various teachings which shall follow; but it is noteworthy that *the entire sum* of these instructions is now designated a Torah, and that this totality ('Torah' as a comprehensive designation) is itself subject to various exegetical clarifications by Moses. Note well that this latter instruction is not the product of either divine inspiration or revelation, but is rather a type of rational pedagogy appropriate to the issues at hand.

This said, we should add that, for the deuteronomic tradition, the Torah corpus is not limited to technical explications of specific laws. It can also serve *in toto* as a spiritual instruction. We may learn this from Deuteronomy 17:18-20, where it is stated that a king should transcribe a copy of this Torah and "read from it all his life, that he may learn to fear the Lord his God, to observe all the words of this Torah . . . , and that he not raise his heart (pridefully) over his compatriots." The emphasis on knowledge of the law and the inducement of proper piety is stressed here, and one may assume that what the Torah is meant to do for the king it is also meant to do for the entire people. The case of the king, and his transcription and study of the Torah, is thus emblematic for everyone.

Hence the study of the Torah and its explication, as well as the piety to be derived from its teachings, are thus all highlighted by the book of Deuteronomy. As the work itself indicates, this Torah-instruction "is not in heaven," far off, but rather "near" to the people, something accessible—to be put in their heart for practical study and religious guidance (Deuteronomy 30:11, 14). In the larger context of Deuteronomy, and its characteristic focus on ratiocinative praxis and wisdom, this coda is not exceptional. But this distinctive ideology of Torah interpretation with its revolutionary potential occurs elsewhere and bears special emphasis. It marks a new path in the development of Torah instruction, and with it a new setting for piety.

The significant shift in these matters is observable in a key post-exilic text, in the book of Ezra. In it, earlier and late traditions of consulting (or 'seeking') a medium-like individual for divine instruction (*torah*) merge with the practice of studying Torah and of investigating (or 'seeking explication in') legal or other cases (called both *torah* and *mishpat*) for an actionable verdict. The result is the study or consultation of the Torah as *itself* a medium of divine truths and teachings. This exegetical *transformation* of Torah is strikingly recorded in Ezra 7:9-10, where we learn that Ezra the priest, at the beginning of the people's return from Babylonian exile (following the decree of Cyrus in 539 BCE), "set his heart to consult (*lidrosh*) the Torah of the Lord (*torat YHWH*), to do and to teach law and statute in Israel."[4] The construction is as unexpected as it is striking. Indeed, it is axial in every sense. Two phrases are blended. The first, indicating 'the setting of one's heart' or mind (*hekhin lev*), is found especially in late sources to indicate a pious orientation, as noted for example regarding King Hezekiah, who, we are informed, "set his heart to seek God (*lidrosh ha-elohim*)" (2 Chronicles 30:19). The spiritual aspect of this passage is thus quite clear, and the writer of Ezra 7:10 may capitalize on its resonance. But the particularly innovative element, most surely intended, is the additional use of the verb *darash* in connection with the Torah. Significantly, early mantic sources speak of a person going to "seek" a divine oracle, in connection with some difficult personal or national matter. Thus (leaving aside the consultation of God through Moses for juridical purposes in Exodus 18), we note that Rebecca in her travail goes *lidrosh et YHWH*, "to consult YHWH" (Genesis 25:23); that King Jehoshaphat in his quandary whether to join a military alliance asks the king of Israel to "please consult (*derosh na*) this day the oracle of YHWH" (1 Kings 22:5); and that King Josiah, having initiated Temple repairs in a fit of piety, was informed that a Torah book was found and in his consternation asks the priests

4. See my full discussion in *Biblical Interpretation in Ancient Israel* (Oxford: Clarendon Press, 1985), 245.

to "consult the Lord (*dirshu et YHWH*) . . . regarding words of the scroll" (2 Kings 22:13). Exactly how these oracular consultations were conducted in each case is not altogether clear (but notably, 1 King 22:6 suggests some type of binary inquiry addressed to designated persons; a similar binary form is implied in the mantic queries 'asked' by David of the Lord via the priestly Ephod in 1 Samuel 23:2-4, 8-12), but the plain sense is that the questions were posed to God through some medium.

By contrast with these technical cases of oracular inquiry, the innovative moment found in Ezra 7:10 is that *the inquiry is made of the Torah itself.* To be sure, the ostensive purpose of such an inquiry was to derive new rulings for a new situation; but the significant absence here of terms like "read," "study," "learn," or "explicate" underscores the particular nature of this instance of inquiry. A weak construal of the phrase would suggest that an intense inquiry was made of the words of the Torah so that new divinely authorized explications might result; whereas a stronger one would even suggest a divinatory orientation, whereby the reader-inquirer believed that the exegesis was divinely given and a teaching from the arcane depths of Torah. Either way, we stand before a significantly new cultural moment. For hereby the content of the received divine revelation is the source of further exegetical revelation or learning, such that the God of the written Torah of Moses continues to teach and instruct through oral explications of it by Ezra and his disciples. And if all this is not yet an explicit indication of some pneumatic practice geared to disclose the hidden mysteries of the Torah, it at least conveys the clear sense that pious Torah study could be complemented by divine inspiration (received through a proper exegetical attitude of inquiry). Moreover, if the point of oracular exegesis is still uncertain in Ezra 7:10, such a bold possibility cannot be excluded in other cases. For example, in the contemporary Psalm 119, alongside various 'exoteric' appeals to God to "teach me (*horeni*)" or "cause me to understand (*havineni*)" the words and the path of Torah (cf. verse 32), we find a more 'esoteric' element in the remarkable request (by a Torah adept) that the Lord "open my eyes (*gal eiynai*) that I may perceive wonders (*nifla'ot*) from [the words of] your Torah" (verse 18). Could we presume that this passage is also marked by the transferred use of mantic-visionary terminology in a context of Torah instruction? In positive support, one need merely recall at this point the depiction of the soothsayer Balaam, who, when the "spirit of God" was upon him, called out and said, "This is the oracle of one who hears the words of El, who perceives the visions of Shaddai, who falls [in trance?] *galuy einayim* (his eyes opened)" (Numbers 24:3-4). Unless we are wholly mistaken, it would seem that Psalm 119:18 remarkably indicates that for some people the Torah had become a meditative medium for the disclosure of hidden mysteries. Be this as it may, there is no doubt that certain members of the Dead Sea scroll fellowship (in subsequent centuries) took this verse in precisely such a mantic sense.[5]

TORAH AS SPIRITUAL IDEAL

We shall now turn from such arcana to the *spiritualization* of Torah learning and the new *spiritual relation* to Torah that results. This is the second part of our inquiry; and here again our biblical sources formulate or prefigure striking dimensions of later Jewish religiosity.

To set the parameters, let us begin with the contents of Psalm 1, an important Torah-based composition which undoubtedly reflects the values of the final redactors. In this liturgical piece, highest felicity is accorded one who not only keeps apart from evil persons, sinners, and scoffers (a genuine piece of wisdom advice), but "whose delight (*heftzo*) is the Torah of YHWH, and who recites his Torah day and night" (verse 2). Such a person will be firmly rooted against the hardships of life, and all that he does "shall succeed (*yatzliah*)" (verse 3). In brief, there are practical benefits to Torah study and commitment—marked by a providential reward for such involvement. Our text leaves the matter as such, without a specific application. But later tradents were more specific and produced a striking inner-biblical revision of an earlier case of direct divine mediation. That initial situation involves Moses's stirring exhortation to Joshua as future leader of the conquest. According to the formulation found in Deuteronomy 31:6-7, the aged leader addresses his successor before the national assembly and tells him to "be strong and courageous," for he is soon to enter the land promised by the Lord to their ancestors, and he will enact the inheritance thereof. Moreover, God himself "will go before you and be with you," neither failing nor abandoning you—hence, he repeats: "be not afraid or terrified." The repeated exhortation that frames the reference to divine protection in battle is a clear inducement to military courage in the face of a fearsome enterprise. The leader is told to go forward, knowing that God will aid his activity. Resoluteness is the demand of the hour, nothing more.

By contrast, when this tradition is re-cited (in the same terms) at the beginning of the book of Joshua, it is placed in God's mouth, who first of all tells Joshua that he will be with him, and neither fail nor abandon him. Hence Joshua should be strong and courageous, because he will cause the people to inherit the land which God swore to give to the ancestors (Joshua 1.4-6); and this exhortation to be courageous and not be afraid is repeated for good emphasis one more time

5. See the pneumatic reuses of Psalm 119:18 in 1Q *Serah Ha-Yahad* xi.3 (cf. lines 5-6); and the allusion to it and to Numbers 23:3-4 in 1Q *Hodayot* vii.19 (cf. x.4-7).

(verse 9). However, on closer examination, these military exhortations form a bracket within which another exhortation occurs. In vv. 7-8 Joshua is now told to be strong and mighty (the same terms) "to observe and do all the Torah which Moses my servant commanded you; do not depart from it, to the right or left, that you be successful in all that you do: let the Torah not depart from your mouth, but recite it day and night, that you observe and do all that is written in it, for then you will succeed in all your ways and be successful (*tatzliah*)." It is surely evident here that strong notions of nomos have influenced our final version—specifically, the benefits of Torah study (as articulated in Psalm 1:2-3), and the exhortation to hew to its observance, not veering right or left (as emphasized in Deuteronomy 17:11). But most significantly, divine beneficence is now deemed the bilateral consequence of human obedience and faithfulness to the norms of Torah, not a unilateral guarantee of divine power for military success. To be sure, this is not an outright spiritualization of Torah, but it is certainly a spiritualizing revision of military terms for all that, and the religious revision is more than evident. A decisive shift toward a Scripture-centered religiosity must be presupposed.

Such a shift must have meant a more spiritual valuation of the Torah and its benefits. Famously, such a dimension and its benefits is celebrated in Psalm 19, where, for example, the psalmist exults and expresses the following equations: "The Torah of YHWH is pure: it restores the soul; the Testimony (*edut*) of YHWH is trustworthy: it makes wise the foolish; the Statutes (*pequdei*) of YHWH are upright: they rejoice the heart; [and] the Commandment (*mitzvah*) of YHWH is pure: it enlightens the eyes" (vv. 4-5). Such a series of synonyms for Torah (*edut, pequdim, mitzvah*) recur in the grand celebration of Torah and its learning found in Psalm 119, along with a rich catalogue of similar virtues and benefits. Such encomia are of much cultural value for the window they open to an emergent Torah-based spirituality in ancient Israel. But it is also possible to perceive this point beyond such topical references and remarks. Most notably, spiritual attitudes directed to God in various Psalms and other passages in Scripture are actually applied or addressed *to the Torah itself* in Psalm 119. This does not in any way imply that Torah piety has become a substitute for a God-centered piety, or that the Torah comes to mediate divine benefits and displace spiritual attitudes directed to God alone. It rather serves to disclose how language expressive of the most profound God-oriented piety was transferred to the Torah, where it came to serve as a focus and locus of a deepened religious attachment. To present this point as succinctly as possible, I shall note several instances in which one verse from Scripture expressing a religiously charged verb related to God tracks very closely with another in Psalm 119 where the referent is to the Torah. One could certainly multiply examples; but the following list makes the point:

1. "You shall love (*ve-ahavta*) YHWH, your God" (Deuteronomy 6:4); "How greatly do I love (*ahavti*) your Torah" (Psalm 119:87)
2. "Loving YHWH, your God . . . and cleaving (*le-davqah*) to him" (Deuteronomy 11:22); "O YHWH, I have cleaved (*davaqti*) to your testimonies" (Psalm 119:3)
3. "I have set (*shivviti*) YHWH before me, always" (Psalm 16:8); "I have chosen a path of faith, and set (*shivviti*) your statutes [before me]" (Psalm 119:30)
4. "O Israel, trust (*betah*) in YHWH" (Psalm 115:9); "I have trusted (*batahti*) in your words" (Psalm 119:42)
5. "Raise up (*se'i*) . . . your hands to him (God)" (Lamentations 2:19); "I shall raise (*esa*) my hands to your commandments" (Psalm 119:48)
6. "And they trusted (*va-ya'aminu*) in YHWH" (Exodus 14:31); "I have trusted (*ha'emanti*) in your commandments" (Psalm 119:66)

We should in no way minimize the seismic implications of the expressions found in Psalm 119. They reveal a new spiritual attitude in which the Torah and the commandments have become the object of spiritual veneration, love, and trust. This is more than a piety of study and observance and seems remarkably to open up a relationship to the commandments and Torah which is pious and religious in its own right. With this stunning transformation of Torah study and its teachings, we are close to the characteristic heartbeat of rabbinic Judaism. Psalm 119 is thus an axial document in the history of the religion of Israel—one which sets the course for millennia of Jewish spirituality from late antiquity on. It is at once an ancient formation and a preformation of subsequent types.

Torah as Rabbinic Practice

By way of conclusion, I wish to adduce one striking unit from classical Jewish sources which integrates the great powers of Torah study with a sense of (and belief in) its role as a substitute for other rituals. To my mind, this text is of paradigmatic significance for our understanding of the development of a text-based Jewish spirituality—self-standing and self-sustaining. In this setting, I shall specify one remarkable sequence of exegesis which highlights this fundamental character of Jewish interpretation. The examples are formulated through the medium of midrashic discourse, and thus attest to the attempt to ground the comprehensive nature of Torah study in scriptural exegesis itself. I deem it a fundament of this great innovation in ancient Judaism, whose impact was broad and deep throughout the medieval and early modern periods.

The source at hand is *b. Menahot* 110a, near the conclusion of this tractate in the *Babylonian Talmud*. The pertinent portion begins with an interpretation of

Malachi 1:11, "Everywhere incense is burnt to My Name." In context, the prophet celebrates the worldwide worship of the Lord among the nations as contrasted with ongoing Israelite desecrations. But the rabbis interpret otherwise. Referring to the phrase "everywhere," R. Samuel bar Nahman provides an unexpected twist, reported in the name of R. Yohanan. It is now (exegetically) averred that the passage refers to "students of the wise who are everywhere engaged in Torah study," and that God is said (through this reinterpreted passage) to assert that He "counts [this behavior] as if they [the scholars] actually offered incense to My Name." At first glance this midrash has all the marks of a strong rhetorical flourish—a kind of pious exhortation transforming and enhancing Torah study into a ritual offering, in all the places of study, throughout the diaspora. And this may indeed have been R. Yohanan's original meaning. But R. Yohanan's brother-in-law and celebrated study-partner, R. Simeon ben Lakish (Resh Lakish), turns our exegetical attention in a different direction. He asks: "Why is it stated [in Leviticus 7:37] 'This is the 'torah' for the holocaust (-offering), the meal (-offering), and for the sin (-offering) and the guilt (-offering)'?" And his answer is given forthwith: "Everyone who studies 'the Torah' is *as if* he offered up the holocaust-, meal-, sin-, and guilt-offerings." Now because of its terse formulation it might seem that Resh Lakish is simply giving another version of R. Yohanan's teaching. But this would, I think, decisively under-read the interpretation. For on closer inspection it is certain that Resh Lakish's exegesis turns on the biblical phrase, "This is the *torah* for *x*," and this leads to an extraordinary new reading of the passage. For if, in this primary context, the word 'torah' seems to be distributive and to refer to the various 'torah-instructions' that are enumerated forthwith along the lines of the priestly torahs I noted at the outset, the force of Resh Lakish's exegetical innovation would be to read the older phraseology in a way that boldly supports a new conception of Torah study and its value. Focusing on the reference to Torah in the most comprehensive sense, the sage took the preposition "for" in an instrumental sense, and interpreted the old passage to mean the following: "This is the Torah [whose study serves as an equivalent] for [the actual performance] of the holocaust- etc. offerings." That is, the sage hermeneutically transforms the syntactical weight of the passage, and this transforms the entire instruction. On his re-reading the study of the Torah may functionally substitute "*le-*" (for) the erstwhile offerings, no longer offered in the Temple (due to its destruction). The result is revolutionary.

Admittedly, Resh Lakish's exegesis (as reported in the Talmud) is quite terse and opaque; and it was probably for that reason studied and explicated in the academy over the generations, as we may confirm from the juxtaposition of a teaching of Rava (a later sage in Babylonia) to this tradition—which indeed seems like a subsequent interpretation of it along the lines just proposed. Here, Rava says (and note that he does not quote a text but offers a dictum, suggesting that he is commenting on the previous remark): "Whoever studies Torah has no need of the holocaust- [or sin-] or meal- or guilt-offering." Thus according to Rava, presumably explicating the teaching of Resh Lakish, Torah study is in fact an efficacious act of devotion and offering in the absence of the Temple. For now the study of the Torah passages dealing with the offerings serves as a substitute for their actual performance. The rhetorical 'as if' is reciprocally transformed into a marker of virtual equivalence. And to reinforce this point, the ongoing Talmudic tradition adduces the teaching of R. Yitzhak, who came to the same conclusion by a different textual route. For him, other Scriptural phraseology made the point just as well (and perhaps even better). He asks: "Why is it written [in Leviticus 6:2, 7, 18 and 7:1]: 'This is the torah of *x*' [i.e., *torat ha-olah/ha-minhah*, etc.]?"[6] He answers: "to teach you that whoever engages in the study of the torah dealing with the *olah* (holocaust), etc., is *as if* he offered the *olah* [in fact; etc.]."

Herewith we come to a remarkable cultural moment. Torah is not only the focus of devoted inquiry and interpretation, but more: the Torah that one studies (in the rabbinic manner) as an object of veneration and spiritual trust may now confer benefits otherwise unavailable. Indeed, in the present instance, the study of the sacrifices provides the ritual equivalent of their performance for purification, atonement, or other types of divine-human reconciliation. Torah study is thus deemed a transformed priestly rite, whose sacrificial satisfactions may be achieved *through rabbinic hermeneutics alone*. Here then is one of the secrets of Jewish spiritual survival and, I would add, one of the most compelling inner-Jewish responses to the claim of ancient Christianity and its ongoing contention regarding a quite different model of atonement and forgiveness through sacrificial substitution.

6. His exegetical source (in which the noun *torah* is in a bound genitival relation to the offerings) thus counterpoints the earlier one, which stated, "This is the *torah le-* (for) the holocaust-offering, etc." For R. Yitzhak, the alternative phrasing makes the new exegetical point more effectively, and his rhetorical opening, "Why is it written?," suggests that he may even have believed his interpretation to be a latent assumption of Scripture itself.

7

Leon Kass and the Poets

Paul McHugh

Being one of them, I work and live amongst physicians and surgeons—caring and thoughtful people who strive to help their patients and happily often succeed. For me as for them clinical efforts can be demanding but are seldom hard to justify. The patients are sick, the alleviating measures are available, and doctors like the job. Where's the problem or the need for bioethical oversight?

In most situations there isn't one. The patients get treated, recover their power to flourish, and gain the tranquility of health. This usual and unproblematic sequence, however, can lull us doctors into seeing all medical practice as straightforward and explains why, when occasionally we're asked questions as to the ethics of what we're doing or planning to do, we can think the questions pointless, uninformed, and strangely out of place.

Therefore, many of my colleagues disparaged the suggestions of the President's Council on Bioethics that such matters as the manufacture of human embryonic stem cells or the use of medications for the enhancement of mental and physical powers might be regulated or at least more closely scrutinized and thought about, rather than promptly put into play. On several occasions my friends identified these proposals from the Council as at best impractical and overly scrupulous and at worst meddlesome, wrong-headed, and harmful.

This is just to say that feelings can run high when ethical questions are raised, because doctors can resent interference with their efforts to help the sick, let alone suggestions that they might do harm when they work to do good. But I have also found most of them open-minded enough to at least agree that there can be a touch of personal and professional egotism tied to their resentment. Many of my doctor friends did eventually acknowledge that the misgivings provoked by the Council's work, when given more than a moment's thought, did enlarge the scope of their reflections about what we doctors are striving to do for our patients and what our actions can occasionally involve.

The opportunity to enlarge my own sensibilities as a physician in this way was the finest gift I received from working on the President's Council on Bioethics—a gift I received in one way or another from every one of the council's members but from no one more generously and effectively than from Leon Kass. For you see, Leon—a doctor, scientist, philosopher—also has the sensibility of a poet and gave expression to that sensibility in the many ways he conceived our mission, directed the council, spoke about issues, and inspired its products.

It may seem peculiar, to Leon no less than to those who know him, to say that his sensibility is that of a poet. But as our council and its projects took form I slowly came to think that the work we were doing confirmed the stunning declaration of Percy Bysshe Shelley at the close of his essay, *A Defense of Poetry*, that "poets are the unacknowledged legislators of this world."[1] And as I saw more of the detailed "brush-strokes" of our enterprises—the public achievements of the Council and the specific ways they were brought about—I became convinced as well that Leon Kass serves as the John Keats of the bioethics world.

Keats not only wrote wondrous and inspiring poetry; he also, in extraordinary letters to family and friends, analyzed the poet's mission and the better poets' modes of thought. The letters are touching when we realize how brief Keats's lifespan would be and yet note how happy and inspired he was about the life he was given. Two of his insights about the ways of poets in those letters I came to believe were powerfully if unconsciously played out by Leon Kass on our Council and through his writings.

The first insight is one of method. Keats in his letter to his brothers George and Tom on December 27, 1817, picks out a quality of mind and manner in literary geniuses such as Shakespeare. He says they are "possessed [with] *Negative Capability*" and then explains that this describes a person who "is capable of being in uncertainties, Mysteries, doubts without any irritable reaching after fact and reason."[2] The key expression in Keats's definition is "irritable reaching," because he intends by this idea of Negative Capability to honor minds receptive to the fullness and diversity of reality, a receptive quality that is often overlooked and unappreciated by lesser artists who tend to seize and quickly advance single and narrow assumptions about human experience.

Leon's commitment to Negative Capability and its rejection of "irritable reaching" expressed itself again and again through the procedures of the Council. I believe it is illuminating to see these procedures in the light of this Keatsian conception and so offer three telling examples from Leon's work.

1. Percy Shelley, *A Defense of Poetry* (Indianapolis, Indiana: Bobbs-Merrill, 1904), 90.
2. John Keats, *Selected Letters* (Oxford: Oxford World Classics, 2002), 41-42.

The first is built into the Mission Statement of the Council itself, which Leon helped compose. In it we were charged by the President with several aims, one of which was:

> The Council shall strive to develop a deep and comprehensive understanding of the issues that it considers. In pursuit of this goal the Council shall be guided by the need to articulate fully the complex and often competing moral positions on any given issue rather than by an overriding concern to find consensus. The Council may therefore choose to proceed by offering a variety of views on a particular issue rather than attempt to reach a single consensus position.[3]

What this directive assumed—quite correctly I believe—is that in the domain of bioethics not only might a variety of views be expected but that, as in reality itself, features of justice could reside in many of them and all should be heard so as to help them—when possible—to converge or coalesce. This mission was facilitated of course by Leon choosing as members of this Council such a full cut of people of diverse experience, knowledge, and commitments. They included Democrats, Republicans, Libertarians and Independents, biologists, social scientists, philosophers, lawyers, journalists, and doctors—none of whom failed to express their views, enriching meetings with constrained disagreement.

The second striking expression of devotion to Negative Capability came in the first meeting of the Council where Leon had us read and discuss a short story by Nathaniel Hawthorne, "The Birth-mark." The protagonist, like so many of Hawthorne's characters, is neither fully aware of his motives nor attentive to their effects on others. Dr. Aylmer, an eminent scientist with "faith in man's ultimate control over Nature," had married a beautiful and gracious woman. The story recounts how his love for his bride, "intertwining itself with his love of science," translates itself into a ruling passion for removing by medical design a tiny blemish on her cheek, an enterprise that ultimately leads to her death.

It's an unsettling story, in its emphasis on the possibility that we may sometimes act like monsters in striving to correct some "flaw of humanity." I saw its message as encouraging in all of us a Negative Capability that would approach human life with awe and support a stance that identified that common temptation of egotism, namely, a tendency to rush decisions and clamor for closure on matters of consequence.

I can pick up this theme of the value of Negative Capability in many of the documents of the Council and in Leon's own writings. For our purposes here

3. President George W. Bush, Executive Order 13237, November 28, 2001.

I'll choose two as they are expressed so well and tackle issues of frequent concern in contemporary bioethics.

The first addresses the common presumption that all of ethics and particularly bioethics is ultimately unproblematic given that materialistic bioscience provides all we need to know about the choices we face. Leon's countervailing idea can be discerned in the title of his first collection of essays, *Toward a More Natural Science: Biology and Human Affairs*, and especially in the closing essay of that volume entitled "Looking Good: Nature and Nobility," where he says,

> Skepticism about any connection between nature and good is now more than ever in the saddle, and anyone who breaks silence to reopen these questions must be prepared to ride against the pack. . . . The beautiful and the good are seen not as ideas that the human mind may discover and behold, but as purely human creations, constructs made by the human mind to give order to a chaotic and inhospitable world. . . . The most powerful obstacle to finding humanly meaningful clues from nature is modern science's approach to and assumptions about the nature of nature. . . . The knowledge of nature that science finds . . . embarrasses the ethical claims of traditional philosophical or religious teachings, by contradicting what they say about nature, man and the whole. If one suspects, as I do, that the questions about nature, man, and the human good are not settled once and for all . . . then one must seek some way to have them reopened. If the problem lies with our view of nature, perhaps we need to take another look[,] . . . a fresh look at what is immediately and manifestly evident. Looking toward a more natural science, one more truthful *to* the phenomena of life, as ordinarily lived and encountered, we can do no better than to look *at* the phenomena, literally at the things that appear. . . . We need to . . . open our minds to the possibility that there is more than we think in what meets the eye. . . . We aim to stir the mind to wonder by means of sightings, not quiet it by means of logical deduction.[4]

The essay that follows these initiating paragraphs is rich in the details of animal and human appearances and presentations revealing, as though straight from Keats, how truth and beauty are essentially entwined and inspire our lives together.

Leon expressed similar sentiments imbued with Keatsian Negative Capability in many discussions of the council and in its published volumes. One telling example addressed a frequent criticism from the public (and especially from physicians) that scrupulous hesitation over giving free rein to a controversial and morally vexed treatment injures people waiting on its curative powers. These critical comments commonly addressed delays produced by debating the issues of the

4. Leon R. Kass, *Toward a More Natural Science* (New York: Free Press, 1985), 319-321 (italics in the original).

destructive use of human embryos in such treatments as "stem-cell therapy." The critics claimed that both the debate and any regulatory delays would make us complicit in the suffering and death of others—often friends and relatives. Stanford biologist Irving Weissman, for instance, argued before the Bioethics Council that "those who make the judgment that this research is banned take the responsibility of whatever medical treatments could have derived from it."[5] Leon's response to such criticism is typical of what sets him apart from the narrow vision of the contemporary bioethics 'establishment':

> People sometimes imagine that human beings are responsible for all the harms they could prevent but do not; yet, this cannot be true. When we refuse to achieve a good outcome by doing what is wrong, and thereby perhaps accept some suffering that might have been avoided, we are not guilty of causing that suffering. To say otherwise would mean that sufficiently evil men could always hold us morally hostage. In order to obligate us to do an evil deed, they need only credibly threaten to do great harm unless we comply. Were we actually responsible for all the harm we might have prevented but did not, they would have us in their moral power. If our duty to prevent harm and suffering were always overriding, if it always held moral trump, we could not live nobly and justly. . . . We are human beings and . . . know that relief of suffering, though a great good, is not the greatest good. As highly as we value health and longer life, we know that life itself loses its value if we care only for *how long* we live, and not also for *how* we live.[6]

Again I believe that in this statement one can see the power of Leon's assumption of Negative Capability. He is not being contrary but open to and expressing a wider conception of life and its meanings in discussing a treatment that so many would seize without these reflections.

Negative Capability permits Leon to do proper homage to another insight of Keats expressed in a later letter to his siblings, where he notes that "the common cognomen of this world among the misguided and superstitious is 'a vale of tears' from which we are to be redeemed. . . . What a little circumscribed

5. Weissman made the remark at the council's February 2002 meeting; see bioethics.georgetown.edu/pcbe/transcripts/feb02/feb13session2.html. Two years later, he repeated and sharpened the point before a U.S. Senate committee, telling the senators that "those in a position of advice or authority who participate in the banning or enforced delays of biomedical research that could lead to the saving of lives and the amelioration of suffering are directly and morally responsible for the lives made worse or lost due to the ban." (See Kristen Philipkoski, "Senator Pushes Adult Stem Cells," *Wired*, July 15, 2004.)

6. The President's Council on Bioethics, *Human Cloning and Human Dignity* (Washington, DC: Government Printing Office, 2002), 167-68 (italics in the original). This comment is in a Council report and therefore speaks on behalf of the entire Council, but this particular portion, in its spirit and in its specific expression, was the chairman's work.

straightened notion! Call the world if you Please 'the vale of Soul-making.' Then you will find out [its] use." Later in the same letter, pressing the same point, Keats asks "do you not see how necessary a World of Pains and troubles is to school an intelligence and make it a soul?"[7]

Again I can find many passages from Leon that agree with Keats over the nature of our life and what we should take from it. As a psychiatrist I welcomed this passage in *Beyond Therapy*, in which the Bioethics Council considers the use of psychopharmacological tools such as beta blockers and anti-depressants not for the treatment of disorders but rather to remove distressful memories and moods derived from experience and from decisions:

> What about the pursuit of happy souls and especially of the sort that we might better attain with pharmacological assistance? Painful and shameful memories are disturbing; guilty consciences trouble sleep; low self-esteem, melancholy, and world-weariness besmirch the waking hours. Why not memory-blockers for the former, mood-brighteners for the latter, and a good euphoriant—without risks of hangovers or cirrhosis—when celebratory occasions fail to be jolly? For let us be clear: If it is imbalances of neurotransmitters that are largely responsible for our state of soul, would it not be sheer priggishness to refuse the help of pharmacology for our happiness, when we accept it guiltlessly to correct for an absence of insulin or thyroid hormone?
>
> And yet . . . there seems to be something misguided about the pursuit of utter and unbroken psychic tranquility or the attempt to eliminate all shame, guilt, and painful memories. Traumatic memories, shame, and guilt, are, it is true, psychic pains. In extreme doses, they can be crippling. Yet, short of the extreme, they can also be helpful and fitting. They are appropriate responses to horror, disgraceful conduct, injustice, and sin, and, as such, help teach us to avoid them or fight against them in the future. Witnessing a murder should be remembered as horrible; doing a beastly deed should trouble one's soul. Righteous indignation at injustice depends on being able to feel injustice's sting. And to deprive oneself of one's memory—including and especially its truthfulness of feeling—is to deprive oneself of one's own life and identity.
>
> These feeling states of soul, though perhaps accompaniments of human flourishing, are not its essence. Ersatz pleasure or feelings of self-esteem are not the real McCoy. They are at most shadows divorced from the underlying human activities that are the essence of flourishing. Most people want both to feel good and to feel good about themselves, but only as a result of being good and doing good.[8]

7. Keats, *Selected Letters*, 232-33.

8. The President's Council on Bioethics, *Beyond Therapy* (Washington, DC: Government Printing Office, 2003), 298. Again, while it was endorsed by the entire council as an element of its report, I can attest that this particular passage came from the chairman's pen.

I could go on with these examples but the point is made. Leon is a splendid intellectual leader and companion not only because he knows science and philosophy (and he does) and not only because he is insightful about how religious traditions speak to us today (and he is), but also because his selfless intellect does not strive to tie what he or we know into neat bundles closed to our aspirations. He expresses an expansive view of human life, medical treatments, and the ways we flourish through our activities and enterprises.

He can rejoice with science and grasp what it misses. He can think about brain and mind, body and soul, even sin and salvation, because he sees like Keats how each human life can be a quest for meanings that open before us as we act. In that quest to make our souls Leon, like Keats, upholds Negative Capability so as to give expression to that special feature of humankind, the freedom bought by self-reflection.

As I was reflecting on Leon's thoughts and achievements, I came across a sonnet by a more contemporary philosopher than Keats that deserves an airing in this essay on Leon and his poetic sensibility. In his third sonnet, George Santayana says what I mean:

> O World, thou choosest not the better part!
> It is not wisdom to be only wise,
> And on the inward vision close the eyes,
> But it is wisdom to believe the heart.
> Columbus found a world, and had no chart,
> Save one that faith deciphered in the skies;
> To trust the soul's invincible surmise
> Was all his science and his only art.
> Our knowledge is a torch of smoky pine
> That lights the pathway but one step ahead
> Across a void of mystery and dread.
> Bid, then, the tender light of faith to shine
> By which alone the mortal heart is led
> Unto the thinking of the thought divine.[9]

Amen.

9. George Santayana, *Sonnets and Other Verses* (New York: Duffield, 1906), 4.

8

Toward a Richer Public Bioethics

Rebecca Dresser

At the first meeting of the President's Council on Bioethics in January of 2002, the new Council's chairman, Leon Kass, articulated a vision for its work that broke from the model established by previous national bioethics groups. He called on Council members to go beyond the policy-oriented principlism that characterized much of bioethics, supplementing the Council's "practical duty to shape a responsible public policy" with "careful and wisdom-seeking reflection about the various human goods at stake: both those that may be served and those that may be threatened by twenty-first-century biotechnology." We should use our time on the Council, he said, to search for and advance "the best ideas and the richest approaches" to bioethical issues.[1]

I had the honor and good fortune to serve on the Council with Leon and to join all the Council's members in the intellectual and political adventure of developing a richer bioethics. In this essay I describe how Leon's vision shaped the Council's work and how that vision has influenced my own thinking and scholarship. Leon's call for a richer and deeper bioethical inquiry gave the Council an opportunity to examine the complex human meanings of contemporary scientific and technological advances. Under Leon's leadership, the Council also established education as a core objective of national bioethics groups.

The Council's Beginnings

In late 2001, I received a call from a White House official asking whether I would consider being part of a new President's Council on Bioethics. As a liberal Democrat, I wondered whether administration officials truly wanted someone like me to participate, but the caller assured me they were seeking to

1. President's Council on Bioethics Transcript, Session 1: Welcome and Opening Remarks, January 17, 2002. Transcripts of all of the Council's meetings are available online at bioethics.georgetown.edu/pcbe/transcripts.

assemble a group with diverse views. After surviving the background check, I was appointed to the eighteen-member Council.

The Council chairman was Dr. Leon Kass, someone I knew primarily by his reputation as a founder of American bioethics. Becoming a Council member gave me an opportunity to get to know him much better and to appreciate the qualities he brought to the Council. Leon is a genuine intellectual. His impressive knowledge of literature and the humanities adds breadth to his thinking about bioethical issues. He also likes to be provocative, even polemical. He often (though not always) takes positions that deviate from the popular and the conventional. These arguments provoke strong disagreement, sometimes outrage, from more orthodox bioethical thinkers. But in Council discussions and deliberations, Leon sought engagement with people holding different views. And he often challenged himself, acknowledging his uncertainties and limitations in conversations with others.

These characteristics made Leon a stellar leader for our group. As a teacher, I was in awe of his skill in conducting our "national seminar" on complicated issues involving science and ethics. Leon exhibited the rare ability to keep track of every point speakers made, often returning to earlier comments as they became relevant to later discussion. Everyone who wanted to contribute had a chance to speak; Leon's pointed questions led people to think more deeply about the issues we discussed.

Leon played a significant role in establishing the Council's mission, too. The Executive Order authorizing the Council clearly bore his mark. It assigned to the group the following five functions:

1. to undertake fundamental inquiry into the human and moral significance of developments in biomedical and behavioral science and technology;
2. to explore specific ethical and policy questions related to these developments;
3. to provide a forum for a national discussion of bioethical issues;
4. to facilitate a greater understanding of bioethical issues; and
5. to explore possibilities for useful international collaboration on bioethical issues.[2]

Thus, the Executive Order listed exploration of policy questions as simply one of many assignments for this national bioethics group. As I shall discuss later, one of the distinguishing features of the Council was its far-reaching, in-depth approach to public bioethics.

The Executive Order described another distinctive Council feature. Although earlier bioethics groups had examined an array of different ethical

2. President George W. Bush, Creation of The President's Council on Bioethics, Executive Order 13237, November 28, 2001. Available online at bioethics.georgetown.edu/pcbe/about.

views in their reports, they typically sought to develop consensus judgments and recommendations. This often produced proposals that combined procedural measures with "minimalist" ethical principles that were acceptable to all or at least most of the members.[3] Such an approach may be appropriate in legislative and policy activities, but it can lead to a "plain vanilla" version of bioethics.

The Council's Executive Order urged a different approach, one more conducive to the richer and deeper bioethical inquiry Leon endorsed:

> The Council shall strive to develop a deep and comprehensive understanding of the issues that it considers. In pursuit of this goal, the Council shall be guided by the need to articulate fully the complex and often competing moral positions on any given issue, rather than by an overriding concern to find consensus. The Council may therefore choose to proceed by offering a variety of views on a particular issue, rather than attempt to reach a single consensus position.[4]

The release from consensus substantially contributed to the nature and quality of the analysis in several Council reports.

Leon also had a role in assembling a diverse group of people, most of them from outside the field of bioethics. In opening remarks at the Council's first meeting, he announced, "This is a council on bioethics, not a council of bioethicists."[5] Contrary to claims in the media and elsewhere, this was not a "politically stacked"[6] group, "most" of whose members were "conservatives like Kass . . . unlikely to recommend anything the President would not want to hear."[7] At that first meeting, Leon observed, "We are a diverse and heterogeneous group: by training we are scientists and physicians, lawyers and social scientists, humanists and theologians, by political leaning we are liberals and conservatives, Republicans, Democrats and Independents, and by religion Protestants, Catholics, Jews, and perhaps some who are none of the above."[8]

At Leon's direction, the Council turned to novel sources for ethical insights. As the basis for ethical deliberation, previous national bioethics groups focused on material related to philosophy, science, and medicine. The Council also relied on such material, but under Leon's leadership we considered literature as well.

3. See John Evans, *Playing God? Human Genetic Engineering and the Rationalization of Public Bioethical Analysis* (Chicago: University of Chicago Press, 2002).

4. President George W. Bush, Executive Order 13237.

5. President's Council on Bioethics Transcript, Session 1.

6. See Rick Weiss, "Bush Unveils Bioethics Council," *Washington Post*, January 17, 2002.

7. Jerome Groopman, "Science Fiction," *The New Yorker*, February 4, 2002, at 23, 24.

8. President's Council on Bioethics Transcript, Session 1.

For example, early in the Council's first meeting, we discussed a short story by Nathaniel Hawthorne called "The Birth-mark." In introducing the session, Leon gave three reasons for such an unorthodox beginning. First, the story addressed one force behind modern biology and medicine, the "human aspiration to eliminate defects and to pursue some kind of perfection."[9] Wisdom in thinking about issues like human cloning would come not simply from science but from considering "certain enduring matters and questions," such as the pursuit of perfection. Second, a discussion of the story would encourage us to converse "not as scientists or humanists, but as fellow human beings thoughtful about these matters and reacting responsively to the story." We would be pushed to be creative and to test our thinking in new ways. Third, Leon hoped the discussion would illustrate how texts other than those typically consulted for bioethics inquiry "can be fruitfully used to deepen our understanding of the meaning of biomedical advance."

The Council's first meeting was not the only time we read literary offerings. We read and discussed stories about illness and about organ donation by Richard Seltzer. We discussed *Peter Pan* and the insights it offered about a life of perpetual youth. Probably the most popular Council publication, *Being Human: Readings from the President's Council on Bioethics*, is an anthology of selections from works of literature relevant to bioethical issues.

THE COUNCIL'S "RICHER" REPORTS

Because of Leon's vision, the Council's reports *are* richer than those of comparable groups, in the sense that they go beyond the customary "ethics lite" and policy focus other groups have adopted. In a 2005 article, Leon himself described how the Council's first five reports sought to apply the richer bioethics approach.[10] I cannot improve on that description but will offer my own thoughts on two of those reports.

In 2003, the Council issued *Beyond Therapy: Biotechnology and the Pursuit of Happiness*. It is a powerful and thought-provoking document. It is beautifully written, often moving and at times poetic. Instead of a pared-down account of ethical and policy considerations, it is an expansive and elaborate exploration of ideas bearing on a difficult set of issues.

Beyond Therapy examines a group of currently available interventions, such as Ritalin and other stimulant drugs, prenatal testing and sex selection, and

9. President's Council on Bioethics Transcript, Session 2: Science and the Pursuit of Perfection, January 17, 2002.

10. Leon R. Kass, "Reflections on Public Bioethics: A View from the Trenches," *Kennedy Institute of Ethics Journal* 15 (2005): 221-50.

mood-brightening agents, that can be used "to treat individuals with known diseases, disabilities, or impairments, in an attempt to restore them to a normal state of health and fitness."[11] These interventions also have other potential uses, however, uses that have goals different from those ordinarily embraced by medicine. The interventions may be used in attempts "to alter . . . not disease processes but the 'normal' workings of the human body and psyche, to augment or improve their native capacities and performances."[12] *Beyond Therapy* also considers several "dual-use" measures that might become available in the future, such as genetic engineering, anti-aging interventions, and agents that might soften an individual's memories of violence or other traumatic events.

Beyond Therapy discusses the safety risks and potential benefits of these interventions as well as their potential to promote inequality. These are all matters covered in typical bioethical analyses. But *Beyond Therapy* does much more than that. The report examines how social pressure to conform to notions of the ideal and the excellent could promote enhancement interventions, limiting liberty in the process. It considers whether some enhancement efforts conflict with a "welcome attitude of modesty, restraint, and humility" toward certain features of the "given world."[13] It describes how enhancements could change our identities and aspirations, as self-improvement is transformed from an active endeavor into a passive dependence on biotechnology.

Beyond Therapy is a humanistic examination of serious questions facing wealthy nations with the capacity to pursue previously unimagined alterations of the human condition. Leon's insights about the natural world and human efforts to improve on it, the human life cycle of childhood, parenthood, aging, and mortality, and the proper goals of medicine enrich the analysis, giving it a force and drama absent from other public bioethics reports. Anyone wishing to evaluate the potential consequences of biotechnological innovation will find much to contemplate in *Beyond Therapy*.

The Council took another look at aging and the life cycle in its 2005 report, *Taking Care: Ethical Caregiving in Our Aging Society*.[14] This report addresses a serious problem facing many families today, one that will only become more serious in the near future. With the aging of the baby boom generation, many

11. President's Council on Bioethics, *Beyond Therapy: Biotechnology and the Pursuit of Happiness* (Washington, DC: 2003), 13. This as well as other Council reports are available online at bioethics.georgetown.edu/pcbe/reports.

12. Ibid., 13.

13. Ibid., 289.

14. President's Council on Bioethics, *Taking Care: Ethical Caregiving in Our Aging Society* (Washington, DC: 2005). My remarks on this report are based on those in my personal statement appended to the report.

more individuals will be affected by Alzheimer's disease and other forms of dementia. In this report, the Council added its voice to those calling for more systematic and sustained attention to the caregiving demands presented by an aging society.

Taking Care offers ethical analysis and guidance, as well as a few rules to govern caregiving decisions. Navigating a proper course between extending life and accepting death is never easy, but discerning that course is particularly difficult in the context of dementia care. People with dementia can live for many years after they lose the ability to make their own choices. And they remain conscious and able to experience burdens and benefits from treatment interventions. These facts join to present special challenges to those who must decide on the patients' behalf.

Taking Care reviews the standard ethical and legal approaches to treatment decision-making for incapacitated patients and shows how they are insufficient to guide families and clinicians responsible for dementia patient care. In the dementia setting, for example, living wills are of limited use. Relatively few people make living wills, and the documents that do exist often fail to resolve treatment questions arising in dementia patient care. In the typical situation, families and clinicians must instead evaluate how different treatment options could benefit and burden individual dementia patients. Many dementia patients remain capable of appreciating experiences and interactions with others. At the same time, interventions often create new distress and discomforts for confused and frail patients, and this must be part of the benefit-burden analysis.

To illustrate an appropriate approach to the challenge of deciding on behalf of dementia patients, *Taking Care* offers case studies involving specific treatment questions. The case analyses identify central features of good care and examine a range of permissible choices by those at the bedside. *Taking Care* identifies a general ethical framework for dementia care decision-making: to respect and protect dementia patients while also recognizing medicine's limits and our status as mortal creatures. The report admits that this framework offers no easy answers to specific treatment dilemmas. By examining the unavoidable complexities and uncertainties characterizing individual patients' situations, *Taking Care* offers the richer bioethical analysis Leon hoped the Council would conduct.

THE ROLE OF NATIONAL BIOETHICS ADVISORY GROUPS

Leon's leadership expanded the agenda for public bioethics. Before the Council's creation, bioethics advisory groups were seen primarily as policy advisers.

But that function occupied a less central position in the Executive Order authorizing the Council. Although the Order directed the Council to "explore" policy questions, it placed more emphasis on providing a forum for "fundamental inquiry" and "national discussion." The Executive Order also instructed the Council to promote "a greater understanding of bioethical issues." Thus, education was an important Council mission.

At times, presidents and Congress have assigned national bioethics groups specific policy roles. The clearest case was the 1973 congressional directive to the National Commission for the Protection of Human Subjects of Biomedical and Behavioral Research, which called on the Commission to "develop guidelines which should be followed [in human subject] research to assure that it is conducted in accord with [ethical] principles."[15] Such directives may be appropriate when ethical analysis is central to a specific regulatory need of the federal government. Yet in the absence of this situation, public discussion and education seem to me more suitable functions for a national bioethics group.

The Council took its education mission seriously. Its members and staff produced a wealth of accessible information for interested audiences. The Council deliberated in public, and its meeting transcripts, reports, working papers, and other materials were made available at its website (now archived at bioethics.georgetown.edu/pcbe). Commercial publishers reprinted several Council reports, which meant that the reports could be purchased at local bookstores.[16] College and university teachers brought students to Council meetings and used Council reports as course readings. They invited Council members to lecture and debate at their institutions. One enterprising Mount Holyoke College professor assigned students to play the roles of different Council members and to conduct a mock Council meeting before a large undergraduate biology class.[17]

The Council considered policy matters too, but with a broader-than-usual audience in mind. In my view, this was an appropriate choice. Unless a group is assigned a specific and direct policy role, as was the National Commission, it seems to me unrealistic, as well as immodest, for a bioethics advisory group to see policy advice as its primary function. In many biomedical policy situations, such as health care reform, ethical analysis is relevant to formulating the appropriate rules. But other forms of expertise are usually essential to policy

15. Evans, *Playing God?*, 84-85.

16. Before this time, no national bioethics report had been commercially published.

17. For a description of the exercise, see Rachel Fink, "Cloning, Stem Cells, and the Current National Debate: Incorporating Ethics into a Large Introductory Biology Course," *Cell Biology Education* 1 (2002): 132-44.

development as well. For example, wise and effective health care reform will emerge only after officials consult a wide array of experts and address the political considerations that determine whether any change can be implemented.

Furthermore, in the absence of a direct policy assignment, I think national bioethics groups should adopt a broad concept of policy advice, a concept that includes not simply direct translation of its recommendations into formal regulatory policy but also a number of possible "trickle-down" effects. This would include decisions by other bodies to incorporate a bioethics group's ideas, analysis, or recommendations into government policies developed at a later time, as well as the influence of a bioethics group's work on nongovernmental policies, such as professional or institutional rules and guidelines. It would also include a bioethics group's influence on students and scholars who at some point in their careers write or participate in policy formation. It could even encompass a group's influence on members of the public, whose views can have a significant impact on legislators and other policymakers.

On this model, a bioethics group's policy influence could depend on the extent to which group discussions and deliberations engage important ideas and examine different positions on significant bioethical issues. One could also gauge a bioethics group's influence by considering its record of developing resources for students, scholars, and ordinary people to examine as they form their own positions on bioethical issues.

If one adopts this definition, the quality and richness of an ethics group's deliberations and reports would be important determinants of its ability to influence policy. Also relevant would be the diversity of views represented and analyzed in its discussions and publications. An analysis presenting a range of views could be more useful than one presenting consensus views. From this perspective, Leon's richer approach to bioethical analysis could be more valuable than the conventional approaches to public bioethics work.

The Council's approach, like any other, had its shortcomings. Although many "ordinary" people have told me that they read and appreciated Council reports, the reports' scholarly style probably limits their public readership (although I doubt that many members of the general public have read the more policy-focused reports of other national bioethics groups either). The Council's practice of recognizing a range of views also disturbed individuals and interest groups with a single agenda, such as promoting or opposing human embryonic stem cell research. Then there were the challenges facing a diverse group seeking to develop a collaborative contribution. When policy recommendations are desired, it can be hard to gain agreement among people who see the world quite differently.

The single instance in which President Bush asked the Council for specific policy advice illustrates this difficulty. In *Human Cloning and Human Dignity*, the Council could not agree on one policy proposal. Instead, it offered two different recommendations. Seven members endorsed a proposal to establish "a system of oversight and regulation that would permit cloning-for-biomedical-research to proceed promptly, but only under carefully prescribed limits."[18] Ten members favored a proposal for "a four-year national moratorium (a temporary ban) on human cloning-for-biomedical-research."[19]

Neither of the Council's recommendations became policy. It is not clear that Council consensus would have altered this situation, however, in light of the political division over this issue. Moreover, despite ongoing efforts in the United States and other nations to develop stem cell lines from cloned human embryos, no scientist has yet achieved this goal. This turn of events is a reminder that uncertainty is an inherent feature of bioethical analysis and policy formation. In hindsight, claims that any pause in research cloning efforts would deprive patients of cures and treatments seem overstated. Indeed, later scientific developments suggest that it may be possible to produce satisfactory alternatives using stem cells from other sources.[20] If the Council's cautious position on research cloning contributed to the search for alternatives, this was a positive ethical outcome.

The Council's diversity may have made policy consensus elusive, but diversity contributed to something that could be even more important in a nation long gripped by the so-called Culture Wars. A group of thoughtful scholars bringing diverse disciplinary backgrounds and moral commitments to the bioethics table generates a certain kind of process and product. If a national bioethics group demonstrates that people of good will with different values and positions can join together in civil debate over the bioethics issues that have been so divisive in this country, I would see this as a "successful" bioethics commission. In my view, future national bioethics groups *should* have as one of their goals to show the public that it is possible (and fascinating) to engage in civil discourse with people with very different worldviews. Success in this arena could be at least as valuable as any formal policy contribution.

18. President's Council on Bioethics, *Human Cloning and Human Dignity: An Ethical Inquiry* (Washington, DC: 2002), 218, 227.

19. Ibid., 205, 227. As a lawyer, I thought that the two proposals were not really very different, since establishing an oversight and regulatory system would be time-consuming, given the procedural requirements of the federal regulatory process and the likely controversy over the system's appropriate features.

20. See Constance Holden, "Biologists Change One Cell Type Directly into Another," *Science* 321 (2008): 1143; Rob Stein, "Scientists Report Advance in Stem Cell Alternative," *Washington Post*, September 26, 2008.

IMPACT ON MY SCHOLARSHIP

Before joining the Council, I was becoming a bit bored with my usual approach to analyzing bioethical issues. I was looking for new ways to think about end-of-life treatment, biomedical research, assisted reproduction, genetics, and the other topics about which I teach and write. Leon's vision of a richer bioethics pointed me in new directions. As I said earlier, the Council often considered literary narratives in its deliberations. Although the Council did not formally incorporate personal narrative into Council reports, Leon recognized personal experience as a legitimate knowledge base for the Council. In his statement at the Council's first meeting, Leon said, "Moral positions rooted in religious faith or in philosophy or in ordinary personal experience of life are equally relevant, provided that the arguments and insights offered enter our public discourse in ways that do not appeal to special privilege or authority."[21]

As a result of my participation in the Council, I turned to literary and personal narratives in my own work. After serving on the Council for a few years, I was invited to participate in a symposium on the Theresa Schiavo case. I considered declining, because I had written extensively about the ethics and law of forgoing life-sustaining treatment and thought I had nothing more to say about the topic. But then I remembered the Council's use of literary texts to explore bioethical issues. In work published the same year the Schiavo controversy arose, Marjorie Williams and Joan Didion offered remarkable insights into the human meaning of life-threatening illness. Their personal accounts of death and dying showed how hard it can be to let go of one's life or the life of a loved one. In my own article, I described how Williams and Didion challenged certain contemporary myths about death and dying, such as the idea that death with dignity is easily attainable, as long as people make living wills.[22]

In an essay in the Council's 2008 volume, *Human Dignity and Bioethics*, I subjected my own experience of illness to bioethical analysis. The essay, "Human Dignity and the Seriously Ill Patient," examines dignity from the bottom up, considering how the concept of dignity bears on the treatment of patients with serious illness. The essay argues that if human dignity applies to anyone, it applies to people experiencing serious illness. It explores what constitutes dignified treatment for patients receiving care in today's medical system. The analysis draws on clinicians' accounts of patient care, as well as on my personal experience as a cancer patient.

21. President's Council on Bioethics Transcript, Session 1.

22. Rebecca Dresser, "*Schiavo* and Contemporary Myths about Dying," *University of Miami Law Review* 61 (2007): 821-46.

"Dignity and the Seriously Ill Patient" considers how concerns related to personal privacy, communication, respect for personal knowledge, and responses to dependency affect patients' sense of dignity. The essay describes threats to dignity arising out of the exposure and forced intimacy patients must endure, as well as the isolation, loneliness, and dependence experienced by patients with serious illness. It offers thoughts on how caregivers and ordinary people can promote dignity in their encounters with seriously ill patients.

For patients, dignity is a precious possession. Serious illness threatens one's place in the human community. Ordinary activities fall by the wayside and relationships are no longer the same. How should the patient, clinicians, loved ones, and others respond to this disruption, this new vulnerability? These matters are fertile ground for the inquiry into human dignity. They deserve a high priority in bioethics scholarship and teaching.

I continue to incorporate narrative and personal experience in my work. In a project called, "Cancer and Bioethics: When the Professional Becomes Personal," I am collaborating with others to examine ethical issues related to cancer from the perspective of personal experience. Members of the group are from the bioethics field and all have had cancer themselves, cared for spouses with cancer, or both.

The project group is engaged in case-based analysis that considers ethics from the bottom up. We consider how we were affected by medical and social responses to cancer and reflect on how our personal experiences influenced the views we express in our teaching, writing, and policy work. The project inquiry is conducted within a framework of recognized bioethics topics, but its focus is on the experience of cancer patients and family caregivers. By proceeding from the particular to the general, we seek to capture elements of "cancer ethics" that have not yet been recognized in the clinical or bioethics literature.

My experience on the Council has renewed my interest in bioethics. I have found new directions for my work, and much of this is due to Leon. His vision of a richer public bioethics had the happy side effect of invigorating my own scholarship and teaching.

Personal Reflections

Everyone familiar with the Council knows that it drew hostility from scientists and others, including individuals from the bioethics field. Although certain writers disparaged the Council on grounds that it included "too many" conservatives, in some respects it was the critics who took the more conservative position. As Jonathan Moreno has observed, Leon's appointment to lead the Bioethics Council disturbed "the Great Bioethics Compromise" that emerged in the 1970s. In this compromise, bioethics assumed the following "consensus philosophy and social role": "Keep a close eye on scientific innovation for its societal implications, apply the brakes now and then as needed through regulations or guidelines or just the glare of public discussion, and let the bioethicists be the ones to analyze how all this is going."[23] Scientists and bioethicists comfortable with the status quo were vocal in their opposition to a politically diverse Council that dared to depart from accepted bioethics orthodoxy.

As someone from "mainstream" bioethics, I was disheartened at the narrow-mindedness characterizing some of the criticism. Although there were important exceptions, critics often preferred to rely on media reports and unfounded assertions about the Council rather than the transcripts and reports that constitute its actual work.

Some showed little tolerance for including people outside the field in bioethics deliberations and ridiculed Council members who expressed views that failed to conform to bioethics orthodoxy. Some of the commentary consisted of petty and personal attacks rather than critiques of the Council's substantive work.

In my view, the failure to treat the Council's work seriously deprived bioethics of an opportunity for engagement and intellectual development. People working in the field presumably believe that bioethical issues are important and merit public attention. They therefore ought to welcome previously uninvolved public intellectuals to the bioethics conversation. As in other disciplines, outsiders with fresh perspectives are needed to keep bioethics vibrant and to keep bioethicists from becoming stale and complacent. Bioethicists should observe civility in debates over bioethical issues, too, especially when that debate occurs in public. They should be willing to deliberate with people who see things differently and seek for common ground.

I was also disappointed that bioethicists criticizing the Council seemed to reject the notion that a skeptical and cautionary stance toward scientific advances is acceptable—indeed, appropriate—in analyzing bioethical issues. This rejection was most evident in commentary on the Council's analysis of embryonic stem cell research and research cloning. Most scientists and many bioethicists dismissed the idea that there could be any ethical or policy problems in an exciting area of basic science that might contribute to future health benefits. In the stem cell debate, a field that began by raising questions about science and medicine seemed to abandon this mission.

By failing to engage with the Council's actual transcripts and reports, bioethicists lost an opportunity to learn from others, test their own views, develop

23. Jonathan Moreno, "The End of the Great Bioethics Compromise," *Hastings Center Report* 35(1): 15-16.

a better understanding of differing positions, and make bioethics more diverse, democratic, and representative of the nation in which we live. Being a member of the Council showed me that it can be challenging, stimulating, and fun to talk about bioethics issues with people holding diverse views. Council discussions were spirited and fascinating, and I always came away from our meetings with a sense of exhilaration. Leon's leadership elevated the discussion to a level I have rarely experienced in my life as an academic.

Besides teaching me new ways to think about science, medicine, and bioethics, Leon has become a good and caring friend. We don't see eye-to-eye on many political and policy matters, but this has been no barrier to our friendship. When I was being treated for cancer a few years ago, I was fortunate to have the help and support of many people. But Leon was one of the most attentive. His e-mails and phone calls (sometimes with Amy) were bright spots during a dreary convalescence. In this and many other situations, I have seen Leon live the ethical life, not simply write about it. Although our time as colleagues on the Council has ended, I'm delighted to have Leon as a collaborator on a current bioethics project. I know that I will continue to learn from this deep thinker and gracious individual.

9

Philosophic Anthropology in Rousseau and Elizabeth Marshall Thomas

Nelson Lund

Anyone who knows anything at all about the lives of Leon Kass and Jean-Jacques Rousseau should think instantly of the contrast.[1] Their writings are as different as their conduct, with clarity and sobriety opposed to self-indulgent excess and infuriating paradoxes. But they can also look like brothers in arms, skeptical about modernity and determined to resist some of its most characteristic developments. They also share a philosophic interest in the natural sources and ends of the human soul. This essay seeks to throw some light on Rousseau's search for man "as Nature formed him,"[2] through the work of Elizabeth Marshall Thomas, who has presented new evidence of a kind that Rousseau hoped would come to light.

Introduction

The nature of the soul is a matter of such manifest scientific interest that Aristotle's *De Anima* opens with only a brief explanation of its importance. Aristotle then offers a pointed warning: "In every way, however, reaching any assured conviction about the soul is one of the most difficult undertakings."[3] This is followed by a lengthy and intimidating discussion of the methodological difficulties posed

1. For many gory details about Rousseau's behavior, see his *Confessions*, which has been usefully and painfully supplemented by Maurice Cranston's three-volume biography.

2. Jean-Jacques Rousseau, *Discourse on Inequality* [*Discours sur l'origine et les fondements de l'inégalité parmi les hommes*], in *Oeuvres Complètes*, vol. III, ed. Bernard Gagnebin & Marcel Raymond (Paris: Bibliothèque de la Pléiade, 1959-1995), 122. All page references to Rousseau are to this edition. The translations are my own, but I have borrowed freely from *The Discourses and Other Early Political Writings*, Victor Gourevitch, ed. & trans. (Cambridge: Cambridge University Press, 1997), and from *The First and Second Discourses*, ed. Roger D. Masters, trans. Roger D. and Judith R. Masters (New York: St. Martin's Press, 1964). The Gourevitch edition includes references to the pagination in the Pléiade edition.

3. Aristotle, *De Anima* 402a10-11.

by the inquiry.[4] I will mention only two. It is not immediately apparent whether the soul is divisible or indivisible; nor is it immediately clear how, if at all, the soul is separate from the body. In the course of the methodological discussion, Aristotle also warns against focusing exclusively on the human soul.

In his own way, Rousseau seeks to begin working us through such difficulties in the *Discourse on the Origin and Foundations of Inequality Among Men*. The epigraph to this book is a quotation in Latin from Aristotle's *Politics*: "What is natural must be viewed not in things that are corrupted but in those things that are well-ordered according to nature." The quotation, taken from a discussion of natural and conventional slavery, is immediately preceded in the text of the *Politics* by the assertion that the soul naturally rules the body in *all* living things. The quotation is immediately followed by Aristotle's assertion that what is natural in human beings will be clear in people with the best disposition in both body and soul.[5]

The *Discourse on Inequality* investigates this linkage or analogy between the rulership of human masters and what we might call self-rulership or the soul-body relationship. Rousseau's method is to trace the coming into being of man and his political relations from their pre-political and even pre-human origins up to modern times. The practical importance of this undertaking, according to some of Rousseau's statements, arises from its political implications. For example: "[S]o long as we do not know natural man, we will wish in vain to figure out the Law which he has received or that which best fits his constitution."[6] Those implications are potentially so radical that the truth or falsity of the underlying analysis becomes a matter of significant political importance.[7] But even apart from politics, there could hardly be many propositions whose truth or falsity matter more than Rousseau's claim that "Society no longer offers to the eyes of the wise man anything but an assemblage of artificial men and factitious passions which are the product of all these new [social] relationships, and have no true foundation in Nature."[8]

The presentation of Rousseau's thought in this book is simultaneously daring and cagy.[9] An adequate commentary would have to extract the whole

4. Ibid., 402a11-403b19.

5. Aristotle, *Politics* 1254a34-1254b2.

6. *Discourse on Inequality*, 125.

7. See, e.g., ibid., 180: "[T]he thing to do would have been to begin by clearing the ground and setting aside all the old materials, as Lycurgus did in Sparta, in order afterwards to erect a good Building."

8. Ibid., 192. Observations of great apes that have been raised as pets, or like adopted human children, may give us a glimpse of what Rousseau believed he saw. Cf. Anne Russon, *Orangutans: Wizards of the Rainforest* (Buffalo, New York: Firefly Books, 2004), 104-12; Jane Goodall, *Through a Window: My Thirty Years with the Chimpanzees of Gombe* (Boston and New York: Houghton Mifflin, 1990), 13; and Notes A and B at the end of this essay.

9. In Book IX of the *Confessions*, Rousseau characterizes the *Discourse on Inequality* as the

of Rousseau's considered views from his deliberately paradoxical presentation and assess the truth of those views. In this short essay I offer a few tentative comments on a handful of passages.

THE STATE OF NATURE

As the full title of the *Discourse* suggests, and as the context of the epigraph from Aristotle's *Politics* confirms, Rousseau's focus is on the relation between natural and conventional inequality. Almost at the outset, he defines the former as that which "is established by Nature, and which consists in the differences in age, health, strength of Bodies, and qualities of Mind, or of Soul."[10] This he distinguishes from moral or political inequality, which depends on the consent of men and consists of different privileges that some enjoy, including even the privilege of making themselves obeyed. Rousseau dismisses the possibility that there is some essential correspondence between natural inequalities and disparities of political power or wealth.[11] Later, however, he asserts that "personal merit" or "personal qualities" are the origin of *all* the political and moral forms of inequality.[12]

The statements are not logically inconsistent, and their relationship is illuminated by Rousseau's account of the state of nature. He emphatically denies that the state of nature should be thought of as a set of circumstances in which people essentially like ourselves once existed without laws or governments. Rather, the state of nature was an articulated period of time during which our ancestors made a transition from life as independent, speechless animals roaming in the forests to socialized beings with stable governments and laws. Natural or physical inequalities among individuals would have had little effect when individuals had little to do with one another. "[T]here was neither education nor progress, generations multiplied uselessly; and as everyone always started at the same point, Centuries passed in all the crudeness of the first ages, the species had already grown old, and man remained ever a child."[13] This original condition

place in which he revealed his principles "with the greatest daring, not to say audacity." *Oeuvres Complètes*, vol. I, 407. In an unfinished draft of a response to criticism of the *Discourse on the Sciences and Arts*, written just before he began work on the *Discourse on Inequality*, Rousseau said that he believed he had discovered great things and set them forth with a "somewhat dangerous frankness," but that he had also often "been at great pains to try to condense into a Sentence, into a line, into one word tossed off as if by chance, the result of a long series of reflections." *Preface to a Second Letter to Bordes*, in *Oeuvres Complètes*, vol. III, 103, 106.

10. *Discourse on Inequality*, 131.

11. Ibid., 131-32.

12. Ibid., 189.

13. Ibid., 160.

is sometimes described in rather disparaging terms, as in this quotation, and sometimes more appealingly. Its crucial feature, however, is that it must have ended through "the fortuitous intervention of a number of foreign causes."[14] By this Rousseau means that changes in the natural environment or migration into new environments led individuals to begin cooperating with one another, perhaps in such activities as hunting for the purpose of self-preservation.[15]

Rousseau acknowledges, as he must, that such acts of cooperation—and all of the much more elaborate forms and achievements of society that eventually came to be—must be natural in the sense that nature provided our ancestors with the capacity to bring them about. What he denies—and this seems to be his central contention—is that *any* specific way of life is natural to man in the sense that it corresponds to our natural range of inclinations and powers.

Speaking of the city, Aristotle says: "If one were to look at how affairs (*ta pragmata*) develop from the beginning, one would, in this as in other cases, get the finest view of them. . . . [E]very city exists by nature, if the first communities really also do."[16] Rousseau denies that either cities or the first communities (other than mother-child pairs) exist by nature, at least in the sense that Aristotle is frequently thought to have said they do. Whatever disagreements he may have with Aristotle, which may be fewer and less significant than is commonly supposed, Rousseau does set out to explain how human society must have "developed from the beginning."

What distinguishes man from all other animals is "the faculty of perfecting oneself; a faculty which, with the aid of circumstances, successively develops all the others, and resides among us as much in the species as in the individual."[17] As Rousseau makes clear, however, "perfecting oneself" involves the acquisition of qualities that *conflict* with our underlying natures. We are not like bees or herd animals,[18] where the individual is necessarily "at the end of a few months what it will be for all its life; and its species is after a thousand years what it was in the first year of that thousand."[19] Rather, man is "compensated for the instinct he *perhaps* lacks by faculties capable of making up for it at first, and of raising him afterwards far above nature."[20] Sadly, we might be forced to agree that these faculties "render [man] at length the tyrant of himself and of Nature."[21]

14. Ibid., 162.
15. Ibid., 166-67.
16. Aristotle, *Politics* 1252a24-26, 1252b30-31.
17. *Discourse on Inequality*, 142.
18. Cf. Aristotle, *Politics* 1253a6-8.
19. *Discourse on Inequality*, 142.
20. Ibid., 142-43 (emphasis added).
21. Ibid., 142.

This grossly simplified summary omits Rousseau's supporting arguments and evidence. It also leaves unexplored Rousseau's very complex interweaving of emotional and judgmental rhetoric with dispassionate and even brutally uncompromising reasoning. But it does at least raise a question that invites further attention. Even if no one way of life is natural for man in the way that the lives of bees and herd animals are natural for them, is there a way of life that is naturally best for man?

"THE HAPPIEST EPOCH, AND THE MOST DURABLE"

Rousseau addresses this question directly. In the course of his description of human pre-history—reminiscent of that in Book V of Lucretius's *De Rerum Natura*[22]—he identifies the last stage of the state of nature, or "nascent society," as the best for man. Before drawing this conclusion, however, he describes a transition from the first societies, which resulted from "a first revolution" that united parents and children in a common dwelling.[23] When these families began gradually to unite in larger bands, people began to "acquire ideas of merit and of beauty which produce sentiments of preference."[24] This would have produced sexual jealousy, and thus bloody conflict. More generally, people would have noticed natural differences in beauty, strength, grace, and eloquence. Soon, with everyone wanting to be recognized and respected, vanity and contempt would produce shame and envy, and thus vengeance.

Notwithstanding the new motives for conflict and violence, Rousseau concludes that fully human beings were at home in this condition, prior to agriculture and metallurgy, property and laws:

> [T]his period of the development of human faculties, maintaining a fair mean between the indolence of the primitive state and the petulant activity of our *amour propre*, must have been the happiest epoch, and the most durable. The more one reflects on it, the more one finds that this state was the least subject to revolutions, the best for man (XVI*) and that he must have come out of it only by some fatal accident, which for the common good ought never to have happened. The example of the Savages, who have almost all been found at this point, seems to confirm that Mankind was made to remain in it always; that this state is the World in the prime of its youth; and that all subsequent progress has been in appearance so many steps toward the perfection of the individual, and in fact toward the decrepitude of the species.

22. Unlike Lucretius, Rousseau offers no cosmology.
23. *Discourse on Inequality*, 167-68.
24. Ibid., 169.

> As long as men were content with their rustic huts, as long as they confined themselves to sewing their clothing of skins with thorns or fish bones, to adorning themselves with feathers and shells, to painting their bodies with various colors, perfecting or embellishing their bows and arrows, to carving with sharp stones a few fishing Canoes or a few crude Musical instruments; in a word, as long as they applied themselves only to tasks that one could perform alone and to arts that did not require the cooperation of several hands, they lived free, healthy, good, and happy lives as far as they could by their Nature, and continued to enjoy the gentle pleasures of independent dealings among themselves.[25]

Note XVI supports these claims with evidence of the extreme reluctance that savages often exhibit when offered opportunities to adopt civilized ways of life. Rousseau also notes that Europeans have frequently chosen to join savage communities permanently, and others have experienced nostalgia after they have left such lives behind. The most striking anecdote involves a Hottentot from southern Africa who was raised from infancy as a European and was found to be so intelligent that he was successfully employed in the Indies by a trading company.[26] According to a report from which Rousseau quotes at length, the young man returned to Africa after the death of his employer and visited his Hottentot relatives. After this visit he informed the man responsible for his European education that he had decided to renounce the civilized life and to live in the way of his ancestors. He then ran off and was never seen again. Rousseau puts so much importance on this anecdote that he depicts the Hottentot's renunciation of civilization in the frontispiece of the book and includes cross-references below the picture and in Note XVI.

Rousseau, who has been called the founder of modern anthropology,[27] offers a frankly conjectural description of the human journey through the state of nature to historical times.[28] He consulted the science of his time but he bemoans the unreliability of travelers' reports, and holds out hope that a more complete understanding of primitive people—perhaps including some far more primitive than those who had by his time been reliably observed—might eventually be developed. In principle, his analysis of the way of life best for man,

25. Ibid., 171.

26. The term "Hottentot" appears to have been used at that time for the speakers of several click languages in southern Africa, a group that included the Bushmen discussed below.

27. Claude Lévi-Strauss, "Jean-Jacques Rousseau, Fondateur des sciences de l'homme," in *Jean-Jacques Rousseau* (Neufchatel, France: La Baconnière, 1962), 239-48. An English translation is available in *Structural Anthropology*, vol. 2, trans. Monique Layton (New York: Basic Books, 1976), 33-43.

28. It is important to avoid overstating the conjectural nature of Rousseau's account of human development. He claims to have proven his most important assertion, namely that our kind did not always have language or live in stable groups. The details of the human journey are conjectural, but Rousseau appears to believe that the starting point is not. E.g., *Discourse on Inequality*, 162-63.

and most durable, is subject to enrichment and possible revision on the basis of new evidence. Such evidence exists, and some of it is presented in Elizabeth Marshall Thomas's recent book, *The Old Way: A Story of the First People.*[29]

ELIZABETH MARSHALL THOMAS AND THE BUSHMEN

Thomas's life has some curious parallels with Rousseau's career as a gifted intellectual outsider, non-specialist, and autodidact.[30] Beginning at the age of nineteen in the early 1950s, she accompanied her parents and slightly younger brother on an extraordinary series of expeditions into the Kalahari Desert. These trips were organized by her father, Laurence Marshall, a retired businessman who took his family and several other adults on a dangerous search for people who were thought to be living in a primitive fashion in the interior of the desert. The mission was successful, and the group spent considerable time over several years living among various groups of Bushmen, including especially a group called the Ju/wasi (singular: Ju/wa).[31] Thomas's mother, Lorna Marshall, was a former English teacher who went on to produce a series of ethnographic studies of the people. Thomas's brother, John Marshall, produced films of the Ju/wasi, married a Ju/wa woman, and remained involved in their affairs until his death. Thomas herself wrote a travelogue shortly after the expeditions,[32] and has pursued a variety of literary projects in subsequent years. Her books include an account of a warlike people among whom she lived for a time in northern Uganda,[33] and two novels set in the Stone Age.[34] She has also written a book about cats,[35] and two books about dogs.[36] Her study of dogs included a period of time camped out, alone, near a den of wild wolves on Baffin Island in northern Canada.[37]

The Old Way, written more than half a century after her first encounter with the Bushmen, supplements her youthful first-hand experiences with further reflection and research. The book has some obvious resemblances to the *Discourse*

29. *The Old Way: A Story of the First People* (New York: Farrar, Straus & Giroux, 2006).

30. Cf. Leon R. Kass, "Looking for an Honest Man," *National Affairs*, No. 1, Fall 2009, 160-80.

31. Bushmen are sometimes called !Kung or San. There are controversies over the proper way to refer to these people, and there are different ways to represent the sounds of words in their click language. In this paper, I follow Thomas's usage.

32. *The Harmless People* (New York: Vintage Books, rev. ed., 1989).

33. *Warrior Herdsmen* (New York: W. W. Norton, 1965).

34. *Reindeer Moon* (London: William Collins Sons & Co., 1987); *The Animal Wife* (Boston: Houghton Mifflin, 1990).

35. *The Tribe of Tiger* (New York: Simon & Schuster, 1993).

36. *The Hidden Life of Dogs* (New York: Simon & Schuster, 1993); *The Social Life of Dogs* (New York: Simon & Schuster, 2000).

37. *The Hidden Life of Dogs*, 31.

on Inequality in its general approach or method. Thomas accepts scientific findings where they are well established, but she is willing to make conjectures when facts are uncertain, and to make moral judgments on matters about which modern science is necessarily silent. She is also unwilling to be confined by all of the conventions or prejudices of modern scientists. One example: She notes that the roots of certain plants stop feeding the vine and leaves at certain times, causing them to drop off and blow away, thus leaving the root hidden from herbivores, and concludes by saying, "This was what the root intended."[38]

The Old Way is specifically related to Rousseau's claim that a certain kind of savage society was the most durable because it provided for the optimal, though not ultimate, development of human faculties. Thomas accepts the standard account of modern science, which traces our lineage to arboreal primates living in African rain forests. Climatic changes—an important element in Rousseau's discussion of the "fortuitous intervention of a number of foreign causes"—stimulated adaptations to what became a substantially colder and dryer environment, and our ancestors eventually evolved as terrestrial hunter-gatherers on the relatively open grasslands in eastern or southern Africa that resulted from these climatic changes.[39] Modern human beings (i.e., members of our species) eventually covered the globe and have undergone spectacular cultural evolution. Thomas believes that the people she observed, who lived in the same general area as the first modern humans, are descended from very early people who never left this area and who had by the 1950s undergone less cultural evolution than any other living people.

Recent work in genetic mapping strongly supports this conclusion.[40] So far as modern science has been able to determine, the Bushmen with whom Thomas

38. *The Old Way*, 11. Cf. Aristotle, *De Anima* 415a22-415b7 (offering a preliminary account of the manifest purposiveness of plants); David Bolotin, *An Approach to Aristotle's Physics* (Albany, New York: S.U.N.Y. Press, 1998), especially 31-48, 149-53.

39. For an overview, see Richard G. Klein, *The Human Career: Human Biological and Cultural Origins*, 2nd ed. (Chicago: University of Chicago Press, 1999). Thomas is not especially concerned with the precise details of biological evolution. She makes at least one technical error, when she assumes that human beings are descended from chimpanzees. Chimpanzees do appear to be our closest living relatives, but we are not descended from them. Ibid., 74-75, 130-31. The closest common ancestor of chimpanzees and humans may have been physically similar to modern chimpanzees, but nothing is known about the social life of this extinct species. See ibid., 135-36. Richard Wrangham argues that these animals may have lived in male-bonded territorial communities that engaged in lethal intergroup raiding, like modern chimpanzees. Richard Wrangham and Dale Peterson, *Demonic Males: Apes and the Origins of Human Violence* (Boston: Houghton Mifflin, 1996). The evidence to support this conjecture, however, is inconclusive. Cf. Note B at the end of this essay.

40. See, e.g., Spencer Wells, *The Journey of Man: A Genetic Odyssey* (New York: Random House, 2003), 56-57.

lived in her youth more closely resembled "the first people" than any we will ever know. This means that the Ju/wa way of life may well have been, as Rousseau says, "the least subject to revolutions," and thus might be the very one that he believes was "best for man."[41] It is important to stress that the Bushmen are not necessarily *typical* hunter-gatherers. Other such groups, having adapted to different environments and having different histories, have different social structures. What makes the Bushman people potentially significant is that their culture may be the *most durable* of any that has ever existed. That makes their way of life a plausible candidate for the state that Rousseau would consider the best for man.

Thomas's account focuses on a group of about 550 Bushmen, particularly those who were still living as hunter-gatherers in the Nyae Nyae area of the Kalahari. These people were almost untouched by other cultures. Almost, but not quite. Although some of these people were so isolated that it took several months just to find them, they were aware of the outside world. Not so long ago, the Bushman range had been larger, and it may have extended throughout eastern and southern Africa for a considerable time after the origin of our species.[42] By the time of the Marshall family's expeditions, these people lived in a relatively small area surrounded by Bantu pastoralists and European farmers and ranchers. Some of the Bushmen had been enslaved or employed as servants, or had at least traded with their neighbors. All of them knew about such contacts (some had escaped from servitude and they all knew of others who never came back), and they had some foreign commodities and artifacts. The Marshall family, however, met and lived with individuals who had never seen a vehicle, a white person, or a graphic representation of any kind. Those living in the interior of the desert had a few tools made of metal obtained in trade from Bantus or Europeans, but the people were not dependent on these tools, and they continued to use stone, wood, and bone versions as well.

41. Rousseau anticipated that science might eventually enable us to trace our lineage back to other species, or at least to animals with radically different physical structures, but he concluded that the relevant sciences had not yet advanced sufficiently to make solid reasoning possible. Accordingly, he begins with the provisional and apparently non-essential assumption that man has always had the same general conformation, especially with regard to upright posture. *Discourse on Inequality*, 134 and Note III (196-98). As it happens, modern scientists treat upright posture or bi-pedalism as the defining characteristic of humans in the broadest sense of the term. See, e.g., Klein, *The Human Career*, 190. Rousseau, moreover, provides a proto-Darwinian account of physical evolution when he touches on what might be called racial differences among human beings. *Essay on the Origin of Languages*, chap. 10, in *Oeuvres Complètes*, vol. V, 407.

42. The Bushmen speak one of several extremely unusual click languages. Outside the area where the Bushmen are found, the only other place where this type of language has been found is in east Africa, and skeletal material consistent with Bushman-like people has been found in paleolithic sites in Somalia and Ethiopia. Wells, *The Journey of Man*, 56-57.

Subsequently, the Bushmen have been intensively studied by anthropologists, but the early Marshall expeditions seem to have been unique in the extent to which they involved an extended and deliberate study of isolated groups that had had only minimal contact with the outside world. Though the life Thomas describes is now gone, due to invasions from our world, I will generally discuss it in the present tense. Her account of the Ju/wasi is far too rich to summarize adequately, and I will focus on a few points that seem particularly relevant to Rousseau's discussion of "nascent society."

EQUALITY AND FREEDOM AMONG THE BUSHMEN

There is no rulership here, not even that of men over women. Decisions are reached by group consensus after discussion, or by individuals making their own choices. The semi-nomadic bands in which the people live, moreover, are somewhat fluid. Bands sometimes come together for a variety of reasons, and smaller groups may pay extended visits to other bands. The bands average about twenty-five members, but some are much smaller, and people gather in larger groups at times. Although rulership and law in our sense do not exist, there is a range of personality types and of natural ability, and the Ju/wasi have an elaborate customary social system. This can be illustrated with two related examples, involving the ownership of land and marriage.

At the most simple level, every person begins with the customary right to live in the place where he was born, unless his mother was only passing through at the time. The people with this right are the customary owners, but their ownership claim weakens if they leave or their close relatives are no longer there, and it may fade away entirely. One may not live in a place without permission from the owners, and this principle is scrupulously observed.

Many people, however, do not live where they were born, mostly because of marriage. With some important exceptions, any man and woman may marry if they so choose, and either can divorce the other simply by announcing it (though this is not done lightly or often). Polygamy (including polyandry) is permitted and is practiced to a limited extent,[43] and care is taken to avoid the marriage of close relatives. Virtually everyone marries, and people who are divorced or widowed before they are old usually remarry. In such a small population the number of possible mates is limited, and many marriages are arranged during childhood. Such

43. Thomas observed polygyny, which was considered unremarkable though also relatively uncommon. She was told that polyandry was permitted though rarely practiced, but she never observed it directly. She was also told that polygyny seems to work best when the wives are sisters. *The Old Way*, 179-80.

arrangements, however, do not bind the individuals when they reach marriageable age (which for girls may be as young as eight or so, though husbands do not have intercourse with their wives prior to the menarche). Through hunting, a new husband must contribute to the support of his wife's family until their third child can walk, which is seldom less than fourteen or fifteen years, and he may remain with that family for the rest of his life. Thomas found that about half the people were living where the wife was an owner and about half where the husband was an owner.

While these customs may sound to us like the fundamental elements of social organization, it is better to think of them as particular consequences of a more general and important organizing norm: sharing. Food and even water are frequently quite scarce. As we might expect from our own experience, close relatives share with each other, and the more closely they are related, the more they share. But the customs of the Ju/wasi take them far, far beyond this unsurprising practice.

Food is of two general kinds. Plants and small (or slow) animals like tortoises, rabbits, and snakes—which are gathered primarily but not exclusively by women—belong to the person who gathers them. Gatherers are generally free to eat whatever they find, or to share it with anyone they choose, which they frequently do. These foods are the staples of the Ju/wa diet, and they appear to be sufficient for sustaining life and health. The other category of food consists of large ungulates, such as antelope and giraffe, which are hunted. This meat is intensely craved by the Ju/wasi, and it is more scarce and hard to get than gathered foods (some of which themselves require considerable skill and exertion to obtain). Hunting is carried out exclusively by men, who pursue it very avidly and talk a great deal about it. Its extreme importance is illustrated by the fact that men may not marry until they have hunted successfully.

The distribution of hunted food is governed by an elaborate set of rules and rituals, which ensure that every member of the community gets a share of the kill, and that the shares work out pretty evenly over time. Unlike the simple and intuitive "finders keepers" rule for gathered food, these rules are highly conventional. The right to make the initial distribution of hunted meat, for example, belongs to the person who fashioned the arrow that brought the animal down, who is often not the shooter and may even be a woman or child.

The central importance of sharing is reflected in the fact that the Ju/wasi never trade with each other, though they do with outsiders. Instead, they have a custom of bilateral friendships, called *xaro*, that begin when one person gives another a small gift, usually a luxury item such as a metal knife or ostrich shell necklace. After a time, the recipient reciprocates, and this practice continues as long as the two people continue to find pleasure in the exchanges. Most people have about fifteen such friendships, which may involve people whose homes are a hundred miles distant. These special relationships, which the Ju/wasi never have with outsiders (even when they receive gifts from them), are extremely important, and people often spend three or four months of the year visiting other bands for the purpose of seeing *xaro* friends.

Like almost everything the Ju/wasi do, these friendships promote survival in the Kalahari's hostile environment. For example, the practice of visiting friends effectively widens people's access to food, promotes communication among isolated bands, and provides relief from the stresses that occur when members of a small group spend extended periods of time in each other's company. But there are some subtler effects that are especially relevant to Rousseau's analysis.

One striking feature of Rousseau's discussion of nascent society is how little he has to say about the good and how much about the bad in the social relations of the state he calls "the best for man." Apart from a brief discussion of the awakening of sexual love, the only new pleasures that he mentions are communal song and dance. His discussion thus leaves us to wonder what it is in this savage state that more than compensates for the ills produced by the vanity and jealousy to which he gives more attention.

In Thomas's account of the Ju/wasi, the pleasures associated with food, especially meat, figure prominently, as one might expect among people who are frequently at the edge of starvation. In addition to sexual and family loves, the social pleasures appear mostly to be of a spontaneous kind. Children's games. Music and dance, involving both children and adults, much of which is not organized, planned, or ritualized. Joking and gossiping, also not organized (and also not without a dark undercurrent).

In the constellation of pleasures, *xaro* friendships are unusual. These relationships have a certain obligatory element, for one may not refuse a gift, and one is expected to reciprocate. But one does not reciprocate immediately because that would look too much like trading. More significantly, people take pleasure in preparing gifts for their *xaro* friends, anticipating the good feelings that will result on both sides. This appears to be a custom that promotes social cohesion by cultivating friendships that provide an especially pure form of social pleasure. Unlike the kin relationships that dominate the social life of the Ju/wasi, these friendships are not imbued with necessity, or not to nearly the same extent. People enter these relationships for the sake of pleasing each other, which is why it seems significant that the gifts are luxury items among people who are often deprived of necessities and have very little in the way of luxuries.

Somewhat counterintuitively, and without elaboration, Thomas says that the *xaro* bonds are "perhaps the strongest fibers in the social fabric."[44] If this is

44. *The Old Way*, 223.

true, I think the importance of the bonds must arise from the extent to which these relationships are experienced as existing for their own sake and for the pleasure they bring. People have deeper ties to their kin, but also more burdensome and inescapable obligations. *Xaro* friendships seem to exemplify what Rousseau calls "the gentle pleasures of independent dealings among themselves," the pleasures that he seems to treat as the defining social good of nascent society, the state that was "best for man."

SOCIAL DISCIPLINE AMONG THE BUSHMEN

In contrast to Rousseau's brief description of nascent society, *The Old Way* offers a detailed description of the difficulties and high personal costs that the Ju/wasi experience in maintaining their social life. The principal problem she identifies, however, is exactly the one on which Rousseau puts overwhelming emphasis: jealousy.

It is perfectly possible for large and highly intelligent primates to lead independent and largely solitary lives in the kind of rain forests where our distant ancestors lived. Orangutans offer conclusive evidence for this proposition. Except for sexual behavior and mothers with offspring, these animals typically spend their adult lives as self-sufficient loners.[45] Whether or not Rousseau was right to claim that our own ancestors did live this way,[46] in what he calls the pure state of nature, such a life is not possible in the very harsh environment of the Kalahari. And everything about the Ju/wa culture reflects this dominating necessity.

The Ju/wasi usually have enough food and water to survive, but they never have much more than that, and sometimes they die of starvation or dehydration. They are seldom killed by predators, but if left alone they are likely to be taken by leopards or hyenas before too long. The overwhelming importance of group membership is poignantly captured in the words of a woman who said: "It is bad to die, because when you die you are alone."[47] And the importance of group solidarity is reflected in virtually every aspect of their relations, especially the tremendous emphasis on sharing.

Such solidarity does not occur without strong social discipline. Anything that even resembles stealing is virtually unknown, and the language has no specific word for theft.[48] Children are trained to avoid physical violence, and the

45. For a slightly more elaborate description of orangutan life, see Note A at the end of this essay.

46. The answer to this question may be less important than it first appears to be. See Note B at the end of this essay.

47. *The Old Way*, 213.

48. The one case of stealing reported by Thomas involved a man who took honey from a bee-

Ju/wasi do not have weapons suited for combat. Their famous poisoned hunting arrows, for example, produce wounds that are invariably fatal, but the poison has a delayed and very slow effect; the Ju/wasi, moreover, do not have shields of any kind. Considering the stresses under which the Ju/wasi live, violence is remarkably rare. The few homicides that Thomas knew of suggest how, and with what success, the Ju/wasi have interrupted man's natural progress toward the Hobbesian state of war that Rousseau saw as the final departure from the state of nature.

In one case, a man suddenly and without explanation shot his wife with a poisoned arrow, then returned a few minutes later and shot two other men who were sitting nearby. The next day, the attacker was hunted down and put to death. In another case, a group reluctantly decided to kill a man who had begun to exhibit signs of mental illness. Thomas reports that none of these five homicides was regarded as a crime or as a punishment. Instead, they were all considered tragedies, in much the same way that the Ju/wasi saw a homicide in which a very young child shot a poisoned arrow at a man who was arguing with the child's father. Similarly, Ju/wa mothers are sometimes required by necessity to put a newborn to death, because of deformities or because it would be impossible to support the child along with its older siblings. Such necessary acts of infanticide, rare because the Ju/wasi carefully space the births of their children, are regarded with extreme sadness.

Correlatively, ridicule and social snubbing—especially in the form of refusals to share—are powerful and common sanctions used against those who deviate from social norms. The success of the Ju/wasi in managing natural selfishness, natural assertiveness, and natural inequality can be illustrated with an anecdote.

A man named Short /Kwi, one of his band's most successful and respected hunters, was bitten by a poisonous snake. Gangrene set in, the lower part of his leg fell off, and Short /Kwi appeared to be doomed. Thomas's father decided to use his vehicle to take Short /Kwi and his wife on the long trip to a hospital, where the couple would have to appear in clothing, which they didn't have. The Marshall family dressed the couple in some of their own clothes as they prepared to depart. Thomas was understandably shocked by what happened next.

> We then heard raised voices at Short /Kwi's camp. The other people were erupting. The grief that all had felt turned to jealousy and anger when we gave so much to these people and nothing to anyone else. We went there and found all the people sitting together in a thick circle, recounting in impassioned voices all the slights and stinginess that anyone had ever shown to them or anyone else. *He was supposed to give me*

---

hive that another man had found. This was such an extraordinary event that the original discoverer of the hive killed the thief. This is the only act of vengeance that Thomas reports, and it may not have been understood in quite that way by the killer.

> *a knife. She was going to give the knife to Gao. Where is the blanket you promised my brother? When I gave her a necklace, she should give a gift in return. She never did. The necklace went to her sister. That was wrong. I have nothing. I am empty-handed. They should have controlled that necklace. Others have it now. Those people are selfish. They don't want to give. They won't give the necklace. People don't think of what they should be doing. They are stingy. All this is wrong.*
>
> Surely some of these grievances had been festering for years. In the middle of the circle was Short /Kwi in his starchy khaki shirt and trousers. Not only was he badly damaged by the loss of his leg and therefore in serious need of his people's goodwill for the future, but we were heaping him with gifts that would cause others to envy him for years to come. Already he was trying to give the clothes to other people.[49]

Thomas reaches the same unequivocal conclusion about the way of life she observed that Rousseau reached about nascent society: "We have certainly gone downhill from the social excellence of the Ju/wasi."[50] Unlike the *Discourse on Inequality*, with its brief discussion of the state that was "best for man," *The Old Way* provides a detailed analysis of the social practices that enable the Ju/wasi to control the powerful forces of natural self interest and natural inequality. The most striking difference between her account of the Bushmen and Rousseau's discussion of nascent society is her emphasis on the elaborate and repressive nature of the socialization that the Ju/wasi use to control the violent and vengeful impulses that Rousseau thought would have gone unchecked in nascent society.

This may not be a decisive correction of Rousseau's analysis. It is possible that Rousseau's picture of nascent society accurately corresponds with an early stage of Ju/wa life, while the social system that Thomas observed developed later.[51]

49. *The Old Way*, 241-42. See also 181:

> [Gao Feet] was unfailingly calm and gracious and had the rather rare distinction of being an excellent hunter and also an important healer. Most men were one or the other, seldom both, because no Ju/wa person wants to stand out above the rest or have more of anything than anyone else, including ability. Thus a man such as Gao Feet was in a difficult position. His people needed both his talents. Any group would. Hence to forsake one talent for the other would have been selfish, depriving his people of a service in order not to arouse jealousy. Yet Gao Feet had such a low-key manner and was so modest and unassuming that people did not hold his talents against him. That was how he managed his excellence.

50. Ibid., 224.

51. Among the Ju/wasi Thomas knew, the oldest male owner of a territory had a special title, with somewhat greater obligations to be generous, but no additional rights. Thomas speculates that the title may be a residuum from a time when the roles of men and women were more sharply differentiated than they are now. Ibid., 78-79. The *Discourse on Inequality* is rather cryptic in its discussion of the transitions to and then from the patriarchal family that resulted from the "first revolution." Cf., e.g., *Discourse*, 160 with 167-68. For some speculations about this revolution and the discovery of fatherhood, see Note C at the end of this essay.

There certainly are other primitive societies (some of which Rousseau knew about) that are much more violent and much less egalitarian than that of the Ju/wasi. The differences could be due to variations among physical environments and to cultural accidents. What may be more significant is that the central social problem faced by the Ju/wasi is exactly the one, namely pride and jealousy, that Rousseau identifies as the basis of all social ills. Thomas's account shows that the most durable solution to that problem may in fact have been devised without the rulership and subordination entailed in all forms of political organization.[52] The evidence she presents, therefore, may serve more to enrich Rousseau's analysis than to correct it.

JEALOUSY AND LIONS

In the spirit of Rousseau, Thomas looks for the roots of Ju/wa practices, and some of ours, in earlier times. For example, she conjectures that the dwellings of the Ju/wasi—grass huts that take only a few minutes to construct and are abandoned when the inhabitants move—are slightly modified versions of the nests that other large primates make for themselves.[53] Unlike Rousseau, who focuses almost entirely on the human (and proto-human) soul, Thomas is also intensely interested in understanding intelligent animals other than primates.

Rousseau understands, of course, that we are animals, and he even says that our ability to think differs from that of beasts only in degree.[54] In a tantalizing passage, he begins by claiming that he sees in animals only ingenious machines, programmed by nature to operate in certain ways, whereas men also have the quality of a "free agent," and often deviate from nature's commands, sometimes to their advantage and sometimes to their detriment.[55] But Rousseau quickly drops the claim that human freedom operates through "purely spiritual acts about which one explains nothing through the Laws of Mechanics."[56] In place of this claim, which he says is disputable, he substitutes the faculty of cultural acquisition (or "perfectibility") as the distinctive human quality. Given what everyone knows about the progress of human history, this is more descriptive than explanatory, and it leaves us to wonder whether animals should also be understood as free agents, or whether men can be seen as ingenious machines.

52. Cf. *Discourse on Inequality*, 187-88, where Rousseau contends that government and laws are always an inadequate substitute for sound *mœurs*.

53. *The Old Way*, 8-10.

54. *Discourse on Inequality*, 142.

55. Ibid., 141.

56. Ibid., 142. Compare Rousseau's critique of mechanical explanations of the behavior of animals in the *Essay on the Origin of Languages*, chap. 15, in *Oeuvres Complètes*, vol. V, 417.

Thomas does not pursue this question directly, but she does give considerable thought to the ways in which certain other animals experience their lives, and to the relation between their experience and ours. A striking example involves the lions of the Nyae Nyae area.

Leopards and hyenas hunt the Ju/wasi, but neither presents a serious threat to the survival of the people. Leopards, which hunt alone and by stealth, are afraid of humans and easily discouraged, though they occasionally do succeed in taking a Ju/wa victim. Hyenas, which hunt in groups and do not kill their prey before they begin to feed, are more formidable. However, these nocturnal hunters focus their attention on stragglers, especially those in a weakened condition, which the Ju/wasi try hard not to provide them with.

Lions are a different story. These powerful predators routinely take prey that are much larger, tougher, and faster than human beings. They live near the same water holes on which the Ju/wasi depend. They hunt cooperatively, and they can do so day or night as they please. Their usual prey, moreover, are the same large ungulates prized by the Ju/wasi, and their hunting methods are similar, so the two are competitors for this food. The lions are fully aware of the Ju/wasi, whose camps they frequently approach at night, usually discreetly and apparently out of curiosity. Lions are known to hunt people in other places, but they do not prey on the Ju/wasi. Why not?

Thomas says that only the lions know the answer to that question, but suggests that the Ju/wasi and the lions of the Nyae Nyae area may have come to a kind of coexistence agreement sometime in the very distant past. The lions in this area hunt at night, and the Ju/wasi pursue the same prey during the day. The Ju/wasi also do most of their gathering during the hottest part of the day, when the lions are least active, even though this imposes extra physical stresses on the people.

When the Ju/wasi do encounter a lion in the bush, they ordinarily observe a protocol that involves an affected nonchalance, neither aggressive nor fearful, and a casual departure at an oblique angle. If lions show themselves in camp, men discourage them with fire and with calm but stern commands to leave. Occasionally the Ju/wasi actually face lions down, as one group did when it came upon a pride that was trying to appropriate a wounded wildebeest that the human hunters were tracking after shooting it with a poisoned arrow.[57] Thomas herself once encountered a lion in the bush, and was so awestruck that she simply stared at the animal in spellbound fascination. The lion finally followed the usual protocol, walking calmly off at an oblique angle.

The lions are respected by the Ju/wasi beyond all other animals, but they are not loved. When confronting a lion they address it with the same term of

57. Cf. *Discourse on Inequality*, 136-37.

respect used when speaking of the gods.[58] But when speaking *about* lions, the people use avoidance terms, one of which is "jealousy." Why would this be? Thomas cannot say for sure, but she offers a suggestion. The Ju/wasi sometimes attribute mysterious deaths to the existence of people who, while appearing normal, harbor a nasty combination of jealous secrets and supernatural powers.[59] This could be a metaphor for lions, "out there in the dark not far away from you, able to kill you whenever they felt like it, refraining from killing you for reasons you were not equipped to determine. You hoped that they wouldn't kill you, but you could never be sure."[60] If lions are the greatest living threat in the physical environment, jealous people are like lions in society.

There is obviously a risk of pushing metaphors and speculation too far, but perhaps this connection between jealousy and lions reflects a Ju/wa insight that the most powerfully dangerous elements in their own souls can only be managed, not really subdued. When Thomas asked the Ju/wasi what they would do if lions were to prey on them, they responded that they would not live in such a place. Many years later, when Thomas studied how the Ju/wasi had changed after their lands were invaded and they were forced to alter their way of life, she found that they did not see themselves as a people of the desert, or one defined by their way of life there. Instead, they saw their community with one another as the central and enduring element of their lives. As Rousseau would no doubt have expected, many Ju/wa individuals easily succumbed to the allures and some of the worst vices of civilization, and it is unclear today how much of their ancient social fabric can survive the disappearance of the conditions in which it developed.

PRE-HUMAN HAPPINESS

Rousseau's most succinct description of the distinctive good that people find in nascent society refers to "the gentle pleasures of independent dealings among themselves." The parallel good for "nascent man"[61] in the pure state of nature is described this way: "His soul, which nothing agitates, gives itself over to the sole sentiment of its present existence, without any idea of the future,

58. *The Old Way*, 168.

59. Caution must be exercised in interpreting the meaning of explanations given by the Ju/wasi. Asked where the stars went in the daytime, one man said, "They stay where they are. We just can't see them in the daytime because the sun is too bright." The same man later said that stars were antlions who in the evening went up to the sky and returned to their sandy traps at dawn. Ibid., 245. If one heard only the second story, it would be easy to get a distorted impression of the speaker's understanding of the world.

60. Ibid., 170-71.

61. *Discourse on Inequality*, 164. As Rousseau's use of this term suggests, man in the pure state of nature was not yet human. Cf. Notes A and B at the end of this essay.

however near it may be."[62] This proposition must be among the most arresting in the *Discourse on Inequality*, and perhaps the most baffling. How could Rousseau believe that he had access to the inner experiences of beings so different from ourselves that they did not even have language? And what implications could he think we should draw from this description of self-contemplation, so oddly reminiscent of Aristotle's description of the unmoved mover,[63] and so obviously evocative of the "Celestial and majestic simplicity" that Rousseau promised would be found beneath the outer surface of the statue of Glaucus?[64]

Thomas may offer a suggestion. In *The Hidden Life of Dogs*, she recounts her efforts to understand what she calls dog consciousness, primarily through the careful observation of several pet animals with whom she and her family lived. At one point, the family moved to a new home, where they built a large pen for the dogs next to the house. Although the pen included a variety of shelters built for the animals' comfort, the dogs built their own den in the side of a hill. No ordinary hole in the dirt, the den was fifteen feet deep, ending in a three foot by three foot chamber that was two feet high. The entrance was hidden in a woodpile. Most remarkably, the dogs' project was carried out in perfect secrecy. Although Thomas spent a great deal of time in the pen and frequently checked for problems and evidence of escape attempts, she never even noticed any sign of the six cubic feet of soil that the dogs had excavated.

The effects of this undertaking by the dogs are at least as interesting as its causes and preconditions. Thomas discovered what had happened by accident, when she suddenly arrived just as one of the dogs was entering the den through the woodpile. Once their project had been discovered, the dogs used the den openly, and it became the focus of their lives. The animals stopped interacting with each other in any manner that she could detect, suggesting that they had achieved a high degree of harmony in their social relationships. The dogs also lost interest in the human members of the family, and would not even respond to Thomas beyond a bland acknowledgment of her presence. The dogs' souls had, so to speak, disappeared from her view.

In response to these developments, Thomas started joining the dogs each afternoon to do just what they were doing. Nothing. Here is how she describes the experience:

> To sit idly, not doing, merely experiencing, comes hard to a primate, yet for once I wasn't among primates. At last, as dogs learn to live among our kind, it came to

62. Ibid., 144.
63. See Aristotle, *Metaphysics* 1072a19-1072b31.
64. *Discourse on Inequality*, 122.

> me to live among theirs. In the late afternoon sun we sat in the dust, or lay on our chests resting on our elbows, evenly spaced on the hilltop, all looking calmly down among the trees to see what moved there. No birds sang, just insects. Off in the silent, drying woods a tree would now and then drop something—a pod, perhaps, or a leaf—and we would listen to it scratching down. While the shadows grew long we lay calmly, feeling the moment, the calmness, the warm light of the red sun—each of us happy enough with the others, unworried, each of us quiet and serene. I've been to many places on the earth, to the Arctic, to the African savannah, yet wherever I went, I always traveled in my own bubble of primate energy, primate experience, and so never before or since have I felt as far removed from what seemed familiar as I felt with these dogs, by their den. Primates feel pure, flat immobility as boredom, but dogs feel it as peace.[65]

Dogs and wolves, of course, are highly social animals, and they organize themselves hierarchically. In that respect they are very different from the solitary pre-humans in Rousseau's pure state of nature. Thomas's experience on the hilltop, moreover was not a solitary experience, either for her or for the dogs. Still, even if it is someday proved that Rousseau wrongly conjectured that our direct ancestors lived much like orangutans, he might have been right to suggest that our soul has a craving to be agitated by nothing, to be given over to something like the sole sentiment of its present existence, without any idea of the future, however near it may be. That is not to say that such peacefulness is *the* good for dogs or for humans, for both display another strong craving for activity, for exploration and interaction. But it might still be *an* experience for which we have not entirely lost the desire. And it might be an experience that is one of the aims of social life.[66]

PROTO-POLITICS

The pre-human condition is obviously irrecoverable, and Rousseau does not pretend that there is any going back to the state of nascent society that he calls the best for man.[67] That does not prevent him from concluding that there are better and worse possibilities among the various forms of political organization that have been devised in historical times. The *Discourse on Inequality* is more

65. *The Hidden Life of Dogs*, 121.

66. In the *Essay on the Origin of Languages*, Rousseau says that only the passion for self-preservation is stronger and more primary than the passion for doing nothing, but he also refers to "natural restlessness," and he says that primitive people are subject to boredom. *Oeuvres Complètes*, vol. V, 376, 400 note, 406.

67. E.g., *Discourse on Inequality*, 133, Note IX, 207.

suggestive than definitive about the contribution that its analysis can make to identifying and fostering the better possibilities, though Rousseau does coyly say that "every attentive Reader . . . will find the solution to an infinity of problems in morals and Politics that the Philosophers cannot resolve."[68]

Thomas apparently has little interest in such questions, but her interest in the souls of animals provokes a number of suggestions that recall Aristotle's assertion that "man is a political animal *more* than any bee or any herd animal."[69] Thomas, who sometimes characterizes our pets as slaves (who are suited by their nature to be our slaves in a way that our fellow humans are not[70]), also believes that we can have political relationships with them. She argues, for example, that wolves decided to form partnerships with our kind, contrary to the usual assumption that we have dogs because our ancestors decided to domesticate wolves.[71]

Another kind of political analysis is offered in one of her stories. Dogs typically use seniority as a default rule in determining social dominance, but they also engage in struggles for status. One such struggle took place when Thomas introduced a new dog into her household's complex multi-species society.[72] About a month before this happened, the dominant dog had died after a long and debilitating illness. The second ranking dog had previously struggled hard to obtain her current rank, but had never become completely secure there. Apparently, both she and the third ranking dog recognized that she was unsuited for the dominant position. Accordingly, the third ranking dog, named Pearl, unobtrusively took over as leader during the illness of the dominant dog: "Pearl had occupied Place One in much the same way that a teacher takes charge of a classroom. The teacher doesn't want to suppress and dominate the students—she wants to help them. She takes the leadership because she has more knowledge and experience than they do."[73]

Thomas first noticed Pearl's new status when she brought the new dog, named Sheila, into the house. Sheila was extremely apprehensive, and apparently ready to defend herself from aggression, but Pearl stepped forward to welcome her. A young stray who had been living on the streets, Sheila started at the bottom of the hierarchy, but soon proved politically ambitious. Using threats and physical aggression, she quickly subordinated the two lowest-ranking dogs, and then the insecure second-ranking dog. Still not satisfied, Sheila began trying to intimidate Pearl. Thomas reports:

68. Ibid., 192.

69. Aristotle, *Politics* 1253a7-8.

70. I leave aside the question whether there is some other way or some other sense in which some people might be slaves by nature.

71. *The Social Life of Dogs*, 123-28.

72. In addition to dogs and cats, Thomas's family kept parrots, another highly intelligent animal.

73. Ibid., 204.

> Pearl was like a dedicated teacher who has been insulted by a student for whom the teacher had always done her utmost and with the best of intentions. The student might want to chase away the teacher, but would lack the knowledge or ability to teach the class. . . . Short of getting rid of Sheila, I didn't really know how to help Pearl. The dog politics of the household would boil around me with an energy of their own no matter how much I tried to suppress them. I felt at a loss, unable to solve the problem.[74]

During this period of conflict, Pearl began having troubled dreams—growling, snarling, and crying out in her sleep. Suddenly this stopped, and so did the aggression between Pearl and Sheila. The political problem had apparently been solved, but how? Thomas noticed that Pearl had begun treating Sheila the way female dogs typically treat their daughters, and she believes that Pearl had in effect adopted the other dog.

> Among dogs and wolves and many other kinds of animals including people, the children of high-ranking parents have high rank too. Thus Pearl was solving the problem of Sheila. Sheila was a high-powered dog who wanted significant status, and her adoption by Pearl raised her status. She would have fought for status if she had to, but she didn't have to. Pearl gave it to her, and meanwhile kept her own.[75]

Thomas emphasizes her belief that other dogs—especially males but also other females with a different temperament and less intelligence—would have handled this situation differently, and not nearly as well. I would add the additional observation that these events occurred in a highly artificial environment composed of masters (however benevolent) and slaves, of different species. Dogs are descended from wolves, and show it in many ways, but they are not simply slaves of lupine instinct any more than they are simply the compliant slaves of their human masters.

It would be easy to ridicule the kind of analysis that Thomas offers here, and in many other discussions of her pets. But if this is not all just a lot of anthropomorphic nonsense,[76] perhaps it suggests that more attention should be paid to a point made subtly, almost invisibly, in the *Discourse on Inequality*.

Rousseau finds the source of our social virtues in a primitive sentiment that he calls pity or commiseration, which softens the equally natural desire for self-

74. Ibid., 212.

75. Ibid., 212-13.

76. For a useful short discussion of the perils of trying too hard to avoid anthropomorphism, see Joe Sachs, "The Work of Imagination: Sundry and Summary," in *The Envisioned Life: Essays in Honor of Eva Brann* (Philadelphia: Paul Dry Books, 2007), 280-98.

preservation, and which is "so Natural that the Beasts themselves sometimes give perceptible signs of it."[77] In support of his claim, he offers several pieces of evidence, beginning with maternal tenderness and the bravery mothers display in guarding their young, a conspicuous part of our mammalian nature. The second example is an image of an imprisoned man forced to watch helplessly as a wild beast tears a child from its mother's breast. The next example is an ancient tyrant who dared not attend a tragedy lest others see him sympathizing with the wife and father of the fallen Hector. The last piece of evidence contains the one vivid reference to civilized women in the body of the *Discourse on Inequality*: "In Riots, in Street fights, the populace assembles, the prudent man moves away; it is the rabble, it is the Market women, who separate the combatants and prevent decent people from cutting each other's throats."[78]

The common thread in these examples is maternal love, and its extension by analogy or imagination to other social contexts.[79] In a note appended to his discussion of natural pity, Rousseau says that "Love of oneself is a natural sentiment which inclines every animal to watch out for its own preservation, and which, directed in man by reason and modified by pity, produces humanity and virtue."[80] The story of Pearl and Sheila suggests one way in which something like this might happen even without the guidance of human reason. Perhaps it would not be completely fanciful to think that Pearl's political acumen may have human analogues, not just in family life but also in the work of exceptionally skillful managers of small human groups within modern societies. And maybe even in contexts as politically momentous as Abraham Lincoln's management of his cabinet?[81]

CONCLUSION

The rhetoric of the *Discourse on Inequality* is overwhelmingly aimed at puncturing unexamined assumptions about the superiority of civilized life and civilized

77. *Discourse on Inequality*, 154.

78. Ibid., 156. A blandly disapproving reference to the use of feminine wiles by civilized women occurs shortly thereafter in the text, 158. Outside the body of the *Discourse*, we find a condemnation of abortion and infanticide by civilized women in Note IX, 204, and a vivid statement about the virtue of Spartan women in the Epistle Dedicatory, 119.

79. The importance of this extension is suggested by Rousseau's comment elsewhere that natural pity would remain eternally inactive without imagination to set it in motion. *Essay on the Origin of Languages*, chap. 9, in *Oeuvres Complètes*, vol. V, 395. It may also be significant that Rousseau characterizes conjugal and paternal love, but not maternal love, as the sweetest sentiments that we know. *Discourse on Inequality*, 168. Compare the discussion of *xaro* friendships above.

80. *Discourse on Inequality*, Note XV, 219.

81. For details, see Doris Kearns Goodwin, *Team of Rivals: The Political Genius of Abraham Lincoln* (New York: Simon & Schuster, 2005).

people. Thomas, who does not begin with the usual unexamined assumptions, is nonetheless herself quite different from the Ju/wasi for whom she has so much admiration, and with whom she has found many friendships.

Thomas, for example, differs from the Ju/wasi in her disposition toward non-human animals. The Ju/wasi, who have tremendous practical knowledge about the living things in their environment, are completely indifferent to the suffering of animals, both the large animals they hunt and the smaller animals that they gather.[82] Unlike the Ju/wasi, who have no pets, Thomas keeps animals for the pleasure of their company, powerfully commiserates with them, and feels a strong moral responsibility toward them.

Thomas never assumes an attitude of moral superiority toward the Ju/wasi. She would no doubt observe that there is a crucial difference between killing animals for food, even without a concern to minimize their suffering, and benevolently enslaving animals as pets. And she might therefore conclude that both she and the Ju/wasi implicitly, though for different reasons, respect Rousseau's suggestion that as beasts "share something of our nature through the sensitivity with which they are endowed, one will judge that they should also participate in natural right, and that man is subject to some sort of duties toward them ... [so that perhaps this sensitivity] should at least give the one the right not to be uselessly mistreated by the other."[83]

Apart from questions of natural justice, Thomas's feelings about her pets seem to be inseparable from her efforts to understand them.[84] The same kind of sympathy informs her efforts to understand the Ju/wasi. Although Rousseau declares that we owe what is best as well as worst in civilized life to a "furor to distinguish oneself,"[85] he also says that "natural commiseration . . . no longer dwells in any but a few great Cosmopolitan Souls, who surmount the imaginary barriers that separate peoples and who, following the example of the sovereign being that created them, embrace all Mankind in their benevolence."[86] In her efforts to promote appreciation of a human way of life that may have been the most durable of all social arrangements, Thomas has certainly distinguished

82. See, e.g., *The Harmless People*, 52.

83. *Discourse on Inequality*, 126. The Ju/wasi exhibit the same acceptance of their own physical suffering that they display toward that of the animals. For a striking example involving a young girl who stoically endured several painful and dangerous hours caught in a metal trap that a white man had set in the desert, see *The Old Way*, 216-17.

84. A related phenomenon can be found among scientists who have done field work with great apes. Not infrequently they find that they cannot separate their desire to understand the animals from a desire to protect those they have come to know. Well-known examples include Jane Goodall, Dian Fossey, and Biruté Galdikas.

85. *Discourse on Inequality*, 189.

86. Ibid., 178.

herself as a cosmopolitan—not just from a "furor" for distinction, perhaps, but not without some displays of *thumos* either.[87] And in her sympathetic observations about other animals, she has provided a vivid reminder of the difficulty—stressed by Rousseau and Aristotle alike—of determining with precision what the soul is and how human beings are unique.[88]

AFTERWORD

> *General and abstract truth is the most precious of all goods. . . . Never has moral instinct deceived me. . . . Nothing personal, nothing which concerns the interest of my body, can truly occupy my soul.*
> –Rousseau, *Reveries of a Solitary Walker*[89]

> *[U]nlimited freedom . . . is not the freedom of the dictator, who enforces his own will on the world, but the freedom of the artist, who has no will, who is free of will.*
> –Isak Dinesen, *Out of Africa*[90]

The Old Way reports an encounter that Thomas had with an art collector at a dinner party. Upon learning that Thomas was writing a book about hunter-gatherers, the woman warned her not to romanticize the past or idealize primitive life. The woman was particularly concerned that in such a society, people with artistic genius "would find no means of self-expression."[91] Perhaps a little defensively, Thomas acknowledged that the Ju/wasi did not paint or sculpt or even produce creative beadwork, and the dinner conversation turned to other subjects. At first inclined to dismiss the woman's comments as lightweight chatter, Thomas suddenly found herself more intrigued.

Upon reflection, Thomas mentions music as a Ju/wa art form, but focuses on hunting stories. These are dramatic and detailed accounts of actual hunts, told by men in special voices that resemble chants, delivered to attentive audiences around the fire at night. These she analogizes to Paleolithic cave paintings, which typically depict large mammals, often with projectiles sticking out of them. She concludes:

87. See, e.g., Elizabeth Marshall Thomas, "Reply to Melvin Konner," *New York Review of Books*, vol. 54, no. 5, March 29, 2007.

88. Cf. Aristotle, *De Anima* 402a11-403b19 (discussed above), 432a22-432b3 (noting difficulties in classifying perception with respect to its being rational or not, and in determining the relationship of the imaginative part or aspect of the soul to the others); *Discourse on Inequality*, 141-42.

89. *Oeuvres Complètes*, vol. I, 1026 (Fourth Walk), 1028 (Fourth Walk), 1065 (Seventh Walk).

90. New York: Vintage Books, 1937, 83. This claim is associated with dreaming.

91. *The Old Way*, 102.

> The will to hunt is deep in the brain, down there with art in the cave of the unconscious. That the two would join is not hard to imagine, especially in the minds of those who live with hunger. What better art form could there be than a successful hunt and its result—strong men together in a dark, lumpy line bobbing toward you through the golden grass, carrying a massive head with spiral horns and hundreds of pounds of meat?[92]

This passage treats the hunt itself—at least as much as its dramatic or pictorial retelling—as a work of art, and suggests that both activities (neither of which is necessary for physical well-being) arise from ancient elements of our soul.[93] Perhaps as ancient and natural as the desire to be agitated by nothing, to be given over to the sole sentiment of one's present existence, and perhaps as significant.

Leon Kass, a proponent of civilized life and an opponent of unexamined assumptions, focuses on a different kind of dinner party and a different kind of art when he retells the Isak Dinesen story, "Babette's Feast."[94] Babette is a talented French chef, forced into political exile and given refuge by religiously zealous Norwegian employers who eat only tasteless food. When Babette wins a large sum of money in a lottery, she uses all of it to prepare an extraordinary dinner for her employers, a group of their similarly ascetic friends (who attend only from politeness), and a visiting military officer who happens to be a gourmet. Inspired by the excellence of the meal, General Löwenhielm delivers an eloquent speech about the gift of grace, which leads the others to experience an unaccustomed joy in the food and in each other. Afterwards, the employers are appropriately grateful, but shocked to discover that Babette has re-impoverished herself. Babette denies that she gave the dinner for their sake rather than her own. And she denies that she is now poor, saying, "No, I shall never be poor. I told you that I am a great artist. A great artist, Mesdames, is never poor. We have something, Mesdames, of which other people know nothing."

Kass offers this comment: "Thanks to genius and taste, thanks to the extreme generosity and openness of both host and guest, the visage of the eternal shows itself in the midst of the most temporal, as superb food and wine nourish also the spiritual hungers of the assembled."[95] The artistry displayed by Rousseau and Elizabeth Marshall Thomas offers a mirror image of General Löwenhielm's work in Dinesen's story, bringing to life a kind of "generosity and

92. Ibid., 105.

93. All great apes eat meat, though some have very little access to this food source.

94. Leon R. Kass, *The Hungry Soul: Eating and the Perfecting of Our Nature* (New York: The Free Press, 1994), 183-92.

95. Ibid., 191.

openness" that may no longer quite be attainable, and for which human beings cannot completely cease to hunger.

* * *

Note A

Until recently, very little was known to science about the lives of orangutans. The following brief and simplified summary is based primarily on field work reported in Biruté M. F. Galdikas, *Reflections of Eden: My Years with the Orangutans of Borneo* (Boston: Little, Brown & Co., 1995), and Carel van Schaik, *Among Orangutans: Red Apes and the Rise of Human Culture* (Cambridge, Massachusetts: The Belknap Press of Harvard University Press, 2004).

On average, wild orangutans give birth once every eight years, and the offspring are weaned only when the mother becomes pregnant again. The mother-child relationship is extremely close and intense. Fathers have no role beyond insemination, and offspring may remain with their mothers for several years after the arrival of a sibling (with daughters remaining longer than sons). The animals go through a playful and gregarious phase during the period between infancy and adulthood.

In most environments, orangutans spend almost all of their adult lives foraging alone. Their primary interests are food and sex, and they display a high degree of intelligence, comparable to that of chimpanzees and perhaps greater. Tool use is common, and it differs from place to place, suggesting cultural transmission. Adult females usually have overlapping ranges (typically near their place of birth) and long-lasting dominance relationships, and they sometimes form transitory foraging parties. Males become much larger and stronger than females, and they are substantially more nomadic.

Both sexes compete for desirable mates—males by displays of virility and sometimes by fighting, females by resisting unwanted suitors (frequently without success) and by seductions (also frequently unsuccessful) of attractive males. Dominant males have a distinctive appearance and a distinctive call, and will not tolerate the presence of another male that has these characteristics. Some males appear to delay the development of these secondary sex characteristics (though not the ability or desire to breed) while living near an established dominant.

Orangutans exhibit significant variation in natural aptitude and personality type. Where population density is high (as in especially food-rich forests), the animals have greater social interaction. In captivity they readily form complex social relationships, not only with other orangutans but with humans as well. Indigenous people tell stories of male orangutans abducting human females, and there has been at least one documented case of a semi-wild orangutan forcibly copulating with a woman. One female orangutan at a rehabilitation center effectively became bicultural, acquiring a substantial sign-language vocabulary, living for extended periods in the wild, and acting as a kind of self-appointed ambassador between humans and orangutans.

The lives of wild orangutans thus bear more than a passing resemblance to that of man in Rousseau's pure state of nature, and their nature appears to include a significant element of what Rousseau calls "perfectibility." See *Discourse on Inequality*, 142.

NOTE B

The line of descent leading to orangutans apparently split off from the line that led to human beings earlier than the line of descent that led to chimpanzees and gorillas. See Klein, *The Human Career*, 88, and compare Rousseau's discussion of the inadequacy of the reports available to him about great apes in the *Discourse on Inequality*, Note X, 208-14. It is arresting, and perhaps significant, that the social structures of three extant great apes roughly correspond to the three main stages of human social evolution that Rousseau attributes to the state of nature. Orangutans live much like man in Rousseau's pure state of nature; gorillas generally live in patriarchal family bands, much as Rousseau imagines man must have lived after the "first revolution"; and chimpanzees are cooperative and contentious hunter-gatherers. At the very least, this suggests that our fundamental ape nature lent itself to all these possibilities, even if it is someday established that none of our actual ancestors lived like orangutans or gorillas.

Of course, just as it is possible that our pre-human ancestors once lived solitary lives, so is it possible that the ancestors of modern orangutans were more social, and that these animals later became more solitary as part of an adaptation to new or changed environments. See Robin I. M. Dunbar, "Brains on Two Legs: Group Size and the Evolution of Intelligence," in *Tree of Origin: What Primate Behavior Can Tell Us about Human Social Evolution*, ed. Frans B. M. De Waal (Cambridge, Massachusetts: Harvard University Press, 2001), 270 n. 4. *All* great apes, however, exhibit varying degrees of so-called "fission-fusion sociality," in which groups wax and wane in size, often when resources become more scarce or abundant. Van Schaik, *Among Orangutans*, 171. Thus, based on what we currently know, it apparently would have been possible for human cultural evolution to proceed very much as Rousseau imagined, even if fortuitous causes in fact produced a somewhat different path of development.

NOTE C

One form of natural inequality about which Rousseau says almost nothing in the *Discourse on Inequality* is that between men and women, whom he generally treats as equal in the sense that they are equally independent in the state of nature. But this is misleading in at least two ways. First, women could never have been as independent as men, for women have a natural social relationship with their children that men do not have. See, e.g., *Discourse on Inequality*, 147 (noting the social consequences of the mother's physical need to nurse). Second, women, like other mammals, have extra burdens imposed on them by nature, and women therefore have more incentive to enter into cooperative arrangements with other people.

In order for men to become fathers in more than a biological sense, they must overcome their natural selfishness at least to the extent that they become willing to share their food (a naturally private good) with another human being. A likely explanation for this self-overcoming is the presence of children who are seen as a shared responsibility. In the family, men and women become equal in a sense that is both natural and unnatural. It is natural because they are equally parents by nature. But it is unnatural because this formal equality of parenthood is naturally hidden by the temporal lapse between insemination and birth, and by the greater natural investment that women make in their children.

Similarly, the family is naturally asymmetric because the father is by nature free of the burdens imposed by motherhood. It is not hard to imagine that the earliest families were constituted through a tacit exchange in which men assumed rulership in exchange for food and protection, an exchange that would have been facilitated by a modification of women's natural subservience toward their children.

One implication of all this might be that the most important inequalities between men and women are both natural and unjust, rooted as they are in the division of labor that nature imposes on mammals. This might help to explain why the *Discourse on Inequality* never offers the patriarchal family as a natural model for political society, while repeatedly suggesting that Sparta is a model. See *Discourse on Inequality*, 180, 181, 187-88; compare 119 (praising Spartan women as rulers of their men) with 158 (asserting that women should obey rather than dominate men). And it might help to explain why early Bushmen would have moved from a patriarchal family structure to the extreme egalitarianism that Thomas observed.

10

Self-knowledge and Moral Seriousness in Jane Austen's *Pride and Prejudice*

Adam Schulman

This essay grew out of an impression I have formed while teaching for some years at St. John's College in Annapolis. My sense is that Mr. Fitzwilliam Darcy, the hero of *Pride and Prejudice*, is widely and warmly admired by the women of St. John's, students and tutors alike, to whom he seems a paragon of male virtue, and that if Darcy were to spring to life and ask one of them to marry him, she would—assuming her affections were not otherwise engaged—be hard pressed to refuse him. I have it on good authority that, at a senior oral examination on Jane Austen not long ago, one of the examiners asked, "Is there any woman in this room who is *not* in love with Darcy?" I am told that the ensuing silence spoke volumes.

Even apart from that memorable academic incident, I sense general approval of Elizabeth Bennet's judgment that marriage with Darcy would "teach the admiring multitude what connubial felicity really is" (III.8).[1] It seems to me that most of my students and fellow tutors put down the book with the expectation that Darcy and Elizabeth can look forward to a happy marriage between true equals, who understand one another perfectly and who see eye to eye on all the most important questions. In this essay I would like to call that expectation into question, by pointing to some noteworthy differences between Elizabeth and Darcy, differences that may even be said to reveal Elizabeth as Darcy's superior in the decisive respect. My purpose, I hasten to add, is not to undermine the general affection for Darcy or the belief that he would make an ideal husband, but rather to strengthen and deepen the reader's appreciation of Darcy's virtues by making it more thoughtful and more true to Jane Austen's understanding.

This essay will be divided into four parts: first, a comparison of Elizabeth's and Darcy's opinions on love, friendship, and the pursuit of happiness; second,

1. Parenthetic references are to volume and chapter numbers of the Norton Critical Edition of Jane Austen's *Pride and Prejudice*, 3rd edition, ed. Donald Gray (New York: W. W. Norton, 2001).

Elizabeth Bennet's philosophy; third, the source of her philosophy; and finally, a comparison of the two most important men in Elizabeth's life.

Elizabeth and Darcy on Love, Friendship, and the Pursuit of Happiness

The plot of *Pride and Prejudice* is easy to summarize. Elizabeth, a spirited and intelligent young woman, who is perhaps too confident in her powers of judgment, meets Darcy, a rich, handsome, and clever gentleman, who is perhaps excessively proud of his superiority. Their first meeting does not go well, and obstacles arise, notably the prejudices of one and the pride of the other, that seem destined to keep them apart forever. Only when Elizabeth's prejudices have been corrected, and Darcy's pride humbled, do they realize that they are perfectly suited to each other, and so find love and happiness in marriage.

Darcy and Elizabeth are easily the most attractive and impressive man and woman in *Pride and Prejudice*, and we are quite likely to find ourselves hoping that they will eventually get together. In temperament they are by no means similar: Elizabeth is said to have a "lively, playful disposition, which delighted in anything ridiculous," whereas Darcy is described as "haughty, reserved and fastidious" (I.4). But there are other differences between Darcy and Elizabeth, far deeper than those of temperament, that I believe go to the heart of what Jane Austen is trying to teach us in *Pride and Prejudice*.

The first and most striking difference is that, while Darcy falls ardently, even violently, in love with Elizabeth, Elizabeth never falls in love with Darcy (I.10; II.11; III.2; III.16; III.17; III.18). Soon after meeting her, Darcy finds himself bewitched by Elizabeth's "sweetness and archness" (I.10) and by "the beautiful expression of her dark eyes" (I.6). Elizabeth, for her part, does not like Darcy at all for much of the novel; but when, with the removal of her prejudices, her active dislike for him is softened, it is replaced, not at once by love, but by respect, esteem, and gratitude, by a real interest in his welfare, and by the wish for that welfare to depend upon herself, for the happiness of both (III.2). Austen comments, "If gratitude and esteem are good foundations of affection, Elizabeth's change of sentiment will be neither improbable nor faulty" (III.4). Elizabeth does indeed come to love Darcy, but she does not *fall* in love with him. Instead, her love grows out of milder, steadier feelings of esteem and gratitude, together with the reasoned conviction that she and Darcy could be very happy together.

Now you might suppose that this merely reflects a difference of temperament between Darcy and Elizabeth; that, unlike Darcy, Elizabeth is simply incapable of falling precipitously in love. But that is not quite the case: for

Austen, after referring to love at first sight "even before two words have been exchanged," tells us that Elizabeth had "given somewhat of a trial to the latter method, in her partiality for Wickham" (III.4). Elizabeth seems to have learned from her unfortunate experience with the handsome and dashing Wickham to mistrust this more romantic and interesting mode of attachment.

After recovering from her mild infatuation with Wickham, Elizabeth seeks to conform her conduct, even in love matters, to the pursuit of what Austen calls "rational happiness" (III.7). It appears to be Elizabeth's considered opinion that the lover as such is an irrational creature who cannot be trusted to keep his own good clearly in mind. To her aunt Gardiner, she speaks jokingly of love as a "pure and elevated passion" that drives the jilted lover to "detest [the beloved's] very name and wish him all manner of evil" (II.3). To Darcy, at the end of the novel, Elizabeth says, "You knew no actual good of me—but nobody thinks of *that* when they fall in love" (III.18). When Darcy's friend Bingley, newly engaged to Elizabeth's sister, sings Jane's perfections to Elizabeth and declares how happy he expects her to make him, Austen notes that, "in spite of his being a lover, Elizabeth really believed all his expectations of felicity to be rationally founded" (III.13).

When Jane asks her how long she has loved Darcy, Elizabeth gives the famous answer, "I believe I must date it from my first seeing his beautiful grounds at Pemberley" (III.17). Jane treats this answer as a joke and begs Elizabeth to be serious, whereupon Elizabeth satisfies her sister with "solemn" assurances of her attachment. But the initial, worldly answer contains more than a grain of truth. When Elizabeth saw Pemberley for the first time, Austen commented: "At that moment she felt that to be mistress of Pemberley might be something!" (III.1). Even or especially in love matters, Elizabeth seems unabashedly ready, as she declares to Lady Catherine de Bourgh, to "act in that manner, which will, in my own opinion, constitute my happiness, without reference to you, or to any person so wholly unconnected with me" (III.14).

This is not in fact the first time that Elizabeth has suggested that there is nothing wrong, in matters of love, with pursuing one's own good. Earlier, when her aunt Gardiner suggests that there is something mercenary in Wickham's pursuit of the young heiress Miss King, Elizabeth answers, "Pray, my dear aunt, what is the difference in matrimonial affairs, between the mercenary and the prudent motive? Where does discretion end, and avarice begin?" (II.4). To be sure, Elizabeth was shocked when her friend Charlotte agreed to marry the odious Mr. Collins; she cannot believe that her friend "would have sacrificed every better feeling to worldly advantage" (I.22). Elizabeth does at first seem to find Charlotte's engagement to Collins disgraceful and humiliating. But her objection to Charlotte's conduct is not so much that it was mercenary as that it sacrificed the chance of a *real* happiness for the mere assurance of a comfortable home and a steady income. Elizabeth is left with the distressing conviction that her friend, though possessed of an excellent understanding (II.9), had agreed to marry a stupid man with "not one agreeable quality, and neither manner nor sense to recommend him" (II.4), so that it was "impossible for her friend to be tolerably happy in the lot she had chosen" (I.22).

Now let us consider Darcy's view of love and happiness. We have noted that Darcy is altogether more violently in love with Elizabeth than she is with him. He says so himself: "You must allow me to tell you how ardently I admire and love you" (II. 11). Darcy's proposal does not find favor in Elizabeth's eyes, in part because he has just done his best to ruin the happiness of her beloved sister Jane by discouraging his friend Bingley from marrying her. Darcy freely admits that he did everything in his power to detach Bingley from Jane, moved chiefly by repugnance at the thought of Bingley marrying into a family as ill-mannered as the Bennets have mostly shown themselves to be. To explain how it was that such repugnance did not also prevent Darcy from proposing marriage to Elizabeth, he tells her that "towards [Bingley] I have been kinder than towards myself" (II.11). This revealing remark is worth pondering. Darcy sees himself as prepared to act on an impulse of love that will, in some measure, do him harm. He seems proud of having, in matters of love, looked out for his friend's interest more than for his own. In other words, he appears to view love as in fact a "pure and elevated passion" that leads us beyond and above our own self-interest. Love is for Darcy a devotion to another that, at its most sublime, may require self-sacrifice. Darcy's view of love is, in this respect, the opposite of Elizabeth's. Where he admires love for its transcendence of self-interest, she is prepared to subsume all under the pursuit of rational happiness and to question the distinction between the prudent and the mercenary motive in matrimonial affairs.

Perhaps it is no accident that Darcy, with his exalted view of the purity and elevation of love, also experiences the anticipated requital of that love with a feeling of transcendent happiness. When Elizabeth at last indicates to Darcy that his renewed attentions would be received with pleasure and gratitude, Austen comments, "The happiness which this reply produced, was such as he had probably never felt before; and he expressed himself on the occasion as sensibly and as warmly as a man violently in love can be supposed to do" (III.16). Of Elizabeth, on the contrary, later that evening, Austen tells us that "she rather *knew* herself to be happy, than *felt* herself to be so" (III.17).

These hints that Jane Austen offers of a divergence between Darcy's and Elizabeth's ideas and experience of love help to bring into focus the world of difference between their moral perspectives on life. One of those differences—Darcy's seriousness vs. Elizabeth's playfulness—turns out to have a deeper ground than a mere divergence of temperament. In their first extended conversation at Netherfield Park (I.11), Elizabeth encourages others to tease Darcy and to laugh at him. Darcy expresses concern that "the wisest and best of men, nay, the wisest and best of their actions, may be rendered ridiculous by a person whose first object in life is a joke." Elizabeth assures him that she never intentionally ridicules what is wise or good. Darcy goes on to say that "it has been the study of my life to avoid those weaknesses which often expose a strong understanding to ridicule." When pressed by Elizabeth, he agrees that vanity is one of those weaknesses. Darcy admits to having faults, but he believes they are not faults of understanding, but of temperament or character. Putting all this together, we may say that Darcy considers himself to be a man of "superior mind" who, like other such men, may be tempted by their very superiority to indulge in petty moral vices, including vanity, that would expose them to ridicule. It is the study of Darcy's life to avoid such vices and the ridicule they provoke. Suffice it to say that Darcy takes himself very seriously, and it is a matter of some importance to him that he not act in such a way as to deserve to be laughed at. To borrow a phrase from Aristotle's *Nicomachean Ethics*, Darcy is a perfect exemplar of the *spoudaios* man, i.e., the morally serious man, who considers moral virtue a subject of the utmost seriousness, and who takes himself, as a gentleman, extremely seriously. As Aristotle suggests,[2] it is characteristic of the morally serious man to judge that actions in accordance with virtue are not merely good, i.e., conducive to happiness, but also noble, i.e., worthy of reverence and therefore not to be laughed at. While Elizabeth insists that she is not the sort of person who would laugh at the wise and the good, she does not say whether she would laugh at the noble, or at the self-importance of the morally serious man.

Elizabeth on the whole does not seem to take herself as seriously as Darcy takes himself. After overhearing Darcy make an insulting remark about her looks, Elizabeth is light-hearted enough about the incident to tell the story with great spirit among her friends (I.3) and to say afterward, "I could easily forgive *his* pride, if he had not mortified mine" (I.4). As for vanity, and whether it is a moral failing or a failure of understanding, Elizabeth's view seems quite different from Darcy's, as is quietly suggested in a much later scene when she is tempted to reveal to Jane that Darcy had made her a proposal of marriage. Such a disclosure, Austen tells us, would not only astonish Jane but would "highly gratify whatever of [Elizabeth's] own vanity she had not yet been able

2. Aristotle, *Nicomachean Ethics* I.8 1099a22: "But [actions in accordance with virtue] are also both good, at least, and noble (*kai agathai ge kai kalai*), and each of these most of all, if indeed the morally serious man (*ho spoudaios*) judges nobly (*kalos*) concerning them."

to reason away" (II.16). The difference here is subtle but telling. If vanity can be reasoned away, it is at least in some measure a defect of understanding, requiring instruction, and not simply a moral failing, deserving of reproach. It is notable that here, as elsewhere, Jane Austen appears to share Elizabeth's consciousness and, tacitly at least, to approve of her opinions.

Austen deepens the contrast between Darcy and Elizabeth by showing us their very different attitudes toward friendship. Each of them has one close friend: Bingley is Darcy's, and Elizabeth's is Charlotte. Charlotte is introduced early in the novel as "a sensible, intelligent young woman" who is Elizabeth's "intimate friend" (I.5). Charlotte and Elizabeth treat each other very much as equals, and it is not hard to see why. The core of their relationship is a sustained albeit intermittent conversation about love, friendship, and happiness, to which both contribute many thoughtful observations, speaking frankly and without reservation. The friendship is pleasant and advantageous to both of them, and one would be hard pressed to say who benefits more. Only when Charlotte shocks and disappoints Elizabeth by contriving to secure Mr. Collins as a husband does the friendship falter. Once Charlotte becomes Mrs. Collins, Elizabeth expects their intimate friendship to end, as it will no longer be possible to speak to each other with the same candor, when one friend thinks the other's husband "a conceited, pompous, narrow-minded, silly man" (II.1).

Darcy's friendship with Bingley is of an entirely different kind. Austen describes it as "a very steady friendship, in spite of a great opposition of character" (I.4). Darcy is far superior in understanding and in force of personality; Bingley is endeared to Darcy not by his intellect but by "the easiness, openness, and ductility of his temper." Bingley looks up to Darcy and has complete faith in his benevolence and his superior judgment. And indeed, after Bingley falls in love with Jane, Darcy has very little difficulty persuading his friend first to give up the attachment when Darcy thinks it unwise, and then to renew it once Darcy has given his approval. To Elizabeth, the inequality of their relationship does not reflect well on either of them. She thinks almost with contempt of Bingley's "easiness of temper" and "want of proper resolution" that "made him the slave of his designing friends, and led him to sacrifice his own happiness to the caprice of their inclinations" (II.1). Now if the slave can trust the master to know and do what is best for him, it is clear what he gets out of the relationship; but in the case of Darcy and Bingley, what does the master get out of it? Why would Darcy prize his friendship with Bingley so much as to follow him into Hertfordshire and put up with the worthless company that county has to offer? Perhaps Darcy would say that "men of superior mind" owe it to those of weaker intellect and character to look after them and guide them to such happiness as they are capable of. But one cannot escape the conclusion that Darcy enjoys the sensation of being looked up to as a superior and of being Bingley's noble benefactor instead of being indebted to his friend for his own happiness. At any rate, Darcy seems content with his unequal friendship with Bingley and does not seek out the company of those who are his equals in strength of mind and character. Or perhaps it would be more accurate to say that, until he met Elizabeth, he was never seriously tempted by friendship with an equal.

Elizabeth does come close, at the end of the novel, to suggesting to Darcy that there is more of utility and less of selfless devotion in his friendship with Bingley than he might be ready to acknowledge: "Elizabeth longed to observe that Mr. Bingley had been a most delightful friend; so easily guided that his worth was invaluable; but she checked herself. She remembered that he had yet to learn to be laughed at, and it was rather too early to begin" (III.16). Elizabeth recognizes that, to a man such as Darcy, nothing is so abhorrent as to undermine his dignity (III.13).

Austen shows us other differences between Darcy and Elizabeth on moral questions, as for example on the permissibility of deception. Darcy early on declares that "whatever bears affinity to cunning is despicable," and when he proposes to Elizabeth he tells her that "disguise of every sort is my abhorrence" (II.11). Elizabeth, for her part, on returning home from Rosings where Darcy had made his proposal, says to herself, "how much I shall have to conceal" (II.16). Later, contemplating how she might learn the secret meaning of Darcy's presence at the hastily arranged wedding of Lydia and Wickham, Elizabeth says, once again only to herself, "my dear aunt, if you do not tell me in an honorable manner, I shall certainly be reduced to tricks and stratagems to find it out" (III.9). This is not to say that Elizabeth is a dishonest person comfortable with lies and deception. But she does not share Darcy's visceral repugnance toward disguise and cunning, and she takes an altogether more light-hearted view of the fact that some situations in life demand that we stoop to such stratagems.

But the greatest difference between Elizabeth and Darcy is revealed in the way each of them recovers from the serious errors that all but prevented them from ever coming together. Elizabeth's recovery is presented to us dramatically as she reads and rereads the letter that Darcy wrote in his own defense after she had rejected his proposal. She begins reading the letter with "a strong prejudice against everything he might say" (II.13). But that prejudice is gradually overcome as she starts to see that mere vanity had strongly colored her judgment of the characters and actions of Darcy and Wickham. She begins to understand that her cherished opinion of Wickham's worth had more to do with his dashing good looks and with his flattering attentions to her than with an impartial weighing of the evidence. Elizabeth had once said, of Wickham, that there was "truth in his looks" (I.17). But now she reconsiders: "As to his real character, had information been in her power, she had never felt a wish of enquiring. His countenance, voice, and manner had established him in possession of every virtue" (II.13). As for her contempt for Darcy, she comes to see that it was entirely unreasonable, fed by wounded pride from their very first meeting at the Meryton ball, where Elizabeth had happened to overhear Darcy describing her looks as "tolerable, but not handsome enough to tempt me" (I.3). These reflections are extremely mortifying:

> She grew absolutely ashamed of herself.—Of neither Darcy nor Wickham could she think, without feeling that she had been blind, partial, prejudiced, absurd.
>
> "How despicably have I acted!" she cried.—"I, who have prided myself on my discernment!—I, who have valued myself on my abilities! who have often disdained the generous candour of my sister, and gratified my vanity, in useless or blameable distrust.—How humiliating is this discovery!—Yet, how just a humiliation!—Had I been in love, I could not have been more wretchedly blind. But vanity, not love, has been my folly.—Pleased with the preference of one, and offended by the neglect of the other, on the very beginning of our acquaintance, I have courted prepossession and ignorance, and driven reason away, where either were concerned. Till this moment, I never knew myself." (II.13)

"Blind, partial, prejudiced, absurd"—In this passage, the dramatic peak of the entire novel, Elizabeth sets herself on the road to self-knowledge by realizing that the very ability she had valued most—the faculty of rational and impartial judgment—had failed her when put to the decisive test, and that she had allowed mere vanity, flattered by the attentions of one suitor and insulted by the indifference of the other, to distort her judgment in regard to the most important decisions of her life.

Elizabeth, however, quickly recovers from the shame and mortification of these discoveries about herself. Her statement—"Till this moment, I never knew myself."—is an indication that she sees her fault as, in some measure, an error of understanding. Whatever vexation and regret she feels at her own errors is moderated by the sense that such errors are correctible, through introspection and the calm, rational appraisal of one's opinions and passions. Self-knowledge in this important but limited sense now seems within her reach. Whether Elizabeth achieves self-knowledge in the fullest sense of the term, and what that knowledge would consist of, are questions we shall return to later.

Let us now compare this scene to Darcy's description of his own recovery from moral error, as recounted to Elizabeth shortly after she accepts his renewed professions of love. Darcy tells her that he now sees that he deserved all the abuse with which Elizabeth met his first proposal: "My behavior to you at the time merited the severest reproof. It was unpardonable. I cannot think of it without abhorrence" (III.16). Elizabeth gently tries to steer the conversation away from the fruitless question of who was more to blame for what was said that evening: "The conduct of neither, if strictly examined, will be irreproachable; but since then, we have both, I hope, improved in civility." But Darcy persists in blaming himself severely:

> "I cannot be so easily reconciled to myself. The recollection of what I then said, of my conduct, my manners, my expressions during the whole of it, is now, and has been many months, inexpressibly painful to me. Your reproof, so well applied, I shall never forget: 'had you behaved in a more gentleman-like manner.' Those were your words. You know not, you can scarcely conceive, how they have tortured me;—though it was some time, I confess, before I was reasonable enough to allow their justice." (III.16)

Perhaps it is all the more difficult for Darcy to forgive himself for his errors because to do so would contradict what he had told Elizabeth of his character in their earliest conversation at Netherfield Park: "I cannot forget the follies and vices of others so soon as I ought, nor their offences against myself. . . . My temper would perhaps be called resentful.—My good opinion once lost is lost forever" (I.11). What Elizabeth calls Darcy's "implacable resentment" is an exaggerated inclination to divide the world between the virtuous and the vicious and to despise the latter as irredeemable. Elizabeth takes an entirely more charitable view of what she calls the "follies and nonsense, whims and inconsistencies" of others (I.11; I.4; III.45), so it is less surprising that when she finds these faults in her own opinions she is able to recover quickly from the feelings of mortification and self-reproach.

Darcy also blames himself for the tone of his long letter, which he now believes to have been written in "a dreadful bitterness of spirit." In answer to this, Elizabeth again assures him that she has long ago recovered from her prejudices regarding Darcy; as to the shame and culpability with which Darcy continues to torture himself, she makes the following suggestion:

> "[T]hink no more of the letter. The feelings of the person who wrote, and the person who received it, are now so widely different from what they were then, that every unpleasant circumstance attending it ought to be forgotten. You must learn some of my philosophy. Think only of the past as its remembrance gives you pleasure." (III.16)

One part of Elizabeth's philosophy seems to be the judgment that errors committed in the past in ignorance of what is good for us, of what would truly make us happy, are to be remembered only insofar as we can learn from them how we might better pursue our rational happiness. But Darcy not only rejects this judgment, he "cannot give [Elizabeth] credit for any philosophy of the kind" (III.16). Instead he insists that Elizabeth is able to think of the past with equanimity not because she is *philosophical* but because she is *innocent* and has nothing to feel guilty about. As Darcy puts it, innocence is much better than philosophy. And so, once again, he rebukes himself severely for having been "a selfish being all my life," and such a being he would still be had not Elizabeth taught him a lesson and properly humbled him. Despite Elizabeth's philosophical advice, Darcy is resolved never to forget his failure to behave "in a more gentleman-like manner." Implicit in his self-criticism is the boast that he is, now and for the future, no longer a selfish being. Elizabeth, as we have seen, has given some thought to this question and doubts whether it is possible, let alone obligatory, for a rational being to be fundamentally unselfish. On this occasion, however, she makes no further effort to discourage Darcy from remembering and blaming his past errors, nor does she for the time being attempt to teach Darcy any other part of her philosophy.

ELIZABETH BENNET'S PHILOSOPHY

So far we have seen evidence that Elizabeth Bennet, while still struggling in her own mind for clarity about love, morality, and happiness, is nonetheless a remarkably penetrating and introspective critic of her own prejudices and vanities. Far more than Darcy she seems well on her way toward self-knowledge in this limited sense of the term. Now, however, I would like you to consider the evidence that Elizabeth is thoughtful in a far deeper sense about the biggest questions of human life. She herself speaks of her "philosophy," one part of which could be called her *philosophy of recollection*: *"Think only of the past as its remembrance gives you pleasure."* In this part of my essay, I will elaborate some other important principles of Elizabeth Bennet's philosophy; then, in the next part, I will speculate as to their possible source. By "philosophy" here I mean something like self-knowledge in the fullest sense of the term, not limited to personal introspection and critical self-appraisal, but encompassing and addressing the deepest questions of human life: What is virtue? What is love? What is a gentleman? What is noble? What is the human good? What is the nature of man?

I must confess that I undertake this exposure of the philosophy of Jane Austen's heroine with some trepidation. Austen clothes her most profound insights in unobtrusive remarks offered light-heartedly in casual conversation, and I hesitate to pull away this veil of delicate restraint. Her writing has something of the sweetness and archness that, in Elizabeth, captivated Darcy. Softly and without ostentation, she manages to raise all the important questions that are solemnly disputed in the books of the philosophers. Here, with apologies, are three principles of Elizabeth's philosophy.

First, Elizabeth's thoughts on the use and abuse of memory are matched by some rather profound musings on our hopes for future happiness, which might be called Elizabeth's *philosophy of anticipation*. The occasion that prompts these reflections is the removal of Wickham's regiment from the neighborhood of Meryton, a separation that she had for a number of reasons looked forward to with great expectations of joy. In the event, her life after Wickham's departure does not seem so much happier than before. Austen comments:

> Upon the whole, therefore, she found what has been sometimes found before, that an event to which she had looked forward with impatient desire, did not, in taking place, bring all the satisfaction she had promised herself. It was consequently necessary to name some other period for the commencement of actual felicity; to have some other point on which her wishes and hopes might be fixed, and by again enjoying the pleasure of anticipation, console herself for the present, and prepare for another disappointment. (II.19)

The suggestion is that we mostly live in the future, not the present, believing that, if only our hopes are realized, a period of actual happiness, such as we have never experienced before, will surely commence. On this occasion, Elizabeth tells herself that it is not good to get everything you wish for; for if all your wishes are fulfilled, and you expect perfect bliss as a result, you are bound to be disappointed. In between regret over past failures and hopes for a felicity not yet attained and perhaps unattainable, we are so imprudent, as Pascal put it, "that we wander in times not our own and do not think of the only one that belongs to us"[3]—the present. I find in these reflections of Elizabeth's a sound basis for rational happiness in the present, neither tormented by regrets, nor hoodwinked by false hopes of future bliss. Note, by the way, the typically graceful restraint of Austen's way of writing. Where a philosopher might say, "It is the nature of man, etc.," Austen writes "Upon the whole, she found what has been sometimes found before."

Second, there is Elizabeth's *philosophy of education*. We have seen that, at the end of the novel, Elizabeth is hopeful that Darcy will one day learn to be laughed

3. Blaise Pascal, *Pensées* 172.

at, i.e., learn not to take himself so seriously, but she judges that now is not the time to begin. In general, throughout the book, Elizabeth seems content to observe and reflect on the follies and absurdities of other human beings without trying to instruct them. I believe this reluctance to attempt to teach others is not the fruit of modesty or diffidence but of a considered judgment that Elizabeth expresses to Jane in the following words: "We all love to instruct, though we can teach only what is not worth knowing" (III.12). What she means, I think, is that the most important and difficult questions, those whose answers would bring not only critical self-awareness but self-knowledge in the fullest sense of the term, can only be learned by oneself, to be sure with the helpful guidance of a mentor, but with most of the heavy lifting of introspection and inquiry carried out on one's own. The wisest teacher can accomplish nothing if the student is not motivated to learn, and if he is so motivated, he will need only quiet indications of where to look rather than elaborate and systematic instruction.

Elizabeth's wise observation is, by the way, a remarkably clear and concise statement of the ground on which Socrates declined to be a teacher, on which Plato wrote not treatises but enigmatic dialogues, and on which every philosopher worthy of the name has given his readers at most hints and intimations of his most important teachings. Plato tells us, in his *Seventh Letter*, that his dialogues are intended "for those who are capable of finding things out for themselves, with the help of little indications (*dia smikras endeixeos*)."[4] *We all love to instruct, though we can teach only what is not worth knowing.* Sometimes, in idle moments, it strikes me that this quietly profound remark deserves to be enshrined as the motto of St. John's College, in place of that solemnly boastful and didactic Latin inscription that adorns our official seal: *Facio liberos ex liberis libris libraque*—"I make free men from children by means of books and a balance." Perhaps the men who founded our College had more in common with Fitzwilliam Darcy than with Elizabeth Bennet.

Be that as it may, there is finally what might be called Elizabeth's *philosophy of strength*, once again summed up in a brief remark she makes in a casual conversation. Addressing Darcy on the subject of poetry and love, Elizabeth says, "Everything nourishes what is strong already" (I.31). Let me explain why this remark strikes me as significant. We have seen how, in Elizabeth's estimation, the actions and opinions of most human beings are full of folly, inconsistency, and nonsense. She is not as quick as Darcy to judge bad behavior as a sign of incorrigible vice. One who loses *her* good opinion might gain it back again by returning to the path of prudence and good sense. Indeed it would perhaps not be too strong to say that she interprets most moral

4. Plato, *Seventh Letter* 341E.

failings as blindness and absurdity rather than corruption and moral turpitude. Nonetheless, Elizabeth does not by any means discount the importance of character, and even of something like virtue, for human happiness. But the virtue that she prizes most is a kind of *strength of character*. It is precisely this quality that she finds missing in Bingley, whose softness and irresolution put him in danger of becoming a slave to his designing friends. It is again this quality that she describes in herself when she says to Darcy, once more in a playful vein, "There is a stubbornness about me that never can bear to be frightened at the will of others. My courage always rises with every attempt to intimidate me" (II.8). It is finally this quality that enables Elizabeth to stand up to that formidable dragon Lady Catherine de Bourgh, whose bullying personality overpowers almost everyone else in the book.

Strength and weakness of character, one might say, are what remain of virtue and vice when the ordinary belief in moral responsibility is subjected to searching philosophical scrutiny. Strength of character in this sense is a kind of health of the soul that enables it to respond optimally to whatever comes its way. Hence Elizabeth's dictum, "Everything nourishes what is strong already." I believe that Elizabeth is here articulating a thought not unlike what Aristotle intends in the *Posterior Analytics* when he defines greatness of soul as "indifference to fortune good or bad."[5] A strong character will be undone neither by great misfortune nor by great good fortune.

Before Elizabeth can allow herself to love Darcy, she must be certain in her heart that he is strong in this sense. The question Elizabeth is struggling with is, I believe, akin to what Shakespeare was addressing in his sonnet 94, "They that have power to hurt and will do none." Genuine strength in a human being is moderate and restrained, rather than vindictive, petty, and cruel. Which of these is the character of Darcy? I think Elizabeth first begins to form a clear answer to this question when she visits Darcy's estate in Derbyshire. Seeing Pemberley and hearing the character of its master extolled by his housekeeper, Elizabeth reflects in silence:

> As a brother, a landlord, a master, she considered how many people's happiness were in his guardianship!—How much of pleasure or pain it was in his power to bestow!—How much of good or evil must be done by him! Every idea that had been brought forward by the housekeeper was favourable to his character. (III.1)

The impressive sight of Pemberley gives Elizabeth a sense of the power to bestow pleasure or pain, to do good or evil, that a man like Darcy must wield; and the praise of Darcy's housekeeper goes very far toward reassuring Elizabeth

5. Aristotle, *Posterior Analytics* II.13 97b22.

that her master is fit to be the guardian of other people's happiness and, in Shakespeare's phrase, "the lord and owner of his face."

THE SOURCE OF ELIZABETH'S PHILOSOPHY

As for the source of Elizabeth's philosophical understanding, or at any rate the mentor responsible for turning her in the right direction, I would like now to introduce a figure who has hitherto escaped our attention, viz., Elizabeth's father, Mr. Bennet. Mr. Bennet is described for us in the first chapter as "an odd mixture of quick parts, sarcastic humour, reserve, and caprice" (I.1). He seems to divide his time between reading books in his library and making fun of his wife, his daughters, and any other human being whose foolish behavior strikes him as sufficiently amusing. The impropriety of his behavior is one of the reasons Darcy decides to put a stop to the marriage of Bingley and Jane, and his negligence in allowing Lydia to accompany the regiment to Brighton facilitates her elopement with Wickham, with all its disastrous consequences. It would be easy to dismiss Mr. Bennet as a self-indulgent, irresponsible buffoon. But he has an important influence on Elizabeth, and his mind and character deserve a second look.

Jane Austen tells us, late in the book, how Mr. Bennet came to live the way he did:

> [C]aptivated by youth and beauty, and that appearance of good humour which youth and beauty generally give, [he] had married a woman whose weak understanding and illiberal mind had, very early in their marriage, put an end to all real affection for her. Respect, esteem, and confidence had vanished for ever; and all his views of domestic happiness were overthrown.

Mr. Bennet did not seek comfort for his disappointment in disreputable pleasures; instead, writes Austen,

> He was fond of the country and of books; and from these tastes had arisen his principal enjoyments. To his wife he was very little otherwise indebted, than as her ignorance and folly had contributed to his amusement.

Austen explains Mr. Bennet's choice of pastimes as follows:

> This is not the sort of happiness which a man would in general wish to owe to his wife; but where other powers of entertainment are wanting, the true philosopher will derive benefit from such as are given. (II.19)

As far as I know, no other figure in all of Jane Austen's novels is described as "the true philosopher," and it behooves us to consider for a moment whether that description of Elizabeth's father might not in fact be an accurate one. Mr. Bennet's life is the story of a man who fell in love with a beautiful young woman and married her with the expectation of domestic happiness, only to have all his affection extinguished as he came to appreciate her ignorance and folly. One is reminded of Socrates who, according to Xenophon, used to tell his friends that, when a man marries a beautiful woman in order to be happy, it is unclear whether he will not in fact be made miserable because of her.[6] Is Mr. Bennet like Socrates in more fundamental ways? Perhaps so. He resembles the philosopher in that, once his first extravagantly hopeful encounter with the beautiful ends in disappointment, he does not become hopeless and embittered but instead contents himself with such modest pleasures as are genuinely satisfying and realistically attainable. As Austen writes, "with a book [Mr. Bennet] was regardless of time" (I.3), and she tells us of the "leisure and tranquility" he was able to attain in his library, while being prepared to meet with "folly and conceit in every other room of the house" (I.15). Austen later describes his usual demeanor as one of "philosophic composure" (III.6).

If Socrates in the *Phaedo* is right that "philosophy is the practice of dying and being dead,"[7] it seems fitting that Mr. Bennet is the only character in *Pride and Prejudice* who speaks matter-of-factly of his own death and who even jokes about the death of his wife and daughter. When a letter arrives from Mr. Collins, Mr. Bennet blandly refers to him as the man who, "when I am dead, may turn you all out of his house as soon as he pleases" (I.13). Earlier, when Mrs. Bennet rejoices that Jane has caught a cold and will have to spend the night at Netherfield, Mr. Bennet comments that, "if she should die, it would be a comfort to know that it was all in pursuit of Mr. Bingley, and under your orders" (I.7). And later, when his wife is complaining bitterly about the prospect of being evicted from the Longbourn estate by Charlotte Lucas, Mr. Bennet replies, "My dear, do not give way to such gloomy thoughts. Let us hope for better things. Let us flatter ourselves that I may be the survivor" (I.23).

Why do these cheerful references to death by Mr. Bennet strike me as significant? Because the real meaning of Plato's dictum is, I think, that the philosopher, and only the philosopher, honestly faces his death and comes to terms with the meaning of his mortality. He alone has the fortitude to patiently sift through his opinions, reasoning away those vanities and pretensions by which most of us distract ourselves from the fear of death. Only the philosopher lives his life from day to day free of the distortions and diversions by which the rest of us try

6. Xenophon, *Memorabilia* I.1.8.

7. Plato, *Phaedo* 64A.

to disguise and embellish our bleak fate. To quote again from Shakespeare's sonnet 94, "The summer's flower is to the summer sweet, though to itself it only live and die." Chief among those diverting vanities is the specious immortality promised by erotic love and by the virtues of the morally serious man. Vanity of vanities—the theme of all genuinely philosophical literature; and it is no accident that, besides *Pride and Prejudice*, the other great philosophical English novel of the nineteenth century bears the title *Vanity Fair* and the subtitle "A Novel Without a Hero."

I detect the influence of Mr. Bennet's thoughtfulness about death and mortality in a remark Elizabeth makes to herself late in the novel, when she believes that Lydia's elopement has doomed any chance that Darcy will renew his courtship. Elizabeth is imagining how Darcy would react if he were to learn that the woman who had proudly spurned his proposals only four months ago would now receive them gratefully and gladly. "He was as generous, she doubted not, as the most generous of his sex. But while he was mortal, there must be a triumph" (III.8). Here Elizabeth draws a connection between our mortality and our need for a triumph. Her thought seems an echo of Socrates's warning to Phaedo that he himself, on account of his impending death, is "in danger of being in a victory-loving (*philonikos*) rather than a philosophical frame of mind."[8] Elizabeth's suggestion about Darcy seems to be that fear of death, and indignation at the felt injustice of our mortality, could tempt even the most generous of men to feel triumphant at the humiliation of a woman whom he loved without being loved in return. She hints at a dark connection between mortality, eros, and moral indignation that we cannot now pause to explore.

Returning from these awful depths to the comic but negligent behavior of Mr. Bennet, it must be confessed that, while quietly deriving amusement from the behavior of his foolish wife and silly daughters, he displays little sense of responsibility for his children's proper upbringing. As Elizabeth reflects ruefully, "her father, contented with laughing at them, would never exert himself to restrain the wild giddiness of his youngest daughters" (II.14). What is especially reprehensible, Austen tells us, is Mr. Bennet's "continual breach of conjugal obligation and decorum," which "exposed his wife to the contempt of her own children" (II.19). Perhaps as a result, the younger daughters grow "vain, ignorant, idle and absolutely uncontrouled" (II. 18; cf. II.14), and Lydia's elopement with Wickham comes close to bringing ruin upon the entire family, or at any rate on the five daughters.

One might conjecture that the dreary spectacle of their parents' shipwreck of a marriage would have left those daughters mistrustful of love and cynical about the possibility of marital happiness. There may be some truth to that, but Austen takes pains to suggest that a failed marriage does not inevitably

8. Plato, *Phaedo* 91E.

blight the children's view of love. After all, it is Elizabeth's friend Charlotte who expresses the bleakest and least romantic view of marriage: "Happiness in marriage," she says, "is entirely a matter of chance. . . . It is better to know as little as possible of the defects of the person with whom you are to pass your life" (I.6). Later Austen describes how Charlotte, "without thinking highly of either men or matrimony," pursues the goal of marriage not with the hope or expectation of happiness but merely as the most pleasant "preservative from want" (I.22). As for Elizabeth, Austen does tell us that from her own family "she could not have formed a very pleasing picture of conjugal felicity or domestic comfort" (II.19). Nevertheless, somehow Elizabeth does end up thinking highly of both men and matrimony.

To account for his shocking negligence, one could speculate that Mr. Bennet, like a true philosopher, has reached the conclusion that there are limits to the good we can do for others; that to acknowledge these limits is itself a sign of strength; that when all is said and done we are not responsible either for the condition of the world we live in or for the fate of our fellow man; and that most souls fare more or less as they should, whether we interfere in their lives or not. Mr. Bennet may have concluded that there was little hope of correcting the folly and conceit of his wife and younger daughters, and not much point in trying. As for Lydia in particular, with her "wild giddiness," "volatility," and "high animal spirits," certainly no one could teach her what she was unable to learn (II. 14; II.18; I.9). Yet it seems, on the other hand, that Mr. Bennet *has* taken some care for the benefit of others, in the form of the education he has given to his two eldest daughters, and especially to his favorite, Lizzy. With her "delight in anything ridiculous" (I.3), she is truly her father's daughter; and Austen emphasizes that Elizabeth respected her father's abilities (II.19; II.10). Contemplating Elizabeth, the skeptical student of human folly, inconsistency, and absurdity, one cannot help but see a reflection of her father's detached amusement at the human comedy. But I also detect the influence of Mr. Bennet's ideas in the quiet audacity of Elizabeth's statement to Lady Catherine de Bourgh: "I am only resolved to act in that manner, which will, in my own opinion, constitute my happiness, without reference to you, or to any person so wholly unconnected with me" (III.14). That is the philosophy of rational happiness, captured in a sentence. Furthermore, no one appreciates Elizabeth's strength of mind as does Mr. Bennet; after her fears about Lydia's wildness prove prophetic, her father says to her, "Lizzy, I bear you no ill-will for being justified in your advice to me last May, which, considering the event, shews some greatness of mind" (III.6). Clearly Mr. Bennet must have recognized in Elizabeth a young woman of extraordinary discernment and intellectual courage.

My suggestion is that, whatever selfishness and negligence one may censure him for, Elizabeth is indebted above all to her philosophical father for the breadth and depth of her inquiry into the human condition: If she more than any other character in Jane Austen's novels attains something like self-knowledge—regarding love, friendship, morality, and the pursuit of happiness—it is by traveling along an arduous road that her father first invited her to set out on intrepidly. Obviously Mr. Bennet would know that by far the greater part of her education must be carried out by Elizabeth herself, and that whether she truly comes to know herself will depend on the strength of mind and character she is able to bring to bear on all the vicissitudes of a full human life, not least in love and marriage.

There is, finally, the interesting question of Jane Austen herself and her relation to Elizabeth and Elizabeth's philosophy. Sometimes, as we have noted, the author appears to share her protagonist's consciousness and to lend at least tacit assent to her judgments. On rare occasions, Austen offers mild and circumspect criticism of a conclusion reached by Elizabeth. Are we to conclude that the thoughts on love, friendship, morality, and happiness enunciated by Elizabeth are in fact the principles of Jane Austen's philosophy? One is tempted to say that in *Pride and Prejudice* Jane Austen is unfolding for us her own moral and intellectual development, by presenting, in Elizabeth, a younger version of herself, still struggling for self-knowledge and still in the grip of "whatever of her own vanity she had not yet been able to reason away." It is well known that Jane Austen herself never married, but whether that was because no eligible Darcy ever presented himself to her cannot be answered with certainty.

THE TWO MEN IN ELIZABETH'S LIFE

I promised at the start of this essay that I would leave you with a renewed appreciation for the virtues of Darcy, and I hope I will not disappoint you. In *Pride and Prejudice* Elizabeth Bennet is confronted with two very different paradigms of male excellence, in the form of her father, Mr. Bennet, and her eventual husband, Mr. Darcy. Mr. Bennet, I have tried to show, is an exemplar of what might be called "philosophical irresponsibility."[9] He practices

9. The related principle of "scientific irresponsibility" was taught to physicist Richard Feynman by the great mathematician John von Neumann while walking in the canyons of Los Alamos: "Von Neumann gave me an interesting idea: that you don't have to be responsible for the world you're in. So I've developed a very powerful sense of social irresponsibility as a result of von Neumann's advice. It's made me a very happy man ever since. But it was von Neumann who put the seed in that grew into my *active* irresponsibility." Richard P. Feynman, *"Surely You're Joking Mr. Feynman!": Adventures of a Curious Character* (New York: W. W. Norton, 1985).

to a fault Elizabeth's precept—"to act in that manner, which will, in my own opinion, constitute my happiness, without reference to you, or to any person so wholly unconnected with me"—only he leaves out the last part. Or perhaps it would be more accurate to say that Mr. Bennet's solicitude is reserved for those connected to him, not by the accident of biological descent (his children) or by the errors of youthful eros (his wife), but by the genuine bond of a shared openness to philosophy. His lack of concern for the well-being of his wife and his younger children reminds us of the legendary indifference displayed by Socrates toward *his* wife and children while he kept company with the likes of Plato and Xenophon—except that in this novel, Jane Austen has contrived to provide the philosopher with one quite remarkable daughter.

Darcy, on the other hand, takes the principle of moral responsibility to the opposite extreme. Recall his "implacable resentment" not only at the vices but even at the follies of others, to say nothing of their offenses against himself. Darcy's good opinion, once lost, is lost forever (I.11). To his own conduct he applies a standard that is, if anything, even more exacting. One may even say that it is characteristic of Darcy to assert personal moral responsibility for things that he manifestly is not responsible for. Nowhere is this more striking than in his reaction to the elopement of Lydia and Wickham. After he learns of this shocking event, he devotes heroic efforts and considerable expense to tracking down the wayward lovers and persuading Wickham to marry Lydia, even witnessing the revolting wedding ceremony himself, the whole operation being smoothed over by the transfer from Darcy to Wickham of some thousands of pounds sterling. Now there is a grain of truth to Darcy's insistence that, had he not kept his knowledge of Wickham's worthless character mostly to himself, "it would have been impossible for any woman of character to love or confide in him" (III.10). Yet surely the wild behavior of Lydia and Wickham had other causes, and it is quite a stretch for Darcy to "generously impute the whole to his mistaken pride." One might even say that it is in a fit of mistaken pride that he obstinately insists on his sole responsibility for everyone else's misconduct and his obligation to solve their problem entirely on his own. As Elizabeth's aunt puts it, "Nothing was to be done that he did not do himself" (III.10).

In part, Darcy seems to have been moved to act in this transcendently generous manner by his transcendent feeling of the "pure and elevated passion" of love. Mr. Bennet, congratulating himself for the "world of trouble and economy" he was saved by Darcy's gallant expenditures, comments: "These violent young lovers carry everything their own way. I shall offer to pay him tomorrow; he will rant and storm about his love for you, and there will be an end of the matter" (III.17).

If resentment is Darcy's characteristic vice, generosity would seem to be his characteristic virtue, and Austen teaches us through Darcy's example to regard generosity as the habit of treating one's own strength as a source of moral obligation to assume responsibility for the fate of others. The generous man sees himself as the guardian of the happiness of those around him. In so doing, of course, he claims for himself the larger share of the only thing he admires: praiseworthy noble action. As Aristotle puts it in Book IX of the *Ethics*, "in all things that are praised, the morally serious man manifestly distributes more of the noble"—which he takes to be "the greater good"—"to himself," and in this connection Aristotle speaks of the morally serious man as "a lover of self."[10] In the novel, on this occasion, Elizabeth prudently refrains from pointing out these subtleties to her future husband.

After their marriage, Elizabeth seems to have wasted no time in beginning to teach Darcy how to be laughed at. And she finds at Pemberley an even more apt pupil in the person of Georgiana, Darcy's younger sister. Austen writes:

> Georgiana had the highest opinion in the world of Elizabeth; though at first she often listened with an astonishment bordering on alarm at her lively, sportive, manner of talking to her brother. He, who had always inspired in herself a respect which almost overcame her affection, she now saw the object of open pleasantry. *Her mind received knowledge which had never before fallen in her way.* By Elizabeth's instructions, she began to comprehend that a woman may take liberties with her husband which a brother will not always allow in a sister more than ten years younger than himself (III.19; emphasis added).

It is an open question whether, in learning to be laughed at by his wife, Darcy will show himself to be educable in the fundamental sense, i.e., open to questioning his understanding of what a gentleman is.

To return, finally to the question of Darcy's suitability as a husband: It seems evident to me that if the aims of education are self-knowledge and utmost clarity about such rational happiness as is genuinely available to us, then the virtues of Mr. Bennet are exactly what one would want in a teacher. But I suggest that the prouder, more generous, guardian virtues of Mr. Darcy are what an intelligent woman might plausibly want in a husband. Surely there is a place in this world for men willing to step up to the plate, fight for their honor and the honor of their family, and boldly claim responsibility for things, both good and bad, that they may not actually be responsible for. Such characters make the best statesmen, particularly in rough times that demand a

10. Aristotle, *Nicomachean Ethics* IX.8 1169a30-35.

steely eye and a steady hand; in more ordinary times they might also make the best husbands.

* * *

As a postscript to this essay, and an invitation to further reflection, I would like to try to interpret a perplexing passage from the end of the novel that might, on first reading, seem to call my whole argument into question. The passage is from the scene in which Mr. Bennet questions Elizabeth after Darcy has asked him to consent to their marriage:

> "Lizzy," said her father, "I have given him my consent. He is the kind of man, indeed, to whom I should never dare refuse any thing, which he condescended to ask. I now give it to you, if you are resolved on having him. But let me advise you to think better of it. I know your disposition, Lizzy. I know that you could be neither happy nor respectable, unless you truly esteemed your husband; *unless you looked up to him as a superior.* Your lively talents would place you in the greatest danger in an unequal marriage. You could scarcely escape discredit and misery. My child, let me not have the grief of seeing you unable to respect your partner in life. You know not what you are about." (III.17; emphasis added)

If Mr. Bennet is speaking candidly here, what could he mean by telling Elizabeth that she "could be neither happy nor respectable" unless she "looked up to [Darcy] as a superior"? How could Mr. Bennett, in his philosophic wisdom, wish on his daughter an unequal marriage to a superior husband? Very strange. And yet, if we look at the very next sentence we see that that cannot be what he means. "Your lively talents," says Mr. Bennett, "would place you in the greatest danger in an *unequal marriage*." So which is it that her father recommends, a marriage of equals or of unequals?

The solution to this puzzle is, I think, as follows. Mr. Bennet knows that, by law, by social standing, and by "the kind of man" he is or at any rate thinks himself to be, Darcy will inevitably be the superior of any woman who marries him. The only question is whether, in that position of superiority, Elizabeth will really be able to look up to him. Will she find in him qualities of mind and character that earn him her genuine esteem and respect, and not merely her deference and submission? Or will she, with her lively talents, be constantly tempted to mock the pretensions of a cold, arrogant, supercilious husband, thereby risking social disgrace and conjugal misery? Unbeknownst to Mr. Bennet, Elizabeth had already answered that question to her satisfaction:

> His understanding and temper, though unlike her own, would have answered all her wishes. It was an union that must have been to the advantage of both; by her ease and liveliness, his mind might have been softened, his manners improved, and from his judgment, information, and knowledge of the world, she must have received benefit of greater importance. (III.8)

In short, Elizabeth marries Darcy confident that theirs will on the whole be a marriage of equals, each superior to the other in different spheres, each looking up to and benefitting from the strengths of the other. If, in the decisive respect, the superiority of Elizabeth—what her father once called her "greatness of mind"—will remain somewhat eclipsed by the brighter luster of Darcy's guardian virtues, that is a trial that will perhaps nourish a woman who is strong already.

11

From Hearth-Fires to Hell-Fires: Hawthorne and the Cartesian Project

Diana J. Schaub

> *What I desire is man's red fire to make my dreams come true. Give me the power of man's red flower so I can be like you.*
>
> –King Louie, the orangutan, in Disney's *The Jungle Book*

Nathaniel Hawthorne wrote three tales that make explicit reference to fire in their titles: "Fire-Worship," "Earth's Holocaust," and "Ethan Brand."[1] Read in sequence they form an argument of sorts about technology, progress, and modernity.[2] Whether in the ancient myth of Prometheus or the biblical story of Babel or the modern children's fable of Mowgli, fire is central to human identity and aspiration.[3] In the course of discussing the firing of bricks by the tower builders of Babel, Leon Kass notes that

> Fire is universally the symbol of the arts and crafts, of technology. Through the controlled use of fire's transforming power, human beings set about to alter the world, presumably because, as it is, it is insufficient for human need. Imitating God's

1. The first two were written in 1843 and 1844, published in 1846 in *Mosses from an Old Manse*. The last was written in 1850, published in 1852 in *The Snow-Image, and Other Twice-Told Tales*. A "brand" is a burning or partially burned stick. All citations from these stories are from the following edition: Nathaniel Hawthorne, *Tales and Sketches* (New York: Library of America, 1982).

2. There are stories by Hawthorne that explore related topics, such as the scientific mindset, medical experimentation, and the quest for immortality (the most notable being "The Birth-mark," "Rappaccini's Daughter," and "Dr. Heidegger's Experiment"). At the first convening of the President's Council on Bioethics, Chairman Leon Kass led the members in a discussion of Hawthorne's "The Birth-mark"—a memorable moment in the annals of presidential commissions. (See bioethics.georgetown.edu/pcbe/transcripts/jan02/jan17session2.html.)

3. In Kipling's original, Mowgli discovers that he can keep the tiger, Shere Khan, at bay with a burning brand. In the Disney adaptation, King Louie and his troop of monkeys, dwelling in the ruins of a great city, kidnap Mowgli to wrest from him the secret of fire and, thus, dominion.

> creation of man out of the dust of the ground, the human race begins its own project of creation by firing and transforming portions of the earth.[4]

The footnote accompanying this passage refers the reader to Descartes for evidence of "the importance of the controlled use of fire (or heat or energy) for the modern scientific project to master nature."[5] The sections from the *Discourse on Method* cited by Kass (Part V, par. 2 and 4, and Part VI, par. 2) involve Descartes's attempt to understand the nature of fire and its role in creation. As it happens, it is not the transfiguration of clay into brick that fascinates Descartes, but rather the "transmutation of ashes into glass"—a more dramatic conversion by fire that Descartes declares "as awesome as any other that occurs in nature."[6] Burnt earth in the form of glass would understandably be of great interest to a scientific pioneer in the field of optics.

When Descartes subsequently gives his account of the creation of man—according to the Bible, the transmutation of ashes into Adam by means of the breath of life—he understands it on the model he has already presented of inanimate matter. The breath of life can be understood in purely mechanical terms as "heat." Thus, God "kindled in the man's heart one of those fires without light which I had already explained and which I did not at all conceive to be of a nature other than what heats hay when it has been stored before it is dry, or which makes new wines boil when they are left to ferment after crushing."[7] We have been cooked up like compost or fermented like a nice glass of bubbly. There may be a slight problem with the analogies, however, since the damp hay is decomposing, as are the grapes. Can animal life really be understood on the model of heat-generating rot? No wonder the production of lifeless glass—often blown into incomparable shapes by the breath of the artisan—is more impressive to Descartes. This may also explain why medicine is for Descartes the "indispensable" science; we must learn to regulate the heat within, for "[h]eat is the great transmuter, the mediator between death and life."[8] According to Descartes, "the animal spirits" are "like a very pure and lively flame that rises continuously in great abundance from the heart to the brain, and from there goes through the nerves into the muscles, and gives

4. Leon R. Kass, *The Beginning of Wisdom: Reading Genesis* (New York: Free Press, 2003), 226.

5. Ibid.

6. Descartes, *Discourse on Method*, trans. Donald A. Cress (Indianapolis: Hackett, 1998), Part V, par. 2, 25.

7. Ibid., 26.

8. Joseph Cropsey, "On Descartes' *Discourse on Method*," in *Political Philosophy and the Issues of Politics* (Chicago: The University of Chicago Press, 1977), 288.

movement to all the members."[9] The body is a kind of furnace whose pilot light could perhaps be re-engineered to be perpetual. Accordingly, Descartes demands a practical rather than a speculative philosophy, pursuing "the invention of an infinity of devices," directed principally at "the maintenance of health."[10]

Descartes's famous method, which culminates in this project of a "Mechanical Jerusalem,"[11] was conceived, by Descartes's own testimony, while he spent a winter day confined in a *poêle* or stove-heated room.[12] It would not have surprised Nathaniel Hawthorne to learn that this audacious project to make men "the masters and possessors of nature"[13] was concocted by a solitary man cooped up with only caged fire for company. Indeed, the whole point of his first fire fable is to lament the advent of the stove. He traces "a great revolution in social and domestic life" brought about by "this almost universal exchange of the open fire-place for the cheerless and ungenial stove."

HEARTH-LESS

"Fire-Worship" is not so much a story as an essay of social criticism, not unlike an article in *The New Atlantis*[14] that observes the effects of some new device or application (like cell phones or the internet) on the character and quality of human connection. There are today a fair number of people who are either leery of certain technologies (perhaps declining to own a television or regulating their children's exposure to various electronic media) or at least prepared to acknowledge the downsides (such as the explosion in access to pornography via the internet). However, we tend to take our furnaces and central heating for granted. Aware of fuel costs, we are no longer aware of any moral or spiritual costs. "Fire-Worship" is a wonderful time-traveling exercise offering insights as startling as Socrates's complaint in the *Phaedrus* about the perils of the written word. While we are no more likely to return to open hearths than to an oral culture, we can benefit from the remembrance, as Hawthorne indicates by the title of the collection in which "Fire-Worship" appeared: *Mosses from an Old Manse.*

Of the twenty-six tales, essays, and sketches in the volume, two of them, "Fire-Worship" and "Buds and Bird-Voices," are explicitly linked to the autobiographical title piece, "The Old Manse: The Author Makes the Reader Acquainted

9. Descartes, 30.
10. Descartes, 35.
11. Cropsey, 289.
12. Descartes, 6-7.
13. Descartes, 35.
14. *The New Atlantis: A Journal of Technology and Society*, published in Washington, DC, by the Ethics and Public Policy Center.

with His Abode." That abode was a "moss-grown country parsonage" (the ancestral home of the priestly Emerson family), where, for three and a half years, the newly-married Hawthorne lived as the first "lay occupant." "The Old Manse" is a transcendentalist idyll about the house (especially the study—"It was here that Emerson wrote 'Nature'"—and superannuated library) and natural environs ("the river, the battle-field, the orchard, and the garden"). Similar in tone, although without the focus on scholarly productions, "Buds and Bird-Voices" is a paean to the arrival of Spring. By contrast, "Fire-Worship" is an anti-idyll—a wintry meditation on an advancing technological "abomination." The seasonal setting of each piece is distinct: "Buds and Bird-Voices" belongs to "balmy spring"; "The Old Manse" is set in summer and fall; "Fire-Worship" opens in bleakest winter. Both the non-winter essays, however, make brief but pointed reference to the infernal contraption.[15]

So, why is the air-tight stove an "enormity"? Hawthorne grants that the stove is vastly more efficient than the open hearth, consuming fewer cords of wood, generating more heat, with less risk of danger. Indeed, efficiency, comfort, and safety were the motives behind Benjamin Franklin's invention of the cast-iron stove in the 1740s. Whereas Franklin fully subscribed to the Baconian/Cartesian faith in technology, Hawthorne is a dissenter. He challenges all three motives. Another name for the virtue of efficiency is the vice of inhospitality: "grudging the food that kept him cheery and mercurial, we have thrust him into an iron prison, and compel him to smoulder away his life on a daily pittance." The comfort we gain from our stinginess is a "black and cheerless comfort." We are deprived of "the bright face of [an] ancient friend, who was wont to dance upon the hearth, and play the part of a more familiar sunshine." Even our increased safety is quite overrated, according to Hawthorne:

> Nor did it lessen the charm of his soft, familiar courtesy and helpfulness, that the mighty spirit, were opportunity offered him, would run riot through the peaceful house, wrap its inmates in his terrible embrace, and leave nothing of them save their whitened bones. This possibility of mad destruction only made his domestic kindness the more . . . touching.

The gravamen of Hawthorne's complaint, which is a complaint not just about the Franklin stove but about the spirit of Franklin, is that "the inventions of mankind are fast blotting the picturesque, the poetic, and the beautiful out of human life." The stove is a representative instance, but also a special one, since fire is "that quick and subtle spirit whom Prometheus lured from Heaven

15. Hawthorne, 825 and 1144.

to civilize mankind." Fire is both an elemental force of "wild Nature"—"he that comes roaring out of Aetna, and rushes madly up the sky, like a fiend breaking loose from torment"—and our instrument—"he is the great artisan and laborer by whose aid men are enabled to build a world within a world, or, at least, to smoothe down the rough creation which Nature flung to us." But beyond his "terrible might" and "many-sided utility," he was heretofore also our "homely friend." Hawthorne calls fire "the great conservative of Nature!" (exclamation mark in the original) because of his part in all "life-long and age-coeval associations." The hearth is the center of the home, and the home is the foundation of larger enterprises. Hawthorne asserts that "While a man was true to the fireside, so long would he be true to country and law—to the God whom his fathers worshipped—to the wife of his youth—and to all things else which instinct or religion have taught us to consider sacred." The virtues of marital fidelity, patriotism, and piety all take their spark from the domesticated fire.

Hawthorne attaches particular importance to the glowing face of the fire which works sympathetically upon the imagination. For whoever looks into the fire-light, "[h]e pictured forth their very thoughts. To the youthful, he showed the scenes of the adventurous life before them; to the aged, the shadows of departed love and hope; and, if all earthly things had grown distasteful, he could gladden the fireside muser with golden glimpses of a better world"—all the while, "causing the tea-kettle to boil." The stove, of course, retains (and even intensifies) the useful heat. However, it removes our contact with the light. The fire becomes invisible, damaging both communion and contemplation. In the opening sentence, Hawthorne speaks of a revolution not only in "social and domestic life," but also "in the life of the secluded student." Without "that peculiar medium of vision," both fellowship and scholarship will take on a different—less insightful and generous—quality.

"Fire-Worship" is a tightly constructed piece, just eleven paragraphs in length. After the opening four paragraphs (summarized above), in which Hawthorne delineates the multifarious nature of fire, the central three paragraphs offer a description of a day around the hearth of "the good old clergyman, my predecessor in this mansion." Hawthorne imagines him in his prime, decades before he would brick over the fire-place and install the wretched modern convenience. We see him writing a sermon under the influence of "the aspect of the morning fireside"; receiving a parishioner who has "been looking the inclement weather in the face" but to whom "the warmth of benevolence" is now extended. We see him, after making his own daily pastoral rounds, return to the twilight fireside, "a beacon light of humanity." Finally, in the evening, the family gathers, "children tumbled themselves upon the hearth-rug, and grave Puss sat with her back to the fire." After this commemorative portrait, Hawthorne declares: "Heaven forgive the old clergyman!" He notes the reasons that might have led the octogenarian to "bid farewell to the face of his old friend for ever": cutbacks in his monthly allotment of wood and the increasing draftiness of the old house; "but still, it was one of the saddest tokens of the decline and fall of open fire-places, that the grey patriarch should have deigned to warm himself at an air-tight stove."

The final four paragraphs shift to Hawthorne, who, despite his views on the matter, compounded the "shame" by installing three more stoves throughout the house, so now "not a glimpse of this mighty and kindly one will greet your eyes." Hawthorne finds himself in the position of so many technological doubters. His conscience worries and objects, but in point of fact, he allows himself to follow the current. Hawthorne's own complicity may help explain his ironic tone. In the preface to the *Mosses*, he says that these sketches are "often but half in earnest." So while he has no intention of forwarding a rejectionist policy of radical reaction, he does want us to reflect on the moral effects of living with stoves and furnaces. Poetic hyperbole is part of his method. He writes from experience—the experience of his own grudging participation. As a member of the transitional generation, he warns of the coming hearth-lessness.

As he had described the gladsome character of fire's visible presence, Hawthorne in turn describes the malign character of its invisible presence. Though caged, the fire can still be felt in scorched fingers and singed garments; and smelled in the "volumes of smoke and noisome gas" that issue through the cracks; and especially heard—sighing, hissing, and moaning, "burthened with unutterable grief" at "the ingratitude of mankind . . . to whom he taught all their arts, even that of making his own prison-house." In transforming the transformative agent, we live with a "darkened source."[16]

Hawthorne traces the "invaluable moral influences" that will be lost when "the sacred trust of the household-fire . . . transmitted in unbroken succession from the earliest ages" has been extinguished by "physical science." The effects will be most profound for future generations. Those who grew up around the fireside will retain certain salutary habits:

> We shall draw our chairs together, as we and our forefathers have been wont, for thousands of years back, and sit around some blank and empty corner of the room, babbling, with unreal cheerfulness, of topics suitable to the homely fireside.

16. Hawthorne's critique of the truth-obscuring effects of technology seems to anticipate Martin Heidegger's *The Question Concerning Technology* (an essay first published by Heidgger in *Vorträge und Aufsätze* [Pfullingen, Germany: Günther Neske, 1954]).

> A warmth from the past—from the ashes of by-gone years, and the raked-up embers of long ago—will sometimes thaw the ice about our hearts.

For the young, however, raised with either "the sullen stove" or, even worse, "furnace-heat" in "houses which might be fancied to have their foundation over the infernal pit," the mutual bond will be broken. Hawthorne predicts that "[t]here will be nothing to attract these poor children to one centre. . . . Domestic life—if it may still be termed domestic—will seek its separate corners." If Hawthorne is right, it didn't require televisions and personal computers in every room for the family to be atomized. What we call "central heat" is in truth diffused heat. With heat diffused so efficiently into every nook and cranny, there is no necessity for family and friends to gather together, and no special atmosphere (which "melts all humanity into one heart of hearts") to vivify the occasional grouping. Along with the heat, fellow-feeling is diffused. Social intercourse of many types will suffer or even disappear: "easy gossip—the merry, yet unambitious jest—the life-long practical discussion of real matters in a casual way—the soul of truth, which is so often incarnated in a simple fireside word." Instead, "conversation will contract the air of a debate."

As a kind of confirmation of Hawthorne's intuition, it is interesting that for a long time after the advent of whole house heating, homes continued to be built with at least one functioning fireplace, usually in the living room. However, beginning in the 1960s and 70s, new homes were constructed without even that token of tradition. In the last two decades, this trend toward hearthlessness has been dramatically reversed. New homes now have multiple fireplaces, in kitchens, family rooms, and master bedrooms. They are of course often gas or electric, so they are convenient, but they do offer a visible flame (or simulacrum thereof). Wood-burning fire-pits for the deck are also all the rage. Sales of candles increase every year. Perhaps there is an ineradicable human longing for the fireside and fire-light. We seek ways to compensate for the social and psychic disruptions of technological progress. It remains an open question whether these modern versions of the hearth (which are strictly speaking gratuitous) can truly preserve traditional practices and virtues.

In the final paragraph, Hawthorne returns to his opening claim about the linkage between the virtues of the domestic, religious, and political realms. His text is the ancient "exhortation to fight 'pro aris et focis'—for the altars and the hearths." These are the sacred locations—kindred in spirit—that inspire patriotic sacrifice. Hawthorne calls the hearth "a divine idea, embodied in brick and mortar," presided over by mothers rather than priests. The hearth with its chimney, though constructed of the same brick that built the impious tower of

Babel, expresses a very different aspiration. Those who would defile the hearth would stop at nothing:

> The man, who did not put off his shoes upon this holy ground, would have deemed it pastime to trample upon the altar. It has been our task to uproot the hearth. What further reform is left for our children to achieve, unless they overthrow the altar too?

Once hearth and altar are both gone, Hawthorne wonders what patriotism will rest upon or appeal to. "FIGHT FOR YOUR STOVES!" is not a battle cry that will "rouse up native valor."

THE BONFIRE OF MODERNITY

One change begets others. At the close of "The Old Manse," Hawthorne tells of his forced relocation from the Old Manse to the Custom-House (where he would write *The Scarlet Letter*) prompted by the current owner's desire to renovate—not a project of which Hawthorne approves, inasmuch as "the hand that renovates is always more sacrilegious than that which destroys." The renovating, progressive temperament is the main theme of Hawthorne's second fire story, "Earth's Holocaust."

In this satirical allegory we find not a hearth but a bonfire, by means of which Earth's inhabitants plan to rid themselves of "an accumulation of worn-out trumpery." Instead of being "the great conservative," fire will become the cleansing and purging agent of reform. The site of the bonfire, selected by "the Insurance Companies" with a view to safety and accessibility, "was one of the broadest prairies of the West." The account of the fire's progress and the reactions of various bystanders are given by a narrator who hopes that "the illumination of the bonfire might reveal some profundity of moral truth."

After the bonfire is kindled with "yesterday's newspapers," a group of "rough-looking men" hurl all the paraphernalia of aristocracy into the fire, such things as "the blazonry of coat-armor; the crests and devices of illustrious families; pedigrees that extended back . . . into the mist of the dark ages," at the sight of which "the multitude of plebeian spectators set up a joyous shout." The narrator's comment acknowledges the justice of the democratic triumph over the past. After all, the nobility were "creatures of the same clay and same spiritual infirmities, who had dared to assume the privileges due only to Heaven's better workmanship." Nonetheless, Hawthorne, rather like Tocqueville, does not allow the reader to forget the beauty that is lost with the demise of aristocracy. A "gray-haired man, of stately presence," steps forward and lectures the spectators:

> "People, what have you done! This fire is consuming all that marked your advance from barbarism, or that could have prevented your relapse thither. We—the men of the privileged orders—were those who kept alive, from age to age, the old chivalrous spirit; the gentle and generous thought; the higher, the purer, the more refined and delicate life! With the nobles, too, you cast off the poet, the painter, the sculptor—all the beautiful arts;—for we were their patrons, and created the atmosphere in which they flourish. In abolishing the majestic distinctions of rank, society loses not only its grace, but its steadfastness—"

"A rude figure," who threatens to cast the nobleman himself into the fire, responds with a speech in defense of various natural superiorities ("strength of arm . . . wit, wisdom, courage, force of character") but dismissive of the "nonsense" of inherited "place and consideration." The final word on this first reform goes to a "grave observer," with whom the narrator converses, who approves of the burning of this "antiquated trash" but with a caveat: "if no worse nonsense come in its place."[17]

Next upon the pile went all the insignia and pomp of monarchy. The age of "universal manhood" having arrived, no one speaks up for monarchy. The "fallen nobleman," hooted from the scene for defending his prerogatives, has "shrunk back into the crowd." Hawthorne seems to suggest that the fundamental political alternatives are aristocracy and democracy. Monarchy is simply a further refinement of an order built upon hereditary rank. As Montesquieu argued: "the nobility is of the essence of monarchy."[18] Once the notion of rank is discredited, monarchy cannot sustain itself. To escape the smoke and smell of the burning purple wardrobes, the narrator and his acquaintance move to the other side of the bonfire, where another facet of "the general and systematic measures of reform" is underway.

The "votaries of temperance" have collected "the whole world's stock of spirituous liquors" and offered them to the "insatiable thirst of the fire-fiend." Once again, "the multitude gave a shout, as if the broad earth were exulting in its deliverance from the curse of ages." However, "the joy was not universal." In fact, there were "many" who "deemed that human life would be gloomier than ever." The "Last Toper" steps forth as their spokesman:

17. In "My Kinsman, Major Molineux," there is a similar "gentleman" who, while not a participant in the riotous antics of the revolutionaries, seems to be a judicious friend of the new democratic order.

18. Montesquieu, *The Spirit of the Laws* (1748), Book 2, chapter 4.

> "What is this world good for . . . now that we can never be jolly any more? What is to comfort the poor man in sorrow and perplexity?—how is he to keep his heart warm against the cold winds of this cheerless earth?—and what do you propose to give him, in exchange for the solace that you take away? How are old friends to sit together by the fireside, without a cheerful glass between them? A plague upon your reformation! It is a sad world, a cold world, a selfish world, a low world, not worth an honest fellow's living in, now that good-fellowship is gone forever!"

Despite the "great mirth" of the bystanders at this harangue, the narrator "could not help commiserating the forlorn condition of the Last Toper" who had indeed lost his "boon-companions." He had also managed to "filch a bottle of fourth-proof brandy that fell beside the bonfire"—the first concrete act of resistance. The reformers don't notice, however. In their moralistic "zeal," they are casting tea, coffee, and tobacco "upon the heap of inutility." The assault on tobacco, in particular, startles and provokes "an old gentleman" who declares: "Everything rich and racy—all the spice of life—is to be condemned as useless. Now that they have kindled the bonfire, if these nonsensical reformers would fling themselves into it, all would be well enough!" Earlier, the fallen nobleman was told to count himself lucky to have lost his pedigree rather than his life to the fire. Now, the reformers themselves are at least passively wished into the pyre. The final word, however, goes to "a staunch conservative" who seems to warn against such wishes. With grim irony, he predicts the course of the holocaust's relentless logic: "Be patient . . . it will come to that in the end. They will first fling us in, and finally themselves."

The narrator's attention shifts again, "from the general and systematic measures of reform" to "the individual contributions." There is a purely personal animus toward the past. The jilted and the bored toss their love letters, disappointed professionals throw the tools of their trade (e.g., the false teeth of "a hack-politician" defeated for office), and, most striking to the narrator, "a number of ladies, highly respectable in appearance," propose "to fling their gowns and petticoats into the flames, and assume the garb, together with the manners, duties, offices, and responsibilities, of the opposite sex." As the feminist slogan of the 1960s expressed it: "the personal is political." Before the narrator can witness the outcome of this moment in which female dissatisfaction is annealed into feminism, a "poor, deceived, and half-delirious girl" attempts to throw herself into the fire and is rescued by "a good man" who counsels "patience." He attempts to instruct her in the difference between what is fit for the fire—"things of matter, and creations of human fantasy"—and what is not—"a living soul" meant for "Eternity." Insisting, however, that "the sunshine is blotted out," she only sinks from "frenzy" to "deep despondency." While it is possible that a particular reform has driven her mad (say, the one contemplated by the respectable ladies), it seems more likely from the textual evidence that she embraces the fire as a final solution to some earlier trauma (thus, she had rushed toward it, "exclaiming that she was the most worthless thing alive or dead"). Her attempted suicide demonstrates the difficulty of setting any bounds to the fire's destructive use. Regret can extend well beyond yesterday's feelings and actions, well beyond the conventions and choices of the past, to one's very essence and existence. The flame of modernity attracts and consumes the flighty moth of "the self."

The scene shifts dramatically back to politics proper, both foreign and domestic, with the next two reforms targeting the weapons of war and the instruments of capital punishment. Disarmament, the prelude to the abolition of war itself, occasions "great diversity of opinion," with "the hopeful philanthropist" greeting the millennium, while those "in whose view mankind was a breed of bull-dogs . . . prophesied that all the old stoutness, fervor, nobleness, generosity, and magnanimity of the race, would disappear." Despite the doubters, the reform proceeds apace: "It was wonderful to behold, how those terrible instruments of slaughter melted away like playthings of wax." Commentary, in this case, is provided by a "veteran commander" and a man identified only by his "sneer." The commander believes that "all this foolery has only made more work for the armorers and cannon-founderies." Since "the battle-field is the only court" where suits between nations can be tried, the "necessity of war" will return. The narrator speaks up on behalf of universal peace, suggesting that a transnational tribunal of "Reason and Philanthropy" will be constituted. In effect, there will be a new sovereign; international law will replace national sovereignty. In the midst of the discussion between the commander and the narrator, the man with the sneer interjects a comment that reaches deeper than the debate over whether rearmament will occur: "When Cain wished to slay his brother, he was at no loss for a weapon." In other words, guns don't shoot people, people do. The problem is man's heart, not his arms.

While God dealt with Cain in his own way, the descendants of Cain—Cain, remember, was the founder of the first city and the forefather of Noah—have instituted their own method: capital punishment. The reformers, after bringing the whole world under juridical control, seek to make human judgment milder. In casting "those horrible monsters of mechanism"—the headsmen's axes and halters, the guillotine and gallows—into the blaze, they correct "the long and deadly error of human law." Not surprisingly, the executioner, "an ill-looking fellow," defends his livelihood "with brute fury." However, the narrator notes that men consecrated to the benevolent guardianship of society also took "the hangman's view of the question." One of this class declares:

> "You are misled by a false philanthropy!—you know not what you do. The gallows is a heaven-oriented instrument! Bear it back, then, reverently, and set it up in its old place; else the world will fall to speedy ruin and desolation!"

The reformers prevail when one of their leaders counters: "How can human law inculcate benevolence and love, while it persists in setting up the gallows as its chief symbol?" In a pattern that has become familiar, this "triumph of the earth's redemption" is hedged about with doubts. Although the narrator declares the act "well-done," the "thoughtful observer" is more cautious: "well done, if the world be good enough for the measure. Death, however, is an idea that cannot easily be dispensed with, in any condition between the primal innocence and that other purity and perfection, which, perchance, we are destined to attain." Still, he thinks "the experiment" is worth trying.

The next rash of moral reforms serves as a verdict of sorts on the experiment. With the most fearsome bulwark of society gone, the crowd is caught up in more radical measures: burning marriage-certificates, currency, title-deeds, statute-books, and written constitutions. The narrator himself finally balks at this assault on the institutions of marriage, private property, and government. The growth of radicalism can be seen by comparing the first phase of "individual contributions" to the bonfire to this second phase. Earlier, disappointed lovers rejected the past, burning old "bundles of perfumed letters and enamored sonnets." Now, in burning "their marriage certificates" and other instruments of fixed commitments, they are in some sense burning the future, or at least the link between present and future. Each of these institutions depends on a present promise (or agreement or contract) that binds and determines the shape of the future. Such promises, however voluntary, can be experienced as a restriction on freedom. Accordingly, the very notions of promise-keeping and law-abidingness must be abolished, so that each moment will be left radically undetermined. The "good people around the bonfire" are pursuing a powerfully antinomian version of autonomy. For the self to be absolutely sovereign, it must be above all law, even those laws that it gives to itself. The arbitrary self scorns the rigors of self-government.

Interestingly, the reformers expect not only the fullest freedom but the widest fellowship as well. Free love will yield "a higher, holier, and more comprehensive union"; once property claims are destroyed, "the whole soil of the earth [will] revert to the public." Belonging will be universal rather than exclusive or specific. In a "consummated world," freedom and fraternity will be conjoined. Departing from his usual practice, Hawthorne does not provide any expressions of doubt or debate on these reforms, other than the narrator's opening remark that "I was hardly prepared to keep them company."[19] Perhaps he assumes that most readers—even relatively naïve ones like the narrator—will part company with the enthusiasts at this point.

The narrator's attention is now drawn to matters that "concerned my sympathies more nearly." The book burning has begun. "The world's entire mass of printed paper, bound or in sheets" is to be consigned to the fire. It isn't just written law that oppresses, but the written word of all types. "A modern philosopher" heartily approves, since we need to "get rid of the weight of dead men's thought." There follows a delightful excursus upon literature, as the narrator is able to judge the quality of each author's (or nation's or genre's) writing by how it burns. Some authors generate "a brilliant shower of sparkles" (Voltaire, for instance); others "smouldered away to ashes, like rotten wood" (the class of commentators); the Germans emit "a scent of brimstone"; while "the English standard authors made excellent fuel, generally exhibiting the properties of sound oak logs." Special mention is made of Milton ("a powerful blaze") and Shakespeare, from whom

> there gushed a flame of such marvelous splendor, that men shaded their eyes as against the sun's meridian glory; nor, even when the works of his own elucidators were flung upon him, did he cease to flash forth a dazzling radiance, from beneath the ponderous heap. It is my belief, that he is still blazing as fervidly as ever.

The burning of Shakespeare occasions a debate between the narrator and "a critic"—doubtless a follower of Emerson—about poetic originality and the anxiety of influence. The critic favors self-reliance, whereas the narrator argues for standing on the shoulders of ancient giants: "It is not every one that can steal the fire from Heaven, like Prometheus; but when once he had done the deed, a thousand hearths were kindled by it." Appropriately, the narrator goes on to praise humble works like "Mother Goose's Melodies," "the single sheet of an old ballad," and "an unregarded ditty of some nameless bard," which he observes burn brighter and longer than many more acclaimed works. As in "Fire-Worship," Hawthorne links the poetic and the prosaic; the Promethean genius Shakespeare lights the way for more homely, domesticated writers. This fire of imagination, whether heavenly or hearth-ly, is profoundly different from the bonfire of progress.

19. Three years before writing "Earth's Holocaust," Hawthorne spent eight months at Brook Farm, a socialistic, utopian community that would provide the critical inspiration for *The Blithedale Romance.*

In "Fire-Worship," Hawthorne spoke of the fiendish, riotous form of fire "to whose ravenous maw, it is said, the universe shall one day be given as a final feast." Here the narrator fears that the apocalypse may be the next item on the reform agenda: "Unless we set fire to the earth itself, and then leap boldly off into infinite space, I know not that we can carry reform to any further point." His friend, however, realizes there is still fuel to come "that will startle many persons, who have lent a willing hand thus far." The fresh fuel turns out to be the accoutrements of religion: surplices, mitres, crosses, baptismal fonts, everything from the "undecorated pulpits" of New England to the "spoils" of St. Peter's. Despite the narrator's initial "astonishment," he reconciles himself to this latest reformation with the thought that the purging of external emblems may render faith "more sublime in its simplicity" and that "the wood-paths shall be the aisles of our cathedral—the firmament itself shall be its ceiling!"

The reform, however, is not complete. There is a final consummation. The Bible, which we learn had been spared during the "general destruction of books," is now sacrificed by "the Titan of innovation." Reform is its own religion. Here is how Hawthorne describes the apotheosis:

> But the Titan of innovation—angel or fiend, double in his nature, and capable of deeds befitting both characters—at first shaking down only the old and rotten shapes of things, had now, as it appeared, laid his terrible hand upon the main pillars, which supported the whole edifice of our moral and spiritual state. The inhabitants of the earth had grown too enlightened to define their faith within a form of words, or to limit the spiritual by any analogy to our material existence. Truths, which the Heavens trembled at, were now but a fable of the world's infancy. Therefore, as the final sacrifice of human error, what else remained, to be thrown upon the embers of that awful pile, except the Book, which, though a celestial revelation to past ages, was but a voice from a lower sphere, as regarded the present race of man? It was done!

The Church-Bible, family-Bible, and bosom-Bible are all flung in. As in "Fire-Worship," the institutional structures of society are linked. Tearing down one prepares the way for the demolition of others. The titanic spirit of reform, which is hostile to tradition qua tradition, is incapable of making distinctions between unsound and sound, between the superannuated and the timeless.

In his easygoing way, the narrator has adjusted to most of the reforms, arguing for instance that the general book-burning would open "an enviable field for the authors of the next generation" and counseling "the desperate book-worm" to consider whether "Nature" is not "better than a book." At the Bible-burning, however, he grows pale. Somewhat surprisingly, his distress—and the distress of the other onlookers—is not shared by the man who has been at his side throughout. With "singular calmness," the unnamed man assures him that "there is far less both of good and evil, in the effect of this bonfire, than the world might be willing to believe." The culture-warriors on both sides of the reform question are apparently mistaken. Perplexed, the narrator wonders how the world will continue with "every human or divine appendage of our mortal state" gone. His "grave friend" claims that in the morning "you will find among the ashes everything really valuable . . . not a truth is destroyed—nor buried so deep among the ashes, but it will be raked up at last"—a proof of which is already visible in the pages of Holy Scripture, which had not "blackened into tinder" but instead "assumed a more dazzling whiteness." The narrator leaps to the happy conclusion that the fire purifies. If so—"if only what is evil can feel the action of the fire"—then the fire must have been "of inestimable utility." The philosophic observer, however, directs him to "Listen to the talk of these worthies"—a distinctive group gathered in front of the pile—to learn "something useful." The "profundity of moral truth" that the narrator had sought in the fire's illumination is to be found instead in the conversation of a party formed by the hangman, the Last Thief, the Last Murderer, and the Last Toper.

They are despondent, passing the filched bottle of spirits. The hangman offers to dispatch them all, including himself, from the nearest tree (no fiery death for them). A new figure joins them: "a dark-complexioned personage" whose eyes "glowed with a redder light than that of the bonfire." He confidently informs them that they "shall see good days yet" since the conflagration begun by "these wiseacres" amounts to "just nothing at all." This figure, whom the narrator dubs "The Evil Principle," has spent the entire evening laughing at the reform project, since it overlooked "the human heart"—"that foul cavern" from which "will re-issue all the shapes of wrong and misery. . . . Oh, take my word for it, it will be the old world yet!"

The narrator has been helped to the thought—"how sad a truth"—that "Man's age-long endeavor for perfection" is fundamentally misguided, since it is a project of "the Intellect" that doesn't reach "the Heart— . . . the little, yet boundless sphere, wherein existed the original wrong." Hawthorne does not suggest how (or whether) one could "purify the inner sphere." Certainly, the strategy of "Earth's Holocaust" applied to human beings themselves—tried in the last century by the most zealous of purging reformers, both fascist and communist—does not work. Hawthorne's teaching is anti-millenarian and anti-utopian. There is a hint that the revealed word—or even a human "pen of inspiration" like Shakespeare's—can touch the Heart. But politics can never be re-formative in the deep sense. With sadness rather than glee, Hawthorne joins the Devil in his dismissal of ideological agendas. Miles Coverdale, the skeptical narrator from *The Blithedale Romance* sums up Hawthorne's view of his Transcendentalist colleagues: "No sagacious man," says Coverdale, "will long retain his sagacity, if he live exclusively among reformers and progressive people, without periodically returning to the settled system of things, to correct himself by a new observation from that old stand-point."[20] Political expectations need to be moderated. Hawthorne is not a movement conservative any more than he is a movement liberal. His message, however, circles back around to defend the traditional institutions of the social order (family and property, even war and capital punishment). He defends them not as fine accomplishments, but rather as somewhat unfortunate necessities, themselves involving cruelty, hypocrisy, and corruption. Yet, they serve as restraints upon the worst of us and the worst in each of us.

THE BURNING BRAND

"Earth's Holocaust" closes with the devil's laughter; "Ethan Brand" opens with a disconcerting "roar of laughter" and closes with a "frightful peal of laughter" from another fiendish figure. The last of Hawthorne's fire tales is an inquiry into the perversion of the Intellect in a man who starts with "love and sympathy for mankind" but finishes "a cold observer, looking on mankind as the subject of his experiment." The prediction of the "staunch conservative" in "Earth's Holocaust"—that those who fed the bonfire would ultimately fling themselves into it—comes to pass in "Ethan Brand."

The setting for the story—which with a protagonist, a plot, and third-person narration is more of a story than either "Fire-Worship" or "Earth's Holocaust"—is a lime-kiln, a special kind of furnace. There, Brand conceives his unique quest for the Unpardonable Sin—some human act that will, Brand believes, "extend man's possible guilt beyond the scope of Heaven's else infinite mercy." There, too, after an eighteen-year pursuit, Brand returns, having discovered within himself what he sought, intent on completing his mission by suicide.

We are told that tending a lime-kiln is a lonesome occupation and, for those few so inclined, like Ethan Brand, "an intensely thoughtful" one. From "Fire-Worship" we know the sympathetic power of fire to reflect the inner man. In Brand's case that communion produced "the IDEA." His already "dark thoughts" were "melted" into "the one thought that took possession of his life": a quest for the Unpardonable Sin. The kiln, of course, has nothing of the forgiving quality of a hearth-fire. Indeed, Hawthorne, with reference to *Pilgrim's Progress*, compares the kiln to "the private entrance to the infernal regions, which the shepherds of the Delectable Mountains were accustomed to show to pilgrims." When Bartram—the ordinary, unthinking man

20. Nathaniel Hawthorne, *Collected Novels* (New York: Library of America, 1983), 755.

who now serves as lime-burner—keeps watch upon the fire, he does so "turning his face from the insufferable glare." Brand, however, immediately upon returning from his impious pilgrimage, "fixed his eyes, which were very bright, intently upon the brightness of the furnace, as if he beheld, or expected to behold, some object worthy of note within it." Later in the story, he "bent forward to gaze into the hollow prison-house of the fire, regardless of the fierce glow." Later still, "he sat looking into the fire, as if he fancied pictures among the coals." Just as Brand is transfixed by the "lurid blaze," so little Joe—the sensitive son of the insensitive Bartram—is transfixed by Brand's face, which mirrors the kiln. (Brand's eyes "gleamed like fires within the entrance of a mysterious cavern.") Wisely, the child begs his father to shut the furnace door to break the spell.

Even the "dull and torpid" Bartram, unconsciously reminded of his own sins, begins to sense the horror of Brand's "Master Sin." Bartram's fears take a conventionally supernatural shape, as he remembers the stories told about Ethan Brand: how he "conversed with Satan himself" and summoned a fiend from the furnace "to share in the dreadful task" of finding the sin that surpasses God's understanding. What Bartram doesn't understand is that Brand now regards himself as beyond good and evil. Thus, Brand rebukes him, saying: "what need have I of the devil? I have left him behind me on my track. It is with such half-way sinners as you that he busies himself." Whereas Bartram had been frightened by a heartfelt kinship based on universal human sinfulness, Brand denies the connection. On his reckoning, his sin is not of the same "family." Asked by Bartram what "the Unpardonable Sin" is, he answers: "The sin of an intellect that triumphed over the sense of brotherhood with man, and reverence for God, and sacrificed everything to its own mighty claims!" Brand speaks "with the pride that distinguishes all enthusiasts of his stamp"—a textual indication that Brand's sin is perhaps not as special as he believes. His pride may indeed be the "Master Sin" (or the original sin), without being the "Unpardonable Sin."

Nonetheless, there is a sense in which Brand's sin, especially his self-murder, is unpardonable. One suspects that, for Brand, self-murder was a feasible substitute for the murder of all mankind. His interactions with the townspeople who assemble on the forlorn hillside on the news of his return indicate as much. Calling them "brute beasts," he commands them to "Get ye gone!" To the "Jew of Nuremberg"—the traveling showman who tellingly mocks the nihilism of Brand's quest—his instruction is more explicit: "get thee into the furnace yonder!" Through suicide, Brand murders the world he despises, along with the self. Moreover, suicide is a form of murder by which he willfully removes himself from the realm of remorse and redemption. Perhaps because it was understood as a declaration of the most profound and radical alienation, suicide was long punished under the civil law, and suicides were denied the solace of the church graveyard, populated with fellow-sinners.

Not surprisingly, "Brand" is a name rich in religious significance. There are Old Testament references to Israel being "a brand plucked from the burning" (Zachariah 3:2 and Amos 4:11). In America, the phrase was made famous by Cotton Mather in his books about redeeming women from witchcraft, *A Brand Pluck'd Out of the Burning* and *Another Brand Pluckt Out of the Burning*,[21] and then by John Wesley who adopted the biblical phrase as a description of his own deliverance from danger (he was rescued from an arsonist's blaze as a child) and as a metaphor for spiritual salvation. Wesley requested the phrase "A brand plucked out of the burning" as his epitaph.

In Hawthorne's version, there is no plucking out, no rescue, no redemption. The narrative convention is aborted or reversed; hence the subtitle of the story: "A Chapter from an Abortive Romance." Hawthorne's Brand, claiming to have fulfilled his impious quest for the "Unpardonable Sin," triumphantly throws himself into the flames. His first name "Ethan" means "steadfast," and he does indeed hold to his world-obliterating intention.

How did Ethan Brand arrive at this paroxysm of misanthropy? Hawthorne suggests a surprising genealogy, tracing the development of misanthropy out of philanthropy. We are told that Brand began with "love and sympathy for mankind," and more especially with "pity for human guilt and woe." Like the reformers of "Earth's Holocaust," he sought to free men from their burdens. In Brand's case, it was human guilt in particular that he wanted to assuage or remove. The quest for the unpardonable sin was conceived as instrumental to that goal. While Hawthorne does not reveal the precise steps in Brand's reasoning, we might speculate that Brand was led to the thought that men will be plagued by guilt so long as they believe in the need for divine pardon. If there were an unpardonable act, one might move beyond guilt, beyond good and evil, beyond God. What Hawthorne does tell us is that Brand's quest (initially entered upon with reluctance) triggered a "vast intellectual development" which "disturbed the counterpoise between his mind and heart." He becomes "a cold observer, looking on mankind as the subject of his experiment, and, at length, converting man and woman to be his puppets, and pulling the wires that moved them to such degrees of crime as were demanded for his study." Whatever their crimes, they pale in comparison to Brand's. It is he, the manipulator, who becomes "a fiend."

In his ruthlessness and monomania, Ethan Brand is similar to Hawthorne's other experimenters and men of science. Aylmer in "The Birth-mark" and

21. For Hawthorne's knowledge of Mather, see John McElroy, "The Brand Metaphor in 'Ethan Brand,'" *American Literature*, Vol. 43, No. 4 (January 1972), 636 n. 5.

Rappaccini in "Rappaccini's Daughter" both put science before all else, conducting lethal experiments upon those dearest to them—a wife in one case, a daughter in the other. The only experiment of Brand's about which we learn any details involved a girl whom Brand "had made the subject of a psychological experiment, and wasted, absorbed, and perhaps annihilated her soul, in the process." In these men of science, even erotic and paternal love is subordinated to *libido sciendi*. As Hawthorne describes in the opening paragraph of "The Birth-mark," such ardent intellects believe that their pursuit "would ascend from one step of powerful intelligence to another, until the philosopher should lay his hand on the secret of creative force, and perhaps make new worlds for himself." While "The Birth-mark" and "Rappaccini's Daughter" trace the course of the experiments and the disastrous effects on the research subjects, "Ethan Brand" offers a more interior look at the consequences of "faith in man's ultimate control over nature." What does this ardency of intellect do to the scientist himself? As a result of the shift in perspective, one feels a compassion for Ethan Brand that one does not feel for Aylmer or Rappaccini. When Bartram and his son retire for the evening, leaving Brand to watch the fire, the boy "looked back to the wayfarer, and the tears came into his eyes; for his tender spirit had an intuition of the bleak and terrible loneliness in which this man had enveloped himself."

The climax confirms the boy's intuition. As the atheistic descendant of the Puritans, Brand embraces the hell-fire of the lime-kiln as the only element that will receive him. He no longer belongs to the human or natural order. The earth is no longer his "mother." His "frame" will not return to ashes and dust within her bosom. He no longer shares brotherhood with the rest of mankind. The "stars of Heaven" no longer draw him "onward and upward." The next morning, when the lime-burner checks his kiln, fearing that five-hundred bushels of lime have been spoilt by Brand's dereliction, he finds instead that "the marble was all burnt into perfect, snow-white lime," and "on its surface . . . —snow-white too, and thoroughly converted into lime—lay a human skeleton" with "the shape of a human heart" visible "within the ribs." Although perplexed that a man could have a marble heart, the practical Bartram judges that Brand's heart was "burnt into what looks like special good lime" and that he is "half a bushel the richer for him."

Hawthorne has chosen Brand's ironic fate carefully. The furnace has processed Brand into lime, one of mankind's oldest chemicals and a key ingredient in the manufacture of bricks. Brand has become the matter of technological production, rather than its master. Hawthorne's presentation of the literal reductionism of the scientific outlook anticipates C. S. Lewis, who spoke of a class of men he called "Conditioners":

> It is not that they are bad men. They are not men at all. Stepping outside the *Tao*, they have stepped into the void. . . . Man's final conquest has proved to be the abolition of Man.[22]

> [I]f man chooses to treat himself as raw material, raw material he will be.[23]

Hawthorne provides a brief sketch of an alternative vision of man, nature, and providence in his description of a restored and refreshed world on the morning after Brand's suicide:

> [Bartram] issued from the hut, followed by little Joe, who kept fast hold of his father's hand. The early sunshine was already pouring its gold upon the mountain-tops, and though the valleys were still in shadow, they smiled cheerfully in the promise of the bright day that was hastening onward. The village, completely shut in by hills, which swelled away gently about it, looked as if it had rested peacefully in the hollow of the great hand of Providence. Every dwelling was distinctly visible; the little spires of the two churches pointed upward, and caught a fore-glimmering of brightness from the sun-gilt skies upon their gilded weathercocks. The tavern was astir, and the figure of the old, smoke-dried stage-agent, cigar in mouth, was seen beneath the stoop. Old Graylock was glorified with a golden cloud upon his head. Scattered, likewise, over the breasts of the surrounding mountains, there were heaps of hoary mist, in fantastic shapes, some of them far down into the valley, others high up towards the summits, and still others, of the same family of mist or cloud, hovering in the gold radiance of the upper atmosphere. Stepping from one to another of the clouds that rested on the hills, and thence to the loftier brotherhood that sailed in air, it seemed almost as if a mortal man might thus ascend into the heavenly regions. Earth was so mingled with sky that it was a daydream to look at it.
>
> To supply that charm of the familiar and homely, which Nature so readily adopts into a scene like this, the stage-coach was rattling down the mountain-road, and the driver sounded his horn; while echo caught up the notes and intertwined them into a rich, and varied, and elaborate harmony, of which the original performer could lay claim to little share. The great hills played a concert among themselves, each contributing a strain of airy sweetness.

Here, instead of a man-made tower (or Cartesian project) to assault the heavens, we have a natural stairway to heaven amid the clouds and hills. Ascent is

22. C. S. Lewis, *The Abolition of Man* (New York: Harper Collins, 2001), 64. The "*Tao*" is Lewis's shorthand for the moral law.

23. Ibid., 72.

accomplished by poetic imagination rather than construction or dominion. The human world with its institutions—family, village, churches (note the plural), and tavern (complete with smokers)—fits within an encompassing natural order. Post-Babel, the communities of men have indeed been scattered, but they are in communication with one another—hence, the stage-coach. Men are not without devices and appliances, but they work in concert with nature, establishing a "rich, and varied, and elaborate harmony."

RING OF FIRE

The ancients spoke of a quarrel between the poets and the philosophers. In these three fire tales, Hawthorne enters that fray. Like Aristophanes ridiculing the "pre-Socratic" Socrates,[24] Hawthorne exposes the limitations of our modern votaries of science and technology. He uncovers the human costs of technological advance, the fallacy of the utopian belief in universal enlightenment, and the nihilism of the autarchic intellect. In each round, he reveals the threat to the Beautiful, at the same time that he defends common life and morality.[25] For Hawthorne, beauty and decency are allied. Henry James, in his wonderful biography of Hawthorne, says that "like almost all people who possess in a strong degree the story-telling faculty, Hawthorne had a democratic strain in his composition and a relish for the commoner stuff of human nature."[26] We today—the heirs of Romanticism—tend to think of the artist as a bohemian disdainful of bourgeois conventions. Hawthorne, however, belongs to an earlier and more ambitious tradition in which poetic wisdom argues for its superiority to philosophy and science and seeks to convey, through the craft of popular story, the truths of the human condition.

24. The Socrates of Aristophanes's *Clouds* is not the Platonic Socrates. He is a natural scientist, a thorough-going materialist who investigates such weighty matters as "how many of its own feet a flea could leap" and whether "gnats hum through their mouth or through their behind."

25. In one of his greatest stories, "The Artist of the Beautiful," Hawthorne delves deeply into the artistic temperament, its attitude toward ordinary life, and its chances for survival in a democratic age. While there is indeed a rivalry and profound spiritual difference between the two artisans of the story—one, the delicate "artist of the beautiful," the other the "Man of Iron," a brawny blacksmith—throughout, the real antagonist of the artist of the beautiful is not the simple mechanic but the sneering materialist: the blacksmith's father-in-law, a watchmaker by trade. One is tempted to read this father and son pair as emblems of science and technology (note, they are paired not by blood, but by law; in other words, their alliance is ratified by a specific political order). In the end, it is the grandson—in whom is combined the acrid skepticism of the grandfather and the raw strength of the father—who destroys the artist's production, endowed as it was with the "Mystery of Beauty."

26. Henry James, *Hawthorne*, in *Henry James: Literary Criticism, Essays on Literature, American Writers, English Writers* (New York: Library of America, 1984), 354.

12

Fraternity in *Antigone*

Paul W. Ludwig

I was born to join in love, not in enmity.

–Antigone to Creon

Students of Leon Kass will remember him saying (probably on more than one occasion) that the first brothers in the Hebrew Bible ended up in fratricide, and that Cain, the killer, founded the first city—just as Romulus killed Remus and founded Rome. In a similar way, the reciprocal fratricide of Antigone's brothers, Polyneices and Eteocles, fighting over the kingship of Thebes, sets the stage for the action of Sophocles's *Antigone*, a play in which a sister's love emerges as even more tragic than her brothers' rivalry. A clear-eyed view of the limitations of family love has always informed Leon Kass's public advocacy of the family's sanctity. It is with gratitude for his inspiration and teaching that I offer this exploration touching on one of his important themes.

What is brotherly love? Paradoxically, familial loves tie us to people whom we may not even like. Brothers are often not the people we take the most pleasure in being with. Yet we claim we "love" them. Fraternity is not primarily a friendship in the modern sense. The bond is often less affectionate than it is obligatory. We do not mind asking our brother for a favor where we would not wish to inconvenience a friend. A brother is obligated to help us in difficult circumstances, whereas we sometimes shrink from jeopardizing the freedom of a friendship. Crucially, brotherly love does not ask whether its object merits our love. It is an inclusive love, no respecter of persons—the brother may be bad or useless to himself and others, but we remain loyal to and stick up for a brother "because he is my brother." This inclusiveness of brotherly love is its great strength.

Perhaps because of this inclusiveness, fraternity has become a political metaphor.[1] Brotherhood can have universal connotations (e.g., the "brotherhood

1. E.g., "*Liberté, égalité, fraternité*," the slogan of the French Revolution. Compare Aristotle,

of man"), or it can be local or parochial. Muslims can say "sister" of strangers they meet who are Muslim, and evangelicals can say "our brother in Christ"; both refer to groups with insiders and outsiders. This tension between the universal and the parochial gives rise to a suspicion: Could fraternity's ability to love regardless of individual merit actually be predicated on its parochialness? That is, its apparent inclusiveness or openness may actually rely on exclusivity: members of the club are acceptable because they are insiders. Even the universal brotherhood of man may rely on "species pride." Sophocles's *Antigone* shows grave problems with fraternity that effectually place limits on what we can hope for from fraternity as a political metaphor, while at the same time vindicating the necessity—though not the goodness—of brotherly love.

The fratricide which generates the play's action would be enough to give us pause about brotherly love if it were not eclipsed by the beautiful example of Antigone's sisterly love. Yet the play carefully dissects her love. While the political metaphor of fraternity must take account of male rivalry, a sister's love for her brother is less rivalrous. Antigone's love better isolates—or provides a stricter test case for—the greatest possible love between siblings. Without looking at sisterly love, we might have believed that Polyneices's and Eteocles's sibling rivalry—perhaps artificially exaggerated by politics—clouded or masked the possibilities for fraternity. Yet Antigone's heroic love will prove to be an equally unworthy basis for the political metaphor. In the *Antigone*, two entities, the family and the polity, make incompatible claims, each vying for first place in citizens' hearts. Familial fraternity emerges as more basic and natural than political fraternity: the drama confers a partial vindication upon Antigone that Creon does not receive. But the play also exhibits the full horror of fraternal love when left to itself, untutored by civics. Antigone's embrace of her family spirals down into a black hole of Siamese twinship, incest, and suicide.

Civic Friendship

Creon in his maiden speech offers a theory of civic *philia*:

> Whoever thinks he has a better friend than his own fatherland, I hold him of no account. . . . I would never establish a man as my friend who was an enemy of the

---

Nicomachean Ethics 8.10, 1161a4-7, 8.11, 1161a25-31, where brotherly love is characteristic of citizens under a broad-based regime with a property qualification. Aristotle draws two more analogies between regimes and family loves: married couples' love is like the love between citizens in aristocracies, and parent-child love is like the love between king and subject.

> land. For I know that this [ship of state] is what saves us, and that it is through sailing upon her, upright, that we create friends for ourselves. (*Antigone*, 182-90)

The polis or fatherland is our "first friend," and our lesser friends—like the phantom friends of Plato's *Lysis*[2]—are determined by their instrumentality toward helping this first friend. Creon, thinking civically, says that we "make" (*poieumetha*) or "establish" (*theimên*) friends and loved ones. His language smacks of legislation or a business deal. Friendship is conventional, contractual. "Making" friends seems true of friendship proper but untrue of Greek *philia* in its larger sense. It leaves out brothers, sisters and other family members that we grow up stuck with. These are *philia*-relations, too. We cannot drop our fraternity when our brother joins the wrong side of a political question, or even when he raises an army and attacks our polity. We remain his brother, even if we disown him, in the sense that public opinion will still tie us to him.[3] Does Creon ignore the political fact that we are likewise stuck with our fellow citizens, whom we do not truly choose or make?

But Creon's blindness is sophisticated. Civic friendship may begin as a given we are stuck with, but it must become an active choice. It is true that the traitor grew up among us; he was one of us. But he revealed himself as someone we do not choose. For Creon, we make friends for ourselves "by means of our sailing" (*pleontes*, 190; the participle is ambiguous but richest if taken instrumentally) upon the upright ship of state.[4] We are doing more than passively riding a giant Leviathan, a beast which, if it goes under, we go under with it. We are working the oars. The peacefully working state is a condition for having friends, as Thucydides's description of Corcyra's descent into civil strife bears out.[5]

But in Hobbes's and Thucydides's accounts, private friends can free-ride, as it were, on the state. Creon's account goes further by disallowing the free ride: it is only by working together at the oars and the sails that we see who is helping the ship of state, who is not, who is loyal and who is a slacker. We actively deem them friends and enemies accordingly.

Such active choice is in tension with the passivity of family love. A brother is always already a part of us. Only dire circumstances introduce active choice into the fraternal relation, as when we are called to acknowledge our brother, or disown him. If your brother is the Unabomber, what do you do? Turn him

2. Plato, *Lysis* 219c-d. As we shall see, the view of *philia* arising out of the *Lysis* has many resonances with the *Antigone*, and may be the single best philosophic source for understanding both Antigone's fraternal love and Creon's civic friendship.

3. In anthropology, the common technical distinction is between "achieved" and "ascribed" relationships. Fraternity is ascriptive rather than achieved.

4. Cf. 158, 541, 715-17.

5. Thucydides 3.82-84.

in? Even today, when the ethic of helping friends (instead of, say, helping all "Others") seems parochial, many siblings would try to remonstrate with their brother first, get him to stop bombing, even if he already had blood on his hands. Partiality seems inherent in fraternity.

To combat this ethic, Creon proceeds to make his theory of friendship into a new law or custom (191). Citizens will henceforth be judged on whether they hold the polis to be the highest friend, and lesser friendships to be merely instrumental to it. This is strange because Creon seems to admit that at least one friendship (the "first friend") can be absolute, not relative. The polis requires absolute loyalty. Why cannot other friendships make absolute claims as well? His argument for the absoluteness of the polis-friendship is that the polis is what saves us (189). But is not the polis, conceived as a savior, merely instrumental to something else: each person's own salvation and security? In which case, the "first friend" of each individual would be himself or herself. Each maintains a "friendship" with the polis to preserve his or her life. On such assumptions, one could imagine a "secondary" friend whom an individual loves more than the polis, on whose behalf he might even betray the polis.

From this more individualistic perspective, the free-rider problem arises, although Antigone herself is too noble to recognize it. The polis is going to provide security for citizens no matter what any one citizen does. Why not piggy-back on the civic-mindedness of others, while privately valuing one's own friends even when they contribute nothing to the polis? This free-riding, broadly construed, is what Creon most fears. He anticipates that each citizen will be tempted to put his private welfare ahead of the public good. Although it is easy to forget, Creon happens to be blood kin to Polyneices, too. Creon leads by example; by forbidding burial of his own kin, Creon follows his own legal theory of civic friendship: civic allegiances first, family second. His later harshness toward Antigone stems in part from the fact that Antigone is his niece (659-62).[6] Creon must make an example of himself and her: his civic friendship entails an anti-nepotism campaign (cf. 486-90). Such nepotism is the main way he conceives of the conflict between public and private. In a way reminiscent of the economic assumptions that generated much of the modern literature on political free-riding, Creon is obsessed with monetary corruption.[7] Whenever he smells privacy being placed ahead of the commonweal, he falls into a paradigm of private "gain" in the narrow,

6. Though not, it must be noted, in the paternal line. Creon is Jocasta's brother, so Antigone and Creon can be considered as belonging to different kin groups. A wife marries out of her family into another family. We must consider the extent to which Antigone's love for her brother is her way of vindicating her father Oedipus and his line.

7. E.g., 221-22, 293-314, 1037, 1047, 1055, 1062.

economic sense. In his tirade at 293-314, Creon's words betray him because he wants to teach the guards that they should not "love" gain (*kerdainein philein*). But of course *love*—of something beyond gain—is actually what is behind the burial, not bribery, not corruption. Creon's political theory of public friendship has led him to an inadequate conception of private friendship.[8] He neglects the fact that private loves do not stay private but open out onto public concerns.

Creon's blindness to the larger dimensions of privacy becomes almost comical when he is confronted with Antigone, for whom graft and corruption are meaningless, obliterated by the blinding white light of her private fraternal bond. Creon's anti-corruption initiative does, however, adequately address the motives of some of his fellow citizens, e.g., the guard, who admits he would sell a friend (434-40). Antigone's outright confession gets the guard off the hook for negligence or corruption. The guard avers: "to have escaped from evils oneself is most pleasant; but to lead *philoi* into evils is painful. But it's in my nature to value all that less than my own salvation." The guard represents a Hobbesian lowest common denominator. He is a type which any political theory must account for. He acts out of fear and interest. Friendship counts a little too, but not enough to bank on. Only in a sense does the guard do what Creon's theory called for: he betrays his lesser friend when that friendship comes in conflict with the "first friend"—not the polity, but his own skin.

But in his way, the guard loves Antigone. Everyone loves a strong lover. The people of Thebes know she took care of her father in his exile. So long as the guard's interests are not threatened, he is free to admire devotion like hers, and he does. The whole city honors Antigone for burying her traitor brother (692-700). The chorus of nobles is pleased by her disobedience (504-505). Sticking up for our loved ones against the public good is publicly held to be admirable. This is a paradox that Creon cannot abide. People love her for doing the precise opposite of what Creon's program—and natural self-interest—jointly demand: they love her precisely for putting her private bonds ahead of the public. In this way, private loves are shown to transcend economics: in the minds of Antigone and others, some things (and people) are not for sale. Political theory must make room for these more idealistic passions that go beyond economics—and beyond safety.[9]

8. Tellingly, Creon casts acceptance of his rule not in terms merely of the relatively emotion-free civic friendship (*philia*) but even in terms of passionate affection, *storgê*: some men in the city "do not love me" (*stergein eme*; 292). Aristotle would later distinguish merely social *philia* without *storgê* from more personal *philia* with *storgê* (*Nicomachean Ethics* 4.6, 1126b20-24). It should be noted that *stergein* may also denote a less passionate sense of "bear with" or "acquiesce in."

9. Creon's city as "savior" shows other Hobbesian features in its implicit bargain. Citizens must risk their lives in defense of the city because it alone saves them. At 672, "anarchy" is the greatest evil. At 676, obedience to authority (*peitharchia*) saves the greatest number of bodies (*sômata*).

As if to emphasize the tension between Creon's new law of love and the fraternal love he inadequately conceives, Sophocles gives Creon a line dripping with dramatic irony: "And now, as brothers to these [laws], I have heralded proclamations" (192). If laws have brothers in the metaphoric sense (i.e., corollaries they cannot be separated from), do not people have brothers in the literal sense? The latter sense of fraternity is real and tangible; the legal sense is merely an analogy. The proclamations are that a literal brother, Eteocles, will be eternally separated from his brother, Polyneices. Is not real fraternity the basis for Creon's hopes about civic friendship? Unwittingly, Creon shows what is on his mind, shows his dim awareness of the opponent his new theory is going up against.

Families, it can be argued, are building-blocks of the polity; and therefore familial bonds must take precedence over civic ones. By contrast, if we adduce the quintessential republican act—Brutus's killing of his own sons when they betray the republic—we can muster more sympathy for what Creon is trying to do. Yet Creon's own title to rule is based on his nearness (174) of kinship to the deceased. The royal succession keeps the crown within the ruling household. Family life remains determinative of political life. Blood (*haima*) and its importance are, in fact, all over Creon's civic-friendship speech. Creon is led to mention the shared blood of all Thebans: Polyneices "wanted to feast on our common blood" (*haimatos koinou*; 201-202). The founding myth of Thebes is that all Thebans are related by blood. The dragon's teeth sown by Cadmus that sprang up into men (cf. 1124-25) mean that Thebans are autochthonous, sharing the earth as their mother. They are literally brothers. This is civic fraternity in the most concrete sense. But how real is it? From a rationalistic perspective perhaps alien to the play (although Sophocles was certainly familiar with it), the Theban belief in civic fraternity is "mythical" in the narrow sense of being literally untrue. But the mere fact that Thebes must make up a fictional blood tie for itself would give the lie to Creon's legal theory of contracting in and out of friendships according as they are useful to the polity.

If Creon hopes to lead the way toward civic virtue even when that entails sacrificing his relative Antigone, the play will force him to give up a nearer blood relative, his own son Haimon.[10] Fittingly, as though to remind Creon of what his friendship theory neglects, Haimon's name contains within it the notion of blood (*haima*).

Creon is unfazed by Haimon's contemplating suicide because, he opines, suicide would be superhuman (768). Death is the worst thing Creon can imagine. But how can he expect citizens to risk death in battle if death is the worst thing?

10. Intriguingly, Creon has already given up an elder son, Megareus (cf. 1303), who was literally sacrificed or sacrificed himself, on Teiresias's advice, to save Thebes. Creon is not simply a hypocrite unable to sacrifice.

FRATERNAL TOGETHERNESS

The things of friends are held in common.

–Greek proverb

When I read this play with students, I get caught in a bind. I want to point out the pathologies of Antigone's love. My students are all too ready to see her in the terms of modern psychology (e.g., she is "controlling"). But this prevents them from recognizing that Antigone is a *hero*. She makes lesser mortals like ourselves uncomfortable. You would not want Antigone for a sister (unless you were dead). In the same way you would not want Achilles or Heracles as a friend (or worse, as a husband—the problem in Sophocles's *Women of Trachis*). Heroes are divine or holy monsters. People around them tend to get crushed. Whose fault is that? So we have to prepare ourselves to see her pathologies as good—as aspects of her love. We should all love as Antigone loves, even though that would lead us to tragedy. The fact that our loves are "healthier" than hers just means we are ignoble. Antigone is the limiting case of fraternal love. She shows where our own lesser loves lead; she reveals what fraternal love is.

"Would real love kick a sister out of the family?" my students ask. For that is what Antigone does to Ismene. So I have to point out: "If you doubt it, then you disagree with Ismene herself." Ismene of all people has reason to find Antigone unloving; she bears the brunt of Antigone's anger. But what does Ismene say, right after Antigone has read her out of the family? For doing this, "you're rightly dear to your dear ones" (98-99). That is, for loving so much, it is right that your family love you back. Ismene still loves Antigone. She loves her more *because* Antigone now hates her. This is not virtue on Ismene's part. This is Ismene responding to virtue on Antigone's part.

Antigone's problem is evident from her opening line. She speaks of her sister's head as common (*koinon*) to the two of them. Young Antigone addresses her sister not by name alone but with a formal term of endearment: "head of Ismene." The head is the kissable part of a sister, the part one wishes to get close to by hugging. "Dear head" is the analogue in older English idiom. Antigone loves her sister very much, enough to pretend they share one head. This sharing is the very sign of friendship (or other *philia*), according to the proverb. The things of dear ones (*philoi*) are common (*koina*). When two people are that close, ownership does not fade away but becomes joint: what is mine is yours and what is yours is mine. Antigone goes beyond transferable property to body parts and selves.[11]

11. Mark Griffith *ad loc.* misses that "head of Ismene" is endearing, while correctly pointing out

But heads cannot be shared in common. Only Siamese twins are sometimes—horrifically—connected at the head. Imagery of monstrously-connected siblings is in fact ubiquitous in the play. Ismene's upcoming description of the deaths of the girls' brothers, Polyneices and Eteocles, who killed one another, will show that she (or more likely Antigone) conceives of them as one compound entity—a single, whole person that slew itself in a kind of suicide. The literalism of sharing body parts is not Sophocles's own but belongs to his characters. The ordinary feeling that "we sisters are in this together" becomes, for Antigone, "we sisters are one." Her language, at the very least, points up a problem with friendly and familial love: *philia* desires a togetherness which is thwarted by the physical separateness of bodies. Strong love like Antigone's will, in the limit, try to override those natural boundaries, or will cease to recognize them. She continues to regard Polyneices's remains as one with herself and Ismene. What can be said of Antigone from her opening line is that she loved much.

It might be objected that a prickly (not loving) Antigone takes her stand on principle and performs her heroic action not primarily out of familial love and loyalty (motivations especially proper to Greek women and girls), but rather on the principle that tyranny must be resisted, a motivation proper to all human beings but, for the Greeks, an especially masculine motivation. From a technical point of view, there is no reason to think of Greek fraternity as being loving at all. Modern anthropology distinguishes between ascriptive and achieved relationships. For Antigone and for the audience that viewed her, fraternity is clearly ascriptive. Greeks had to stand up for the philoi ascribed to them, as well as for philoi with whom they had achieved their relationships. This objection has much to recommend it and, taken together with the "strong love" interpretation (instead of in opposition to it), it will lead into the heart of the *Antigone*. Her attempt to "achieve" what is already ascribed to her is what makes Antigone unique. She takes her stand on the principle of kinship love.[12]

that the formula "head of X" is periphrastic for the whole self. The fact that such formulas indicate an elevated register in boilerplate tragic—or heroic—speech is not enough to exhaust Sophocles's intention: of the five Sophoclean usages Griffith cites, all but one occur in contexts explicitly laden with *philia*-language. *Oedipus at Colonus* 321, in particular, may be said to convey almost inexpressible longing for a loved one. Cf. *Antigone* 899. Some physicality seems to be implied by the head, and not merely "the marriage of true minds." See Mark Griffith, *Sophocles: Antigone* (Cambridge: Cambridge University Press, 1999).

12. Creon, at least, so interprets her stand, contemptuously relegating her to the Zeus of blood-kinship (*Dia xunaimon*, 658-59; for love see especially 523-25). It might be objected that Antigone takes her stand not so much on family love as upon the divine law. The source of the play's action would then be the conflict between divine law and Creon's human positive law (e.g., 449-60), rather than the conflict between family love and civic friendship. But the two readings do not conflict

Antigone's angry repudiation of her sister when the latter violates the principle of kinship love is in fact quite in keeping with the great, open secret about family love: its connectedness to angry passion.

This connection between anger and *philia* is only one of several grave indictments in the play's presentation of Antigone's sisterly love. Scholars have been slow to see how the play could criticize Antigone at all: her evident nobility and Creon's evident tyranny have made it seem obvious that the play is "on Antigone's side," however complex its championing of her might be. At their most critical, scholars who admire Antigone for her heroism perceive that she—like such male heroes as Heracles and Achilles—has a nature difficult for lesser mortals to love. I will argue that her unlovableness needs to be connected, philosophically, with her ardently loving nature.[13] What is the connection between loving much and becoming unlovable?

---

as much as appears: the content of the divine law Antigone upholds is kinship loyalty. The content of Creon's positive law is civic friendship. It is true that Teiresias partially vindicates Antigone's claims about the unwritten laws of the gods: Creon has mixed up above and below, burying a live person and keeping a corpse up here that belongs to the gods below (1068-70). "You [Creon] have no business with such things, nor do the upper gods" (1072-73). Teiresias clearly demarcates spheres of influence. The chthonic gods mind burials and family matters, while the Olympians' sphere is civic; Creon has confused these. "Therefore the maimers, late-destroying Furies of Hades and the gods lie in wait for you" (1074-75). But Teiresias's own theology shows that the claims of neither sphere can override the other's. In other circumstances we see the Olympians enforcing their claims over the chthonic gods, even putting them in their place. For example, in Aeschylus's *Eumenides* those same Furies who avenge family murders are literally sent underground—given a new job—by Athena, who subordinates them to a new civic order. It is not clear that Antigone's claims, if followed to their logical conclusion, would not represent an encroachment by the chthonic gods on the civic gods' sphere just as problematic as Creon's reverse encroachment. As Creon rightly exclaims of the civic gods: "Could they honor as a benefactor/ . . . this man who came to burn the pillars of their temples and their votive offerings,/ to scatter their land and their laws?" (284-87). Creon has gods on his side, too. Thus the religious struggle—between the two types of gods—seems not so much to eclipse the struggle between family love and civic friendship as to show another dimension of it. The gods are divided over this tension just as humans are. The basic tension between polis and household is inscribed into Greek theology itself.

13. Ruby Blondell tries out different ways of resolving this problem. First, she sees historical differences between Greek *philia* and our modern concept of love: the Greek concept need not imply any tender feeling, and Antigone does not love her brother as an individual (Ruby Blondell, *Sophocles' Antigone* [Newburyport, Massachusetts: Focus, 1998], 76-77). But as we shall argue, the play itself points out that fraternal love is not a love of the individual. This latter turns out to be a problem with all *philia*, as the *Lysis* also implies (205b9). It would be a historicist error to assume, without proof, that Greek love was never for individuals while we ourselves have achieved that aspiration. The truth may be that Greeks, like us, wished for *philia* to become a love for individuals while Greek authors were more honest about the human inability to achieve it (cf. Pascal, *Pensées*, 688 [323], "*Q'est-ce que le moi?*"). Later, Blondell sees Antigone's prickliness as adding "complexity" (90-91). The latter explanation would assume that theatrical verisimilitude trumps the revealing of human nature in Sophocles's intention. Needless to say, accurately revealing human nature might be a way of achieving theatrical verisimilitude anyway.

"You can never lose your family." This oft-heard sentiment captures Ismene's sensible opinion about their dead brother. Ismene thinks she will still be Polyneices's brother even if she does not come to his aid. Conventionality continues to link the names of brothers even after they kill each other, as Polyneices and Eteocles did. Cain is forever the brother of Abel whom he killed. The fraternal tie does not require active choice. If they fail to bury Polyneices, even if they betray his memory, they can still sue for his forgiveness in the land of the dead (65-67). On a spectrum of activity and passivity, Creon's "making *philoi*" occupies the active pole, while Ismene's assurance that *philia* endures regardless of action or inaction represents the passive pole.

Does the fraternal tie compel us to acts of brotherly love? Or does the very strength of the bond render active love unnecessary? Antigone believes that brothers and sisters are tied together; that is why betrayal is unthinkable. Ismene agrees with the premise but draws the opposite conclusion. We remain tied even if we do nothing. Attitudes such as hers can be made ridiculous with examples such as, "You can throw your daughter out on the street, but she is still your daughter." Unloving behavior un-sisters us; it makes us less than family towards our loved ones. Antigone's own contradiction is something like the following. A brother is a brother no matter what he did; fraternity is independent of actions. But I cannot be a sister unless I take action; fraternity (sorority) is dependent on actions. So fraternity is both dependent on and independent of actions.

Their descriptions of the brothers' deaths contain the most telling information about the sisters' assumptions, especially in comparison to Creon's descriptions of the same event. Ismene and Antigone emphatically use the grammatical dual number to describe the brothers (a pair of brothers) and to refer to themselves: a pair of sisters.[14] The two hands with which the brothers struck each other merge into one "double hand" in Ismene's language (*diplêi kheri*). Creon's account unwittingly goes further: the brothers used the "same hand" to murder themselves (*autokheir*; 172). Sophocles plays upon ordinary Greek usage, which made little distinction between murdering kinfolk and committing suicide (cf. 1175, 1315).[15] Creon wishes to point out that Polyneices

14. Perhaps it would be more accurate to say that Ismene falls in with Antigone's way of speaking about pairs; cf. line 3 with lines 12-14; cf. 21.

15. *Autokheir* is not enough to distinguish suicide from kin-murder, as when the messenger announces: "Haimon is dead; and by that very hand (*autokheir*) his blood is shed." But "very hand" is not enough to denote a suicide for the Chorus, who need more information: "By which hand—his father's or his own (*oikeias*)"? To get at what is really Haimon's own hand, the Chorus are forced to resort to "one's own," the language of the household (the adjective *oikeios* is cognate with *oikos* and *oikia*, house and home). If the reader is sensitive to the etymology, this new

and Eteocles simultaneously incurred pollution, each one by slaying a brother "with same hand *miasma*." Without modifiers *autokheir* often denotes "acting alone."[16] Greek popular opinion wanted to know which physical hand incurred the pollution.[17] But Sophocles's etymologizing poetry[18] gets at something quite different. The mutual fratricide was actually a joint suicide. Relatives are so close, the language implies, they might as well be you. Brothers are invisibly joined at the hip, or at the head. Brothers are part and parcel of one another; they are a family's "members." It was not two people who slew each other at all, but rather a single, composite entity that slew itself. Polyneices and Eteocles can no more be separated in burial than if they were Siamese twins. Creon, crucially, avoids the grammatical dual number in describing the brothers. The dual would make them a pair, so Creon speaks instead in the plural. Brothers are not so joined at the hip that they must always be considered together, he seems to imply. Witness their own strife against one another. But the dualness or doubleness (*diplês*) of their fate seems to join them even as it divides them.[19]

This imagery of doubles and sames, taken together with Antigone's "common head," reminds modern readers of the circle-people in Aristophanes's myth in the *Symposium*. The circle-people were also double people, pairs or combinations of male-male, male-female and female-female persons melded together. They had faces front and back, and double the number of hands, feet, and limbs. The origin of love occurred when Zeus punished the circle-people for hubris by splitting them into individual humans as we know them today. Each half of the original pair longs to rejoin with its other half, restlessly seeking and finding peace only in bonding with a person like that half.

---

adjective merely multiplies the possible culprits by spreading the blame throughout the whole household, with the father, of course, as the prime suspect. Finally, to settle the question once for all, the messenger repairs to the original language of self and same: "He himself [did it] of his own self, enraged at his father" (*autos pros hautou*; 1175-77). But from the standpoint of the cognates Sophocles is punning on, the *autos* can hardly be said to clear up the matter of who is guilty of striking the actual blow: the original ambiguity lay precisely in the *autos* (of *autokheir*).

16. For blame or credit: at line 900, Antigone uses *autokheir* to claim all the credit, in the afterlife, for the burial: *sc.* "I and no other did it." Hence Seth Benardete plays with interpreting line 1's curious "*autadelphon*" and its subsequent occurrences as "sister [or brother] and nothing but." If Ismene turns out to be anything other than a sister, she will be no sister at all in Antigone's eyes. Seth Benardete, *Sacred Transgressions* (South Bend, Indiana: St. Augustine's Press, 1998).

17. E.g., Creon rejects the report that his wife Eurydice killed herself *autokheir* (1315), saying "No, it was I, I killed her. . . . / I really truly affirm it" (1319-20). His repetitions show the weight of the popular opinion, interested in individual pollution, which he must argue against.

18. See Nicolas Gross's commentary on lines 51 and 52 for Sophocles's "etymologizing" of *auto*-cognates. Nicolas P. Gross, *Bryn Mawr Commentaries: Sophocles' Antigone* (Bryn Mawr, Pennsylvania: Thomas Library, 1988).

19. Creon, too, is forced to recognize this doubleness in them. He says that the brothers "from a double fate on one and the same day, die, both striking and being struck" (170-72).

Antigone's conception of brotherly love is very like the "togetherness" of the circle-people before being split into two, except that in seeking an image for family togetherness, she happens on an image appropriate for eros.

A moment's reflection on duality and doubleness reveals deep problems with the fraternal unity or solidarity to which Antigone's conversation with her sister aspires. Although duality means connectedness, it does not mean unity. Rather, duality implies difference. Things that go together in pairs could not be said to go together at all unless they first were two. When making her proposal to Ismene that they bury their brother together, Antigone speaks in the language of *sun-* cognates (literally "with"), implying the joining of two things together to make one—rather than finding them already existing as a pair. "See if you will join in the labor and join in the deed" (41). When Ismene fails to see or feigns failure to see what Antigone is driving at, Antigone spells it out: "If you will raise up the dead [*sc.* for burial], joining with this hand" (43). The actor playing Antigone at this point probably raised a hand. The allegedly natural pair of brothers worked with a "double hand," the "same hand" and each other's hands, but what was one double and joint hand for the brothers is comprised of two, separate single hands for the sisters. Antigone needs Ismene to join hands with her, to *make* the doubleness (just as Creon said we "make" or create friends). Sisters' hands do not naturally exist as pairs with each other, any more than brothers' do. Will and choice are needed to make one conjoined or double hand out of two single ones.

Antigone asserts that Creon has no part in "keeping me from my own [*sc.* family]" (*tôn emôn*, 48). But external enemies and resistance (like Creon or the city) are the least of the problems of familial love. What about when family members themselves refuse to be "her own" anymore? Ismene is this minute resisting Antigone, failing to live up to what Antigone thinks family loyalty entails—to say nothing of Eteocles's resistance against Polyneices. The supreme irony is that Polyneices himself has already crossed each of Antigone's sacred moral thresholds. Polyneices betrayed and slew his brother. How can it be true that brothers are a part of us, or that we and our siblings make up a larger whole, if such self-division and internecine strife is possible? Of what importance are blood ties, when Polyneices could be so different from the blood he shared? He wanted to feast on that blood (as Creon hyperbolically points out; 201-202), to eat his own blood. Blood emerges as next to worthless for keeping behavior in line. Family members' wills are crucial, because they can move out, never write, never call.

Ismene, as if to retort, Your own! Let me tell you about your own—*our* own!—launches into a desperate and impassioned diatribe against their family ties. By cataloguing the Labdacids' self-inflicted tragedies, Ismene hopes to make Antigone see reason (49, 58, 61, 68). She stresses the illicit dualness, the illicit togetherness of their family—the closeness which became incestuous. "Think, sister, about our father [Oedipus]"—Ismene uses the dual for "our"—"How he died hated and infamous,/ For self-detected misdeeds striking his two-fold (*diplas*)/ Organs of sight by himself with self-working hand (*autos autourgôi kheri*)" (49-52), referring to Oedipus's self-blinding.[20] Still unspoken is the incest that was half the motivation for Oedipus's action. But first comes suicide in Ismene's crescendo: "Next, [Jocasta] . . . with/ Plaited fastenings disfigured her life." Jocasta hanged herself only in response to a far graver misdeed among kin, which Ismene glances at with a shudder. "[His] mother and [his] wife—a double name" (*sc.* for the same person; *diploun*, 53-54). Doubleness or dualness stems here from Oedipus's unwitting marriage to his mother. Ismene levels a broadside right at Antigone's embrace of pairing and togetherness. The sisters share a brother who was never supposed to be a brother to them: their own father. So much for your brotherhood, Ismene implies.

Oedipus's brothers Eteocles and Polyneices bear the family stamp. Ismene reaches her climax: "[Our] two brothers, a pair, on one and the same day,/ Self-slaughtering, those poor wretches, worked out their/ Common destiny by [using] each another's hands" (55-57). The *auto*-prefix of "self-slaughter" reduces kin-murder to suicide, as per ordinary Greek assumptions: "by killing the other, each killed himself."[21] But here the imagery of double-people takes on a new dimension: not only did they commit suicide, but each used the hand of the other to do it (*epallêloin kheroin*).[22] To use someone else's hand implies a voluntarism or agency over that hand that is not naturally given. I cannot make your hand slay me unless we share a central nervous system. The imagery here is of brothers so monstrously conjoined that even their rivalry bears witness to a single house divided, a single self divided.

Antigone's brotherly love causes her to embrace a fratricide. The principle of loyalty to a brother becomes questionable—and theoretically interesting—when the loyalty is toward a disloyal brother, a kin-murderer, a traitor to the family as well as to the state. In this way, the play radically undercuts the normal

20. Here the word "double" (*diplas*) is finally used of an unequivocally natural pair, eyes. Unlike sisters, eyes come in pairs without the need for human will or intervention. But their natural duality only throws into relief the unnatural wish and human intervention required to poke out both at once. "Self-working" carries a connotation of rudeness or rusticity (farmers work with their own hands): like a farmer, Oedipus willingly stooped to "get his hands dirty" in the gore from his own eyes.

21. Blondell's translation captures this: "both killed /themselves in one another."

22. Here I follow Gross's translation in the Bryn Mawr commentary over Kamerbeek and Jebb.

reasons for burying a brother: he requited our love, he was good, he served his family and country well, we want to preserve the memory of his actions. All such motives could as well apply to forms of *philia* other than brotherhood. By removing or reversing these red herrings, the play isolates fraternal love *per se*, or gets at the heart of brotherly love in itself.

What are brothers and on what does our love for them depend? It emerges that they are mere members of a shared commonality (much as citizens are). Their essence or brotherness is predicated on nothing other than their membership in the family. This calls into question the natural ground of brotherhood. No attraction necessarily exists to form the link between siblings. Common upbringing, time spent together, closeness in age, and biological similarities may lead them to cherish the same things, and each other. But brothers remain brothers regardless of whether this further "friendship" develops or not.[23] This is especially revealing insofar as brothers are given to one another by the most natural of means. Birth marks the beginning and the end of nature's work in fraternity, and this shows the largely conventional nature of brotherhood. We deem people brothers and sisters merely because of accident of birth. Regardless of what develops after birth, we continue to deem them brothers or sisters. Brotherhood *per se*, brotherhood without friendship in addition, is almost as conventional as citizenship.

Will conventionality be enough for Antigone's fraternal love? Or will she seek some more natural tie to vindicate her blood connection? To repeat: her attempt to achieve what is already ascribed to her is what makes Antigone unique.[24] Most people never have to face such an overwhelming reason to repudiate their own. Our families are just givens. Antigone's active position is that brotherhood must be achieved, vindicated. But in her attempt to find a

23. To these considerations, Aristotle adds that "All kinship love derives from paternal love. . . . [B]rothers [love] each other because they sprang from the same [parents]. Their sameness with [the parents] makes them the same as each other" (*Nicomachean Ethics* 8.12, 1161b17-32; cf. 1162a9-16). In context, Aristotle implies that parents love children most, children love parents some but less, and children love each other only to the extent they first love their parents. As we shall see, Antigone's love for Polyneices will have everything to do with vindicating her love for Oedipus and Jocasta, her ill-fated parents.

24. As Benardete points out, Antigone is unique in that she wants to prove "by deed" "her right to be . . . what she already is by birth. She reconstitutes the family as something into which one freely enters. The love of her own almost becomes a matter of choice." Seth Benardete, *Sacred Transgressions*, 12-13. But one wonders if the love of one's own is ever found in such a pure form as Benardete imagines it. Do not most humans have to affirm their belongings—at some point—in order to keep them, vindicate their tie to them? Nothing is mine so much as my foot or hand, and only dire circumstance can lead me to want them amputated. But brothers are less my own than that. At some point one has to make them one's own. The pure love of one's own may be a thought-experiment, a category of analysis rather than a real existent.

deeper core of brotherhood, Antigone will arguably leave the realm of brotherly love behind. I will argue that this is what all *philia* wants without being able to deliver: to love by choice rather than as a result of happenstance belonging. For all her strangeness, Antigone's desire is paradigmatic. No human being can be fully comfortable with loving *philoi* merely because they are ascribed to us as "ours." We want them to be good, to be lovable, attractive. Her wish to make family into real friends, though extreme in her own case, is not atypical and speaks volumes about the limitedness of familial love.

ANGER AND MANLINESS

Ismene considers Antigone's plan to be masculine, the theme so interesting to modern readers. "You must get it into your head . . . that we are a pair of women/ In our nature not intended to fight against men" (61-62). Ismene's appeal to the (collective) nature of women answers Antigone's demand that Ismene show whether her (individual) nature is noble or base (38). You are judging me by a masculine standard, Ismene implies. I am no worse than the next woman, and you should not try to be more than woman—more than what you are. There is no suggestion in the text that Antigone sees herself as striking a blow for women as such. This is important because her antagonist Creon certainly does cast their conflict into anti-woman, battle-of-the-sexes terms repeatedly. Good order for him means not letting women get the upper hand: in this he merely follows a lesser-known Delphic rule (e.g., 679-80, 578-79, 746, 756).[25] The play's feminism, if such it is, was thus far more highly provocative for its original audience than it is for us: Creon in "keeping woman under rule" is *doing the right thing* in the minds of the intended viewers. A far finer discernment on Creon's part would be required to enable him to accede to this feminine request.

Antigone in her singlemindedness finds all such class or identity-group considerations irrelevant. She does not vindicate the capacities or nature of women except obliquely, insofar as she shows what one woman is capable of. The stand Antigone takes is not a stand on behalf of any group: not women, not families, certainly not "the family."[26] Her stand is wholly peculiar to *her own* family (see again *tôn emôn*, line 48). She claims her conduct is "a beautiful thing (*kalon*)—for me to die doing this" (72).[27]

25. "Know thyself. Nothing overmuch. Keep woman under rule." Blondell brings out beautifully how Creon becomes feminized in his tragedy—he who wanted to remain masculine (103).

26. I disagree with Peter Euben's attempt to make Antigone a modern class-representative ("Antigone and the Languages of Politics"). See J. Peter Euben, *Corrupting Youth* (Princeton: Princeton University Press, 1997), 139-78.

27. Note the similarity with patriotic language: cf. Tyrtaeus, *tethnamenai gar kalon*. See M. L.

Here her intention approaches the standard of male heroes, who usually oriented their conduct by what was considered *kalon* and what would win them honor in the polis. Her intention of "lying down" (73) with the dead has nothing conscious to do with incest (on which see below) but rather echoes Achilles's resolve to die—and "lie down"—after having first won glory.[28] She desires to win immortal fame (e.g., 97, 501-504; *eukleesteron kleos* 502, cf. 695). *Kleos* is the Homeric hero's motivation par excellence. For men, helping *philoi* went beyond mere kin to include comrades in battle and civic "friends" in political and economic alliances. Merely familial loyalty was considered dangerous and anti-republican, the cause of nepotism, factionalism, and the privileging of private gain over public loyalty (Creon's chief worry). Spartan women were forbidden to mourn in public for their lost loved ones after the Spartan defeat at Leuctra; the private losses were not to overshadow the public exigencies. For similar reasons Pericles in his funeral oration enjoins the women of Athens to keep silence, in part to prevent public mourning. The same *topos* becomes explicit in the *Antigone* at 1246-50, when the messenger hopes Eurydice will not mourn her son in public but will keep it indoors: the queen has too much experience and judgment to make such a mistake, he opines. Thus the position of women within the polis was ambiguous: women were thought capable of sharing in some measure the masculine goals of restraint and conditional love, but the very fact that the Spartans, Pericles, and the messenger have to bring this topic up means that women were viewed as being less attached to the public and more attached to the private family. For a man to do what Antigone does—on behalf of a traitor brother—would be far more questionable than for a woman. Antigone is showing loyalty and love towards an immediate family member, just as women are supposed to. She believes that the polis—meaning primarily the males of the polis—will honor her, not for being a masculine woman (why would they do that?) but precisely for being all that a woman should be toward her family.

Nevertheless, Ismene knows Greek norms as well as anyone, and she perceives what Antigone is proposing to be utterly masculine. To dare all on behalf of a principle, to fight with men—to the death if need be—is manly. Putting one's family ahead of the city may be a feminine thing to do, but taking a stand is in itself masculine. Antigone takes a masculine stand on a feminine principle, and this creates a paradox. Perhaps any single principle—even the feminine principle

West, ed., *Iambi et elegi Graeci* (Oxford: Clarendon Press, 1989-1992).

28. *Keisom' epei ke thanô· nun de kleos esthlon aroimên* (*Iliad* 18.121; Jan Kamerbeek *ad loc.* citing Bernard Knox, *The Heroic Temper*, 51). See Jan C. Kamerbeek, *The Plays of Sophocles. Commentaries. Part III, The Antigone* (Leiden: Brill, 1978).

of kinship love—if asserted over all other moral imperatives, would require manliness (in its primary sense of courage, *andreia*) to stick to it. In this way, masculinity would be the condition that enables feminine principles to exist. But the play will go on to show how the feminine attachments of the household are the condition which makes the political, and masculinity itself, possible.

There are deep connections among ardent love, pride, and anger. Antigone's cold anger in repudiating her sister seems of a piece with her masculine domination of her sister. Everything that could make Antigone seem unloving comes together in a few lines. Ismene concludes that she, at least, will obey authority: to do extravagant deeds is mindless. In Antigone's answer, the door simply shuts. As of this moment, Antigone no longer has a sister:

> I wouldn't even ask you to. And if you were later to wish
> To do it, I wouldn't agree to let you do it with me.
> Be whatever you want. I am going to bury him. (69-72)

One senses the controlled rage underneath Antigone's words. The coldness of her anger shows that her rage is sublimated into steely resolve. The loss of hoped-for support from her sister sharpens, rather than dulls, her spirit. Instead of despairing or breaking down, she sucks it up. Her ability to carry on is predicated on her resentment. Her ability to banish the demons of weakness in her own soul is a concomitant of casting out the weak Ismene who stands before her. Antigone has spirit: she is fed up and she is not going to take it any more.

This is *thumos* in several of Plato's senses.[29] Rage is implicitly connected to manliness in the tradition and, in Plato and Aristotle, explicitly so. The anger (*mênis*) of Achilles is a condition of his winning deathless fame; without getting fed up at the Achaean leadership, Achilles would never have sat out of the Trojan War, turning its tide when he reentered. His anger, first at his fellow Greeks, then at Hector (killer of his *philos*, Patroklos), was the basis of his *kalon* action. Anger at bereavement and anger at injustice are thus further points of comparison between Antigone's heroism and epic male heroism. Anger is also the prickly trait that makes heroes difficult to love.

But why anger at a *philos*? Antigone's anger at Ismene is indicative of love betrayed. As Aristotle argues in *Politics* 7.7, quoting Archilochus, it is not against strangers but "against loved ones (*philoi*) that the heart is choked with rage."

29. The fully political sense of *thumos* is not in the tradition, of course, until Plato's *Republic*. For the word as used in the play, compare 718, 1088, 1254 (anger or rage) with 1097 (soul or proud soul); Blondell's translation correctly conveys that it is Creon's pride that makes it hard for his soul to yield. Plato brings these apparently unrelated senses of anger and pride into relation.

"Those who love excessively will hate excessively too." The reason, he says, is that *thumos* is more aroused against friends than against unknown people, when it deems itself slighted. This is a proof, for Aristotle, that *thumos* actually "creates love; it is the power of soul by which we feel affection." That is, the "indomitable" and "ruling" element in the soul, the element or power responsible for pride and anger, is also responsible for *philia*.

Antigone's love and her honor become intermingled in much the same way as sacrificing for comrades becomes part and parcel of winning honor in the heroic code. She will vindicate her fraternal bond. The suggestion of reactiveness and even vengefulness implicit in our term "vindicating" may be taken as clues to what *philia* is (rather than as a surmountable problem peculiar to one young girl). Antigone's anger at Ismene is only the flip side of her love. As much as Ismene is now hated for betraying the family, just so much would she have been loved for remaining loyal to it. The tight bonds that insiders feel is, from another perspective, the resistance and exclusion that outsiders feel. Strong hate is the concomitant of strong love.

Antigone perhaps misses the irony that she comes close to Creon's position on civic friendship when she casts out the traitor to her family in much the same way as Creon casts out the traitor to the city. Brotherly love is not unconditional love, for Antigone. One has to earn one's keep, merit one's membership. Likewise in Creon's idea of citizenship: mere membership is not enough—working the oars leads to a choice about who belongs and who does not. Here we see both antagonists attempting to transcend the mere "thrownness" of *philia*. But surely Creon is closer to the truth in holding that citizenship involves choice than is Antigone in holding that brotherhood involves choice. In its unconditionality, Antigone's love is quintessentially a woman's: standing up for family members whatever their public wrongdoing. But her conditional stance toward Ismene is just the opposite. Conditional love is a masculine trait: show me, earn my respect. How do the feminine and masculine aspects of Antigone's love fit together?

Antigone's challenge is out of keeping with modern conceptions of love as care or concern, in which the beloved's own best interest (often conceived as comfort) is placed uppermost. Antigone's prickliness here also pushes the envelope of some Greek conceptions of *philia*, which at their most idealistic also aimed to love the friend for his or her own sake.[30] Not comfort but nobility is Ismene's own best interest in the view of Antigone, who challenges her to be noble, to be brave.[31]

30. *Nicomachean Ethics* 8.2, 1155b31-32. Contrast 9.8, 1168a27-1168b11.

31. Cf. *Nicomachean Ethics* 9.8, 1169a32-34, where it is even nobler to be the cause of a friend's

The selfishness inherent in Antigone's pride reveals a contradiction at the heart of *philia*, a contradiction that in turn explains why it is difficult to love someone who loves so ardently. The desire to "take someone in hand" is proper to *philia*. Household *philia* and feminine loving behavior recapitulate, in their smaller sphere, the masculine political goals of honor and recognition. *Philia* makes the subject wish to be useful to her dear ones. She wants to "do for them," in older American dialect. The work mothers and sisters traditionally did for sons and brothers was to all appearances a sacrifice in the interest of the beloved: cooking hot meals, sewing clothing. Each gift expected nothing in return but recognition. But the wish for recognition is a huge string attached. When the food is hot, the loved ones had better be present at the supper table in order to be properly appreciative. The sewing sister has already picked out the style of garment she makes for her brother. Will he wear it? If he does not, it is a rebuke, a slap in the face of her love. The beloved must submit to a gentle yoke of control.

If there is competition among sisters to "do for" the family, the one who loves strongest may push the others aside, or organize them according to her will. Having the honor of being the one to serve is a way of finding recognition even in menial tasks. A modern viewpoint might argue that the strongest love would give the others "space" to do their thing, but that would be strong care or concern rather than strong *philia*. To manifest itself, ordinary *philia* must *sacrifice* for the beloved—"make much of" him, in the language of the *Lysis*.[32] But to sacrifice effectively, *philia* must control certain aspects of the situation, including the beloved.

Thus in a real sense, *philia* promises more than it can deliver. *Philia* wants to put the interest of the beloved uppermost—wishes to be, in this regard, like concern or care in the modern lexicon. Yet in actual practice, *philia* rarely if ever achieves this exalted aim. The self asserts itself, in *philia*-relations, in backdoor ways.[33] *Philia*—no less than eros albeit in very different ways—is a domineering passion.

Antigone's extreme of love shows love's darker side. Only the living retain the power to disappoint our love. This is one reason why she loves her cold, dead brother more than her warm, living sister. The *philos* Polyneices can deliver on his (unspoken) promise to be *semper fi* only in death, only in an afterlife. In life he betrayed her trust, but now that he is safely dead he is forever faithful. If the *Lysis* is any guide, death has a second connection to Antigone's

---

noble action than to perform the noble action all by oneself.

32. *Lysis* 219d5-220a1.

33. The *Nicomachean Ethics* is explicit: all other-love is an extension of self-love (9.8, 1168b5-7).

philia. Our sacrifice—our "making much"—only becomes perfected when the beloved is beyond help. Only when all is in vain—as when the beloved has already died[34]—does our sacrifice fully vindicate our love, show us draining the last drop of our devotion, show us loving for its own sake, for no useful aim. Giving one's life only seems to be the highest form of sacrifice; giving it in vain is truly highest. This is because *philia qua* identity feels perfectly vindicated only when purged of every utilitarian aspect.

Sacrifice is what the law demands, too, including Creon's new law of civic friendship. Eteocles gets full-dress honors for sacrificing himself for Thebes. Never mind that his devotion was shot through and through with his own utility as he hung on to his turn to sit on the throne. Civic memory covers over all such flaws, remembers what it wants to remember. Only failure to remain alive, only giving that "last full measure," can fully vindicate devotion. The Lincolnian language points to the discrepancy between friendship understood as utility and friendship understood as, at bottom, the affirmation of an identity, in this case a civic identity. If you remained alive, you probably sacrificed the commonweal's good to your own utility. Only death can prove your love was the greatest it could be ("Greater love hath no man than this: that he lay down his life for his friend"). The *Lysis*, too, suggests this connection between *philia* and what we would call the "politics of recognition" or "identity politics." Briefly, Socrates is first attracted into a conversation about *philia* when he hears a minor character opine that true love is attracted to a person's individuality (*idion* 205b). Such individuality would be unique to each case and therefore ineffable and impossible to philosophize about. By resolutely attempting to reduce *philia* to utility instead, Socrates isolates the degree to which we all wish to honor our own by making them uniquely valuable or irreplaceable, and to honor ourselves by joining such unique company.

An indication of this is Antigone's open desire to get caught.[35] Ismene, fearing for her sister's life, enjoins her to tell no one else of her plan: "Hide it in

34. We see a similar thought in Phaedrus's speech in the *Symposium*: dying "on behalf of" (*huper-*) someone is noble, but dying "after someone" (*ep'-*) is truly excellent (180a1-2). The prefixes to *apothanein* show Phaedrus's fine distinctions in self-sacrifice. I am indebted to Philip Stadter for this point.

35. In her private justification of her Sisyphean task to Ismene, she says she will do all she can, and the limits of what she can do will only reveal themselves in the moment of truth. "Whenever my strength fails me, [there] I will have stopped" (91). The future perfect tense and aspect look to the uncertainty—*ex ante*—of how far she can get, together with an admission of the absoluteness of that unknown boundary which she will only know when she comes up against it, i.e., *ex post*. But Ismene nails her with "Yet it's unseemly to look for things [to do] that are impossible from the beginning (*archên*)—i.e., things they both know *ex ante* are impossible (92). Antigone's eros for the impossible is a death wish. Her wish to express her *philia* is a death wish. Only by giving her life can she recoup the family honor, get her own back.

secrecy, and I will do likewise." But Antigone is seething by this point and replies: "Tell it out! Much more my enemy will you be/ By keeping silent, if you do not announce it to all and sundry" (86-87). This is doubly perverse because secrecy is doubly crucial. Obviously, the only way Antigone can escape punishment is through secrecy, but the very success of her enterprise also demands secrecy. Her first sprinkling of dust over the corpse is possible only because the body is inadequately guarded, i.e., no one really expected anyone to attempt burial. After the authorities efface her first burial, her capture—in attempting a second burial—is virtually certain. And then her burial will be effaced again, this time permanently. Without secrecy, Antigone will fail. Antigone wants to fail. She should plot and scheme, but Antigone is seeing red. She wants to get caught: only through total self-sacrifice can she adequately "make much of" Polyneices. Like the father whose son drank hemlock in the *Lysis*, she needs to show herself and everyone else that the beloved is "worth everything"[36]—even when he is not. The utility view of *philia* would say "Make the most of the time you have left with Ismene—and with Haemon." The identity or recognition view of *philia* says: "Sacrifice yourself and show by your death how much you loved."

SUICIDE AND INCEST

The Chorus witlessly opine that no one is so stupid as "to be in love with death" (*erais thanein*). The wages of disobedience, as Creon says, is death (220-21). But to Ismene, Antigone is already "in love with the impossible" (*amêchanôn erais*; 90), and the Chorus are so surprised to see Antigone led in as the culprit that she first appears to them as a "holy monster" or prodigy (376). Such a creature as Antigone will show herself to be has never been dreamt of in their philosophy. She says (559-60): "My soul has been dead a long time, so as to help the dead." Jebb and Kamerbeek relativize *palai* to make it long only "since the edict." But perhaps Antigone means to suggest that this is who she is and has been, for long before the edict. Has Antigone merely been biding her time, waiting for an opportunity like this one? Doing so would fit with her self-sacrifice for Oedipus in his exile, and it might befit her, too, as a reaction to the horror of her birth and family. She awaited an occasion to vindicate them. That is the way Creon takes it in the immediate sequel: her "long time" goes back to her birth. He says Antigone has been mindless—if not bloodyminded—"since birth" (*ta prot' ephu*; 562, cf. 471-72). And Creon's line at 567, "She is already

36. *Lysis* 219e1. Cf. Benardete, "On Plato's Lysis," 224, in Seth Benardete, *The Argument of the Action: Essays on Greek Poetry and Philosophy*, ed. Ronna Burger and Michael Davis (Chicago: University of Chicago Press, 2000).

dead," is deepened with the greater *gravitas* of dramatic irony if we take his limited meaning (*sc.* "She's dead because I've already passed sentence") to point toward a larger truth: she is already dead because her desire for self-sacrifice is a kind of death-in-life.

Why is it appropriate that Antigone be buried alive? Because she is acting as if she were already dead. Burial is her life. Ismene sees hope that the two of them can still get out of this, live their lives. Antigone wants to die. Her preference for the dead over the living is evident when we consider her repeated assertions that she goes to her death "unwept by friends" (846; cf. 919). She is unwept again and friendless at 876, and no friend groans at 882. Yet the Chorus wept, and she cannot be so clueless as to ignore the fact that Haimon is around somewhere. Digging frantically into her living tomb as a rescuer, he will come (seconds? minutes?) too late and embrace her corpse in his own self-sacrifice. Antigone is loved. She regrets that, because she will be buried alive, she will only be a metic with the dead, a resident alien—implying that she prefers the full status of citizenship in the land of the dead (850-51; cf. 890). Antigone says she is going "to my own" (*pros tous emautês*), into a "dwelling" (*oikêsis*) which she equates with her tomb (891-95). Her hope is that she will arrive down there as her father's "dear," "endeared to you, mother" (*prosphilês*) and "dear to you, brotherly head" (897-99).[37] The only way to escape the inference that Antigone simply prefers the dead to the living is to contend that she was driven to this desperate preference by events. In her public justification of her death wish, Antigone does indeed appeal to the evils that beset her and twice calls it a "gain" (*kerdos*) to die early, falling into Creon's language of profit and loss (460-64). But this seems like a translation of her passions into language that

37. If reunion with the dead is Antigone's motive, her admission ticket is to have upheld the family honor. By giving her all, Antigone wishes to recoup the family honor, thus winning her own back. This is partly because of the horror that is her family. Unlike Ismene, who shows herself to be ashamed of Oedipus's legacy, Antigone's words "from good [parents]" (38) show that she is *proud* of Oedipus and Jocasta—or wishes to be proud. Both parents repudiated their incest and, in a sense, their very lives in their self-blinding and suicide, respectively. Yet that incest produced Antigone and Ismene, and if the girls are to have a shred of self-respect, if they are to consider themselves good, they must project at least some of their goodness back onto that dark deed. Otherwise, they are simply the accursed products of incest, lives that should never have been. In a weak moment, Antigone confesses what she really feels about her parents, and it accords pretty much with conventional wisdom and Ismene's view (859-66). She bewails as "the most painful of my cares" "our whole fate, the famous Labdacids," the facts that her father slept in her mother's bed, where he himself had been generated. "What kind [of parents] I am sprung from!" (866). Antigone believes what everyone believes about their family; she has no extra information that could save Oedipus and Jocasta's nobility. She finally admits everything that Ismene tried to get her to admit in the opening scene. She is accursed, she says (869)—but if so, why go on attempting to vindicate such a horrific family? Because only in doing so can she make her own life—and theirs—worth living.

he—and we—can understand. She is attracted—not just goaded—into death and dying. The interpretation that events force her into suicide perhaps humanizes Antigone, but it loses more than it gains: it diminishes her heroism and refuses to recognize her status as a holy monster. Without at all removing her *pathos* and our sympathy, the holy-monster interpretation simultaneously brings her near to us while keeping her far, incorporating our revulsion as well as our admiration.

Does Antigone chicken out by taking the easy path to death—suicide—once she has been immured in the cave? Why not starve to death, as Creon hoped: would that not constitute an even greater sacrifice? Her death by her own hand is marked for gender, in the Greek context. Hanging oneself is a woman's way out, less manly than falling on one's sword, as Deianeira did. Jocasta, effeminately, hanged herself: she "disfigured her own life." But Eurydice, Creon's wife and Haimon's mother, took the more manly way: with a knife she struck up from under into her liver (1315-16). In the *Women of Trachis*, the wife Deianeira's manly suicide reverses the poles of masculinity and femininity when contrasted with her husband Heracles's raving, screaming, begging feminine death. In a somewhat similar way, the *Antigone* feminizes Creon in his agony—he who set so much store by gender and keeping woman under rule. For his wife Eurydice to be masculinized or to achieve masculine courage at the end further feminizes her husband and reveals another dimension of the poverty of his ruling conception. We suppose that Sophocles could have contrived to smuggle a sword into the cave for Antigone if he had wanted to mark her suicide as manly.[38]

If Antigone's end shows her nature, then her feminine ending is appropriate for her embrace of kinship love—but not appropriate for her masculine stand. Antigone loves so ardently that she wishes to hasten the hour of her arrival below and her reunion with her family. Suicide is what she wants: she is not overwhelmed by despair at the suffering that awaits her in the cave. Like a hero, she remains steadfast in her purpose: reunion. By her suicide she fights her way into greater (quicker) happiness. But her heroism is also feminine; she is a heroine. The "weak" woman's way out contains nothing undesirable *per se*. Rather, it is *desirably* feminine: Haimon embraces her hanging body in a kind of *Liebestod* (1234-41). By contrast, Deianeira's and Eurydice's suicides could be said to represent impossible gestures at masculinization. Antigone's manly resolve constantly leads back to her femininity rather than away from it.

38. Blondell (101) offers a different social mapping: sword/noose maps onto married/unmarried, respectively, because the noose leaves the unmarried female body unpenetrated even in death. We note that the married woman Jocasta did resort to the noose, however. It seems that the masculine/feminine social map is operative along with the married/unmarried female social map and sometimes distorts its expectations.

How does her love become incestuous? We have argued that Antigone is the *Lysis*'s identity *philia* incarnate: she "makes much of" the burial (which is instrumental, like the cup that holds the antidote to the hemlock) "for the sake of believing" that her brother is "worth everything" (even though he is not). In the *Lysis*, hers is what unphilosophic *philia* simply is. It is beautiful and a horror at once. Her love is not choiceworthy, but it is admirable—or at least wonderful. *Philia* is largely the love of one's own (*oikeion*). We have seen this in Antigone's own language; she is emphatic that she is doing this for her own: *tôn emôn, pros tous emautês*. We can see, then, how the seeds of inwardness might be sown in an extreme love of one's own. But *philia*, unlike eros, is *supposed* to be a love of one's own: fraternal *philia*, for example, looks inside the family for its objects—however much it might wish to look outside, to encompass all fellow citizens. Among the various loves, only eros is forbidden from looking inside the family for its objects; only eros is supposed to seek among the wider pool of fellow citizens. How does the love of one's own become erotic?

We earlier argued that Antigone seeks the missing connection, a natural love that could fill the void found at the core of conventional brotherhood. Antigone (like all sisters and brothers) needs a reason to love—and to like—her sibling. Affection (*philia* with Aristotle's *storgê*[39]) would be the natural candidate for attraction between friends. Biological similarities and especially time spent growing up together are the natural bases of *storgê* among siblings. But Antigone's shared biology with Polyneices is a horror. And she spent her childhood in exile with her father, while the two adult sons lived in Thebes.[40] It is clear that Polyneices was not a loving person nor, in light of what he did, particularly lovable. In the absence of *storgê*, the one passion left that could fulfill her longing is eros. This would be in keeping with the family tradition. Incest is the quintessential way that families become closed in on themselves. In ruling households, incest is the preferred means for keeping the crown in-house. Oedipus unwittingly followed that pattern when he joined with his mother to form an unnatural whole; and the brothers by the manner of their death have shown themselves to form a different kind of unnatural whole.

"Dear with him I will lie, with my dear [brother]" (73). Eros is mentioned explicitly for the first time at line 90. In the context of asserting that Antigone is "in love" (with the impossible), Ismene says "You have a hot heart for cold things" (88). In the first instance the reference is to the *sang-froid* needed to carry out such daring. But the cold things must also refer to the corpse Antigone

39. See footnote 8.

40. They also connive in their father's exile in *Oedipus at Colonus*, 337-56, 427-30.

sets such store by, as opposed to her living, warm sister. She seems to have a death-wish or to be in love with death or with the dead.

A sexual overtone is likely in Antigone's answer: "I know that I am pleasing those whom I ought most to satisfy" (89).[41] Kamerbeek writes: "it is certainly preposterous to read an incestous intention into the words, whatever insinuation may be heard in some utterances of Creon's."[42] But by making the incest intentional, Kamerbeek sidesteps the traditional question of tragic irony. Does Antigone speak more wisely than she is aware of?[43]

41. Why gratify the dead more than the living? Antigone has already given her rationale (at lines 74-76): "Because for a longer time must I please those below than those here [in this life]./ There I will always lie." Her logic is impeccable: the time we spend down with the dead—and dead ourselves—is infinitely longer than the time we spend alive with the living. Granted that we should please the dead at all, the eternity of pleasing them dwarfs the short time of pleasing the living. Her intransigent logic highlights the assumed premise that we should please the dead at all. Ismene will have to choose between all or nothing. Antigone chooses to lie in the grave pleasing her brother.

42. Pp. 48-49, *ad loc.* line 73. Creon's insinuation occurs at 523-24, right after Antigone's own curious statement that "My nature is not to join in enmity, but to join in love (*outoi sunekhthein, alla sumphilein ephun*; 523). To which Creon responds with a coarse incest joke: "Go love the ones down there" (*sc.* in the underworld, 524-25; cf. 654). Superficially, Antigone's statement is a badge of womanliness: "whatever politics may say, I love." Her nature does not return hate for hate but returns love for love. As Jebb (Richard Jebb, *Sophocles: The Plays and Fragments. Part III. The Antigone* [Cambridge: Cambridge University Press, 1900]) reads it (following the scholiast), Antigone ignores her brothers' mutual hatred and returns each brother's love as he loved her. But did they? Their love was nothing compared to hers. Perhaps sensing the disparity, Kamerbeek christianizes it: Antigone returns love even for hate. The more one looks at the line, the stranger it becomes. We earlier saw the connotation of "unite" in the *sun*-prefixes. "Join with loved ones" seems the likely meaning of *sumphilein*. "Join sexually with loved ones" is the way Creon interprets it. However shallow his view of it is (and however Antigone might not want to mean it that way), we will see evidence in favor of Creon's interpretation.

43. It is crucial that Antigone becomes an uncanny prodigy only because of her eros. The famous Eros chorus clarifies the (even more famous) *polla ta deina* chorus, which argues that man is uncanny. The Eros chorus (which the Chorus breaks into after Haimon's love for Antigone pits him against his father's love, 781-99) shows *why* man is uncanny or what in man makes for his uncanniness: his eros. When news arrives that the body has been buried, the Chorus first suspect the deed was god-driven, a miracle or something only gods would do (278-79). But then they realize how uncanny is man in his daring achievements and transgressions. They do not know it yet, but Antigone is the uncanny "man" who buried the body against the proclamation: she is the hidden reason the Chorus break into the *polla ta deina* chorus. By the time we get to the Eros chorus (781-99), we have been sensitized to certain phrases by the *polla ta deina* chorus, prepared to hear their echoes. Just as uncanny man crosses the seas in stormy season (335-37), so Eros himself ranges over the sea (785). Just as uncanny man escaped the bad open places by teaching himself town-law tempers (355-59), so Eros ranges through wild rural open places (785). Man cannot escape Eros by repairing to the city because Eros is inside him: Eros haunts the highest offices of the land no less than the cheeks of a well-bedded bride (795-98). Antigone was to have been that bride (she was Haimon's bride who became instead the bride of Death). It is the eros in man that attracts him into uncanny achievements and transgressions like the burial. Extreme *philia* is not enough to explain Antigone's transgression; eros must be added to it.

On the one hand, Antigone flees incest—and all eros. She wishes to purify her family precisely from the stain of incest. Her flight from her parents' eros leads her to embrace those family loves that are without sexuality: fraternity and, in Oedipus's lifetime, filial piety. This is evident in Antigone's hard words that she would not have defied Thebes to bury a husband or a child, for she could always have remarried and had a substitute child (904-20). Husbands are replaceable, as are kids. A brother, on the other hand, is irreplaceable in Antigone's view because the parents are dead that could have replaced him. She views irreplaceability purely in birth-terms. Most people would view the irreplaceability of a loved one in terms of his individuality, a unique or idiosyncratic personality (cf. the *idion* of the *Lysis* 205b7-c2). Her shift to birth and blood show that Antigone is obsessed with her birth family in a way that wrenches birth out of its normal place in the hierarchy of affections and places it at the top.[44]

For birth to be Antigone's standard is strange because her name ("born in exchange for" or "born to resist") can also mean "anti-birth." Birth is erotic or the product of eros, but eros for Oedipus's family carries the stain of incest. Antigone, who is all about vindicating her birth family, must thus at once oppose birth and be pro-birth. She is pro-birth insofar as she supports her birth family in everything. But she is anti-birth in that she can never think without pain of the eros that led to her and her father's births. Birth without eros is a kind of anti-birth.

And yet, what if eros returns inevitably like nature driven out with a pitchfork or a rock thrown upwards? We see this when Antigone "adopts" her dead brother as her nestling. When she discovers the corpse unburied for the second time, she makes the piercing cry "of a vindictive bird, as when she sees the bed of her empty couch bereft of nestlings" (423-25). Couch and bed are the places of sexual generation, both in conception and in birth. But Antigone reserves these sexual and motherly feelings not for a husband or nestlings but for her dead brother. She feels about her brother the way she ought to feel about Haimon and the children she will never have. Children are the products of eros, not *philia*. It is as if her *philia* substitutes its own objects for erotic objects. Instead of producing nestlings naturally, by birth, Antigone "adopts." Her *philia* has grown so strong that it bends eros to its own ends rather than natural ends.

44. Instead of rejecting (along with Jebb and a host of editors), Antigone's hard words about irreplaceability as interpolations, or explaining them away as "weak reasoning" (with Kamerbeek), we might explicate their repulsiveness for the light it sheds on Antigone's uncanny character. We find ourselves in the presence of a holy monster. The re-routing of her eros is analogous to that of a saint.

Eros is re-routed toward those who are already "friends," her own (*tôn emôn*; cf. 893), away from strangers—fellow citizens—who would normally be its objects. The brother receives the lavish attentions that only a child or sexual partner should receive. Sexual desire fills the vacuum at the heart of fraternity.

Thus her flight from eros and from incest drives Antigone into their arms. Much as Oedipus in the previous generation fled his hometown to avoid sleeping with his mother, only to find his mother in Thebes, Antigone concentrates on unerotic fraternity and piety only to find in them an erotic desire. The steps she takes to avoid incest involve Antigone in recapitulating the original crime. Her unacknowledged eros is oriented toward her dead *philoi*. Ismene's original assertions that Antigone is in love and has a hot heart for cold things and the Chorus's witless dismissal of the idea that someone could feel eros for death now take on their full freight of meaning.

CONCLUSION

Politically, Antigone's loyalty to her birth family is conditioned by the original incest. She was produced only by her family, not by her polity, because her family was not exogamous. Most people are produced by an alliance between two families: a marriage that unites one kinship group to another kinship group. The polity is instrumental to their alliance, sanctioning and policing the marriage-union. Most people thus owe their generation to the polity working in tandem with families. Antigone owes the polity no loyalty in exchange for her generation because the polity contributed nothing. Her insouciance about all things political thus takes on a larger dimension than the male-female dichotomies discussed earlier. Antigone can ignore the political. She represents a self-sufficient family.

A self-sufficient ruling house, moreover, effectually is a city unto itself. By marrying his own mother, Oedipus unwittingly closed off any avenue to the throne for the offspring of Theban nobles, who would ordinarily want to marry *in* to the royal family. But if the royal family does not marry out, then it becomes proof against any control from without or below. As Aristotle also points out, to be a citizen means to share in rule and office. If only a ruling family or junta shares in office, then its members are the only citizens. Such a group becomes a city within the city.[45] Since the polis is the only truly self-sufficient entity,[46] to make the family self-sufficient is to treat the family as a polis. So (somewhat impressionistically) Antigone's model for the household is actually the polis.

45. *Politics* 3.6, 1278b11; 3.1, 1257a22-23.
46. *Politics* 1.2, 1252b28-31.

Correspondingly, Creon's model for the polis is actually the household.[47] His obsession with private gain, as we argued in section 1, shows a lowmindedness that becomes especially evident in his accusations against the prophet Teiresias. This economism shows that his civic assumptions conform to a household paradigm. Economics is a household concern (*oiko-nomia*)—not a civic concern—on Greek assumptions. His metaphor for political resistance—"heads tossing, necks not rightly under the yoke" (291-92)—envisions himself as farmer or husbandman governing animals. When Haimon warns that a one-man state is no polis at all, Creon's response would be more appropriate for Aristotle's "master" of a household full of children and slaves than for a political ruler: "Is not the polis thought to belong to its ruler?"[48] For Aristotle, household rule is different in kind from political rule; household rule imposed on politics is characteristic of barbarians and tyrants.[49] And finally, of course, even Creon's civic friendship is a form of civic fraternity, a metaphor based on the brotherly love proper to households.

Thus each antagonist unwittingly embraces the other's principle. While demoting the household and real brotherhood, Creon elevates a household paradigm for politics along with contractual brotherhood. Antigone champions the household and blood-kin fraternity at the expense of the polis, while unwittingly treating her family as a polis. Crucially, her own relation to Polyneices lacks the *storgê* that would normally have come from a shared upbringing. Their disparity in age and her exile with Oedipus remove that common source of affection. If shared biology is the other source of affection, their biological connection evokes only horror. Thus Antigone's relation to her brother might as well be considered contractual. It has no natural basis. She is upholding a vision of fraternity that is, in essence, Creon's vision. The family principle and the polis principle thus mutually imply and depend upon each other.

The analogy between brotherhood and political fraternity shows severe limitations in each. We want more choice than we have in our siblings as well as in our fellow citizens. In each case we are stuck with them, but in each case the bond that we share with them seeks more, points beyond itself to a more natural form of friendship, one where attraction governs and where, in the limit, the individual is loved for his or her own sake. Political fraternity and brotherhood are both generic loves that neglect the individual. This gives to each a great strength and flexibility. There is something egalitarian about

47. E.g., 661-62, where he opines: "Whoever is a useful man in household affairs will show himself to be a just man in the city too."

48. Cf. 737-38 with 479; cf. *Politics* 1.3.

49. E.g., *Politics* 1.2, 1252b1-10.

accepting all members in spite of what they are like. But a passage from David Hume illustrates the problem with generic loves: "An *Englishman* in *Italy* is a friend: A *European* in *China*; and perhaps a man wou'd be belov'd as such, were we to meet him in the moon."[50] Generic loves depend for their force on what post-structuralists call a "constitutive outside." Only because they are thrown together in a country of foreigners do two Englishmen *qua* Englishmen like each other. At home, where they do not like each other, their civic "friendship" is dependent on outside enemies. Only the existence of outsiders guarantees bonds among insiders. Kinship brotherhood has natural supports to prop it up, but Sophocles removes these (in Antigone's case) in order to get at brotherhood's essence. Fraternity is a generic love, but this fact merely raises the further question about all *philia*: what is the status of our aspiration to love individuals for their individuality?

50. David Hume, *A Treatise of Human Nature*, ed. D. F. Norton and M. J. Norton (Oxford: Oxford University Press, 2000), 3.2.1.

13

Children of Skeptics

Thomas W. Merrill

Readers of *The Beginning of Wisdom* know that it contains rich materials for reflection on a number of matters of contemporary relevance: the meaning of marriage and parenthood, the tensions between technology and piety, and the complex interplay between human dignity and human shame—to say nothing of our relationship to the divine. Yet as its author himself remarks, *The Beginning of Wisdom* occupies an odd place in the contemporary landscape.[1] Devoted to a wisdom-seeking, anthropological inquiry into the book of Genesis, the book might well seem—in this era of culture war—to be a book without an audience: avowed rationalists might find the whole project either foolish or dangerous; believers who come to the book through one religious tradition of interpretation or another might see no need for it. It is a large question—albeit one more about our contemporary scene than about the book—as to whether there is a constituency for a respectful yet genuinely open-minded reading of Genesis. Would it be too pessimistic to say that our national conversation has gotten to the point where believers and nonbelievers confront each as armed camps between which no conversation is possible? The possibility of conversation, one might guess, is not a given fact naturally occurring in the world; it can only be performed, it must be accomplished by us, here and now. One cannot begin the conversation if one knows from the outset that there can be no response. Let us begin then with the opposite hypothesis—that some sense can be made of this world—not as a thing known in advance but as a promissory note whose proof is, as we say, in the pudding.

In fact *The Beginning of Wisdom* is conceived in just such a spirit. Kass addresses himself in the opening pages of the book to those he calls "the thoughtful children of skeptics."[2] The children of skeptics are the inheritors of the Enlightenment, brought up within a world shaped by modern science and technology. Yet they are aware, as only those with an inside view can be, of the moral-spiritual weakness of

1. Leon R. Kass, *The Beginning of Wisdom: Reading Genesis* (New York: Free Press, 2003), 13-15.
2. *The Beginning of Wisdom*, 1, 8.

that world. The modern scientific project combines great power with ambiguity or confusion about what would constitute a worthy way to exercise that power. The children of skeptics—many of whom Kass encountered in his classes at the University of Chicago—recognize that modern science can hardly be wished away. But they also recognize that it leaves us unsatisfied, in search of something more. The children of skeptics are embroiled in the ambiguities of inheritance, which seems always to enable and restrict at the same time. Needless to say, one does not come to terms with an inheritance, even an ambiguous one, by rejecting it wholesale: one must attempt to think it through, to take it seriously in all of its parts. One way to do that is to investigate it rigorously in the light of a serious alternative: the Bible is one such alternative.

Kass's book, which begins a consideration of the Biblical alternative, takes as primary interlocutors just these children of skeptics. It is plausible to say that the book offers something of a dialogue with them. Any reading of it that attends to what is done as well as what is said will have to keep an eye on how it might appear to those silent (and often, as the many footnotes that engage with Kass's students reveal, not so silent) interlocutors. At least at first glance, Kass asks us to engage in an activity rather than giving us a set of answers. He asks us to suspend our disbelief provisionally with a view to seeing what sense can be made out of the world. The suspension of disbelief is not the end of the activity of trying to reason things through but rather the condition of its possibility.[3] Yet one does not and cannot know in advance where such an inquiry might lead us. It would therefore not be surprising if the book inspires different, perhaps contrary, views of the fundamental issues in different readers. It is not skepticism, it is merely honesty, to acknowledge that there is no readily available answer sheet, no secret knowledge potentially available in advance of inquiry, against which our reading of Genesis may be checked, though there surely are better and worse readings. We shall simply have to look and see what sense can be made of the book, and of the world, for ourselves. How and whether the book succeeds in that endeavor is a question for a different time. Here I offer some observations about a text that illuminates the situation of "children of skeptics" and touches on some Kassian themes. Leo Strauss's "Preface" to his *Spinoza's Critique of Religion* is the closest thing we have to an intellectual autobiography from one of the twentieth century's great thinkers.[4] Written in 1962 for the English translation of Strauss's book on Spinoza (originally published in German in 1930), the Preface provides a tour of the intellectual landscape of a young German Jew coming of age in the Weimar

3. For discussion, see *The Beginning of Wisdom*, 16-17.

4. Page numbers in the text refer to Leo Strauss, *Spinoza's Critique of Religion* (Chicago: University of Chicago Press, 1965).

Republic of the 1920s. It traces Strauss's path from the political problems facing Jews in Germany between the World Wars (problems whose end we know all too well) toward a reopening of the great theological and philosophical questions that underlie our modern situation. Strauss shows himself struggling to come to terms with prominent Jewish and non-Jewish thinkers and actors from Spinoza to Herzl and Pinsker, to Cohen, Rosenzweig, and Heidegger. It describes how Strauss came to write his book on Spinoza, and why his historical studies became pressing and even necessary in light of the situation of German Jews. Yet the text is undoubtedly of interest to audiences beyond Jews and scholars of German thought. While Strauss's reflections are oriented toward Jewish problems, he shows how they raise fundamental questions of general interest: questions about the character and viability of the Enlightenment and of reason more generally; the challenge to rationalism posed by orthodoxies of various kinds; and the roots of modern Enlightenment in spiritedness or will.

My concern here is with the matrix—intellectual, social, political—out of which the questions orienting *The Beginning of Wisdom* become genuine questions. Strauss's essay helps to delineate the fundamental situation of the "children of skeptics"—that is, of anyone grappling with the ambiguous legacy of the Enlightenment. And although the foreground of Strauss's essay is understandably occupied with Jewish thinkers and themes, the questions he raises go well beyond Judaism to the heart of our Enlightenment. This essay attempts to sketch what Strauss has to teach us about that fundamental situation, and to tease out some lessons for our own, somewhat different, historical situation.

Since Strauss's "Preface" is lengthy and dense, it may help to provide an overview at the outset. Strauss published his first book, *Spinoza's Critique of Religion*, in 1930. Strauss's "Preface," written from the vantage point of 1962, provides an account of how he came to write that book. It is first and foremost an intellectual autobiography, rooted in a particular place and time and extending only up to about 1928, when Strauss completed work on the Spinoza book. Strauss presents three main stages in his intellectual development. In the first stage, Strauss roots his narrative firmly in the political situation confronting German Jews in the Weimar Republic in the 1920s, who faced a choice between assimilation to German culture, on the one hand, and various forms of Zionism on the other. Strauss chose Zionism; yet however necessary that choice might have been on practical grounds, the intellectual underpinnings of Zionism appeared to him insufficient and unsatisfactory. In the second stage of Strauss's trajectory, the question thus arose whether the political project of Zionism needed a deeper and more substantive grounding in Jewish thought. The possibility of such a "return" to Judaism was explored by thinkers like

Franz Rosenzweig and Martin Buber, thinkers who were themselves influenced by the critiques of modern philosophy offered by Nietzsche and Heidegger. Strauss found, however, that none of these thinkers achieved their stated goals, because they remained, wittingly or unwittingly, under the spell of modern presuppositions. The main obstacle to such projects of return was a genuine intellectual challenge: the thought of Spinoza and the Enlightenment, which claimed to have refuted or superseded orthodoxy. To come to terms with that challenge, Strauss needed (in the third stage of his narrative) to re-examine the most authoritative recent case against Spinoza, the case made—in the name of the Jewish tradition—by the great Neo-Kantian and Jewish thinker, Hermann Cohen. Yet Cohen, for all the passion of his case against Spinoza, turned out to rely on certain key assumptions shared inherited from and shared with Spinoza: he had still not penetrated to the fundamental question underlying the dispute, the question as to whether Spinoza or orthodoxy had been right. It was this question that occupied Strauss in *Spinoza's Critique of Religion*. In re-opening the dispute between Spinoza and orthodoxy, Strauss had to raise some questions that remain fundamentally important today: Did the Enlightenment and the modern scientific project have good grounds for rejecting religion? Or was that rejection motivated by political or passionate impulses that precluded an impartial consideration of the case? Did the Enlightenment's commitment to rationality and science rest on a disinterested concern for truth or a desire for predictability and control?

Strauss's narrative is not simply autobiography for the sake of autobiography. It has an internal logic, and it illustrates how a particular political problem—the uneasy situation of German Jews in the 1920s—points to, and may finally be unintelligible except in the light of, fundamental philosophical and theological questions. In what follows, I offer some, admittedly preliminary, comments on Strauss's trajectory toward those questions.

The Jewish Problem and the Human Problem

Strauss's point of departure is emphatically political: the situation of a Jew in Germany in the early twentieth century. That political situation was defined by the aspirations, and the weakness, of liberal democracy in Germany. Liberal democracy claimed to have superseded religion: no longer would citizens be defined by this or that religious affiliation. Human beings qua human beings linked by a universal secular morality would live together in peace. Yet the fact was that liberal democracy never fully took hold in Germany. German culture fell under the influence of the powerful critique of modernity, including liberal democracy, given by Jean-Jacques Rousseau. Seen in this light, liberal democracy appeared as a thin rational veneer over darker, more profound, and more dangerous passions. In the light of German romanticism and longing for the lost spiritual unity of the Middle Ages—and German resentment at being defeated in World War I—the rationalism of liberal democracy appeared shallow. It is no surprise then that the German liberal democrats were politically weak and eventually swept away by more illiberal forces.

For a modern, enlightened Jew, this situation was deeply unsettling. Raised to believe that a universal tolerant human society was within reach, and that German society would accept him with open arms, the German Jew found himself betwixt and between. The political reality was that the majority in Germany was suspicious of Jews, whether they attempted to assimilate into German society or remained orthodox. Even the most cosmopolitan of Germans, such as Goethe, harbored objections to the full assimilation of the Jews—to say nothing of less savory thinkers or of the darker impulses that came to light later. Yet the premise of Enlightenment was that traditional Judaism had to be relinquished. For the young Jews of Strauss's generation, the path backward was intellectually blocked by acceptance of the Enlightenment. But the political reality of German society made it impossible for them or her to stop being identified with their fellow Jews as a practical matter.

For Strauss, the primary lesson of the Weimar republic was one of realpolitik: in all societies the majority will, in one way or another, determine who belongs and who does not. At the heart of political society is an act of ruling. That act may be more or less humane; it may be wise; but it remains an expression of power, in which the majority asserts its will over the minority. In the moment of decision, there is no third party to appeal to; and in the controversy between German Jews and the rest of Germany, that decision would necessarily be made by the non-Jewish Germans. Jewish citizens, whether they were believers or not, were thus confronted with a fundamentally untenable situation. To simply appeal to the good sense of the German or to rely on the Enlightenment promise of toleration would be to put oneself and one's community at the mercy of powers beyond one's control. Basic self-preservation, as well as responsibility for one's family and community, compelled Jews to look for another strategy.

Political life proper is born from the recognition of the necessity to act or to assist others who act. For some Jews of Strauss's generation, Zionism—in its original, political form—was the vehicle of that recognition.[5] These Jews saw

5. Strauss himself was a Zionist in the 1920s and an active participant in the debates over the future of Judaism. His Zionist writings have now been translated in *Leo Strauss: The Early Writ-*

that they would have to do for themselves what no one else could or would do for them. The Zionism of Pinsker and Herzl took a hard-headed look at the realities of European politics and recognized that mere moral appeals to the powerful of the world would not be efficacious. In standing up for themselves, in taking on the responsibility for their common fate, the political Zionists took a large step toward vindicating Jewish dignity, honor, and pride. Instead of assimilating as individuals to a promised but elusive post-religious Enlightenment society, the Jews would take their rightful place among the independent nations of the world: political Zionism was a Jewish declaration of independence.

Strauss always held the achievements of political Zionism in high regard. His participation in the Zionist movement was perhaps the most important direct political engagement of his life. Yet ultimately he found the Zionism of Herzl and Pinsker insufficient, even on realpolitik grounds. The political Zionists were simply not numerous enough to found a state without an alliance with other Jews. A more fundamental defect was that the movement's roots were not deep: it had not found an answer to the question: for what do we stand, as opposed to, against what are we reacting? Strauss remarks that the Zionists remembered Rabbi Hillel's saying, "If I am not for myself, who will be for me?" but forgot its companion, "If I am only for myself, what am I?" Without an answer to that question, Zionism, or any political movement, could make a case for itself as a matter of calculation and self-interest but not as a cause worth fighting and dying for in itself. It could not engage the heart as well as the head. Having stood for itself *against* the contempt or indifference of others, political Zionism could not say positively what it stood *for*. Yet politics, however hard-headed and realistic, can never escape the deeper question, what justifies—what sanctifies—political action?

Political calculation in the narrow sense is necessary but not sufficient to form a political community that engages the whole human being. Politics requires a supplement to make sense of itself.[6] Yet once we raise the question of justification, the real trouble begins. For some Jews in the 1920s, the answer lay

ings (1921-1932), ed. Michael Zank (Albany, New York: State University of New York Press, 2002). See also the very helpful volume of collected essays by Strauss, *Jewish Philosophy and the Crisis of Modernity*, ed. Kenneth Hart Green (Albany, New York: State University of New York Press, 1997).

6. In *Democracy in America*, Alexis de Tocqueville provides an American parallel. He famously suggests that one democratic vice is a resignation to what is taken to be the tides of history. Upon examination, Tocqueville's account of the psychology of the democratic belief in history turns out to have the same structure as the logic of the tyranny of the majority in the political realm. Tocqueville seems to think that history in the democratic sense is the cosmological version of the tyranny of the majority. Even democrats, who pride themselves on being pragmatic, anti-theoretical, and anti-theological, seem unable to refrain from interpreting being or the cosmos in light of their fundamental political opinions.

in seeing Judaism as one high culture among others. Culture refers primarily to the habits, mores, and traditions of a people. It appeals to a reverence deeper than the hard-headed calculations of politiques. But the source of culture, in the modern understanding, is merely a people. Culture is the unintended consequence of the aggregate activities of many individuals over a long period of time. One may recognize the importance and value of traditional practices and beliefs and still question the underlying authority of ancestral inheritance. This or that custom may prove useful, but why in principle should we look up to the activity of certain particular human beings, who have no obvious claim to be superior to us?

The appeal to culture *qua* culture is even less appropriate in the case of Judaism, which always staked its claim on its dedication to a universal truth and to justice in a transpolitical and transcultural sense. When cultural Zionism takes itself seriously, Strauss remarks, it turns into religious Zionism: it must take seriously the claim of orthodoxy as orthodoxy. Yet from the point of view of Jewish faith, the attempt by political Zionism to solve the "Jewish problem" through human and political means proves to be misguided and finally blasphemous. Politics needs a supplement, but culture alone cannot offer an ultimately satisfying alternative, while religion requires a reorientation away from politics, in the light of which politics and political action must be subordinated to concerns for justice and purity. Mere political success no longer appears sufficient. Zionism is thus a paradox: even or especially in Israel, a new version of the "Jewish problem" reappears.

Strauss goes so far as to claim that this problem is not unique to the Jews but is paradigmatic for political life as such. In this respect, "the Jewish problem" reflects the continuing absence of a satisfactory resolution to the problems of human life. Strauss comes close to suggesting that the experience of exile, of the Galut, is in fact the human experience as such. The founding of the state of Israel is not the coming of the Messiah, and human beings must still attempt to see their way clearly, and make their way as best they can, in a world of insuperable tensions:

> The establishment of the state of Israel is the most profound modification of the Galut which has occurred, but it is not the end of the Galut: in the religious sense, and perhaps not only in the religious sense, the state of Israel is a part of the Galut. Finite, relative problems can be solved; infinite, absolute problems cannot be solved. In other words, human beings will never create a society which is free of contradictions. From every point of view, it looks as if the Jewish people were the chosen people in the sense, at least, that the Jewish problem is the most manifest symbol of the human problem as a social and political problem.

It is not immediately clear what Strauss means by "the human problem as a social and political problem," or indeed what the contradictions are. Presumably he refers to the tension between the political Zionists and the religious Zionists, between the demands of politics and the demands of religion. It may be the case, for example, that every political society must find a way to negotiate between the circumstantial political realities at any given moment and the higher things to which it looks up and which it reveres. The "Jewish problem" may be paradigmatic because it provides one particularly sharp expression of that question.

Be that as it may, the defects of liberalism must appear in a different light once Zionism has shown itself to be paradoxical. Strauss's original dissatisfaction with liberalism stemmed from its inability or unwillingness to genuinely welcome enlightened Jews: beneath the universalistic pretensions of liberalism lurked the old antipathies. But if *no* society is free of contradictions, the judgment on liberalism is not so simple. At its best, liberalism tries to enforce a distinction between public and private: it attempts to govern the body without intruding on the soul. It therefore cannot eradicate prejudice and discrimination in the private sphere without ceasing to be liberalism. But a polity that respects the private sphere also makes room for political and religious liberty, for Jews as well as others. Another liberalism, one that took itself and its principles seriously, might well be far more defensible and successful than the liberalism of the Weimar Republic. To be sure, such liberty comes at the price of being a primarily political community, one in which the highest things are not shared. The question arises whether the Enlightenment hope for a universal human community, one that combined liberty and a deep community of the heart, was not a false hope born from an unwillingness to see the world as it is.

Religiosity without Religion?

For the young Jew of the 1920s who asked whether a return to or reaffirmation of Judaism was possible, several intellectual-moral alternatives presented themselves. Hermann Cohen, one of the greatest German Jewish thinkers before the World Wars, had argued that Judaism was the paradigmatic "religion of reason." So far from being dependent on a law that could only be known through some greater-than-human revelation, Judaism was, on this view, emphatically rational. Its moral teachings could be verified by reason acting alone, and any alleged miracles and revelations could be seen as merely longstanding self-misunderstandings. Yet it is not clear why such a religion would need a transcendent god like the one spoken about in the Bible or even whether such a God is really compatible with it. In the absence of such a transcendent God, it was unclear what the ultimate basis of the rational morality was. By discarding all the super-rational elements of the Jewish tradition, Cohen came close to reducing Judaism to a mere moral ideal or hope with no grounding in nature or the divine. For many of Cohen's readers, God seemed to be on the verge of evaporating.[7]

Not surprisingly, many thinkers found this profoundly unsatisfying. A deeper and more vibrant attempt at a genuine return to Judaism was made by Franz Rosenzweig and others. According to Rosenzweig, all human beings had or could have an experience of the divine command or "call," as a matter of direct experience, a call that is especially manifest in our awareness of our obligation to our fellows. We can in fact recognize our experience of that call in the Bible. For Rosenzweig, that recognition thus prepared the way for a return, albeit partial, to Judaism. Our awareness of the ethical command, however, is available to human beings as human beings and rests on our experience of a call from the divine, from something absolute and beyond the human. Yet that experience tended to be obscured by the various forms of rationalism from ancient Greek philosophy to Hegel. Rationalism in all its forms, for Rosenzweig, was superficial. It could see the world only through the lens of subjects and objects, as mere things or as pure minds, necessarily abstracted from the living human experience of the absolute. Coming to terms with the call or the absolute experience therefore required the critique of philosophy as hitherto known, what Rosenzweig calls the "old thinking."

Rosenzweig was not the only thinker who called for the replacement of the "old thinking" of Western philosophy with a "new thinking." Martin Heidegger also called for a thoroughgoing critique of traditional philosophy, and he also began with the premise of something like an absolute experience or call, prior to philosophic reason. But Heidegger denied that the Jewish interpretation, or any other interpretation of the fundamental experience, could be known to be the true interpretation. For Heidegger the most important virtue is a kind of probity (*Redlichkeit*), or the resolute willingness to look the ugly reality in the face and not cover it up with mere wishful thinking. He demanded that the fundamental experience be seen as it is in itself, stripped of all merely conventional or believed interpretations. Heidegger argued that all such interpretations had

7. Consider the story Strauss tells elsewhere of Cohen being asked by an orthodox Jew about what has happened to the creator of the world in Cohen's philosophy: "Cohen had no other answer than—to weep, and thus to confess that the gap between his belief and the belief of the tradition is unbridgeable." Leo Strauss, *Philosophy and Law*, trans. Eve Adler (Albany: State University of New York Press, 1995), 50.

the effect of hiding from us the reality of death and our fundamental loneliness in the cosmos. Rosenzweig's "Jewish" interpretation of the experience, the Presence or the Call, could be nothing but an attempt to make that experience bearable; for Heidegger it stems in the last analysis from the human hope to escape mortality into something eternal, a hope that is, according to him, indistinguishable from a spirit of revenge.

Yet Heidegger's objection can be turned back on him, for is it so clear that the atheistic interpretation of the fundamental experience is the correct one? Does not Heidegger's attachment to that interpretation stem from his preference for a world in which human beings must demonstrate courage and fortitude in the face of a hostile cosmos? As Strauss put it, "[J]ust as an assertion does not become true because it is shown to be comforting, so it does not become true because it is shown to be terrifying" (11). Heidegger's view presupposes that what is morally serious in life is to face up to the ugly truth about the world. But one might also say the reverse: Heidegger needed the truth to be ugly so that human beings might be morally serious. In fact, Strauss charges, the source of the thought of Heidegger (and in some measure of Nietzsche as well) about *Redlichkeit* and other matters is an essentially Biblical moral impulse. "Being toward death," "conscience," and "guilt,"—the concepts Heidegger uses to explicate the human in *Being and Time*—are all much more closely tied to the Biblical understanding of human beings than to the Greek.

Rosenzweig's version of the "new thinking" appeared to be a more viable alternative. Yet Rosenzweig did not return to orthodoxy completely. He did not claim to believe all the miracles of the Bible, for example. His standard was not submission to a mysteriously revealed law, but the experience of God's call, which, to be sure, could find echoes of itself in the law. This means, however, that Rosenzweig uses the personal experience of the call to judge the law and not the other way around: in the crucial respect, Rosenzweig remained an individualist. As Strauss put it, "The sacred law, as it were the public temple, which was a reality, thus becomes a potential, a quarry or a storehouse out of which each individual takes the materials for building up his private shelter" (14). Rosenzweig differed from his orthodox contemporaries on two points especially. He wished to replace the orthodox understanding of law as prohibition and denial with one of law as granting and liberation. And he did not, and felt that he could not, believe all the Biblical miracles. Yet, as Strauss points out, there is reason to think that the orthodox might have more insight than Rosenzweig regarding both of these disagreements. For does not the understanding of law as prohibition rest on a "deeper understanding of the power of evil in man" than that possessed by Rosenzweig? And would it not be more consistent—if we find traces of God's call in the Bible—to treat our doubts about miracles as moral failings on our part as the orthodox might do than to judge miracles by our individual ability or inability to believe or not believe?

Rosenzweig's position was thus internally unstable. On his premises, the question inevitably arises: is not a genuine return to orthodoxy both possible and necessary? Does not intellectual consistency require that this possibility be explored? Rosenzweig's inconsistency thus awakened in Strauss a renewed and intensified focus on the question of orthodoxy. Such questioning cannot fail to turn us back to the major obstacle to such a return, viz., the belief that the Enlightenment and modern science had decisively refuted or made obsolete all religious belief. For Jews—and not just for Jews—that belief was entangled with their ambivalent views of Spinoza, the Jew who became one of the founders of the Enlightenment and whose excommunication from the Jewish community in 1656 was a defining moment in the origins of the modern age. Strauss remarks that a return to orthodoxy was possible "only if Spinoza was wrong in every respect" (15).

The case of Spinoza's excommunication had in fact been reconsidered by Hermann Cohen. Whatever the defects of the "religion of reason," Strauss concluded that Cohen had given the most sober and impressive consideration of Spinoza's case up until that time. Cohen had affirmed the excommunication, although on somewhat different grounds from the original judgment. Strauss's extended examination of Cohen's case against Spinoza is the last stage before his turn to a direct consideration of Spinoza. This is not the place to give that reconsideration all the attention it deserves; three summary points will have to suffice. First, Strauss confirms and even provides deeper grounds for Cohen's judgment, and thus affirms the original excommunication, albeit on the basis of a somewhat different interpretation of Spinoza. Second, Strauss judged that Cohen failed to recognize some harsh political realities that both Spinoza and the Jewish tradition saw clearly. This led Cohen to misunderstand the character of Spinoza's rhetoric, especially Spinoza's need to appeal to the premises of his Christian audience, premises that Spinoza did not share. Cohen's blindness with regard to politics also led to an excessive utopianism. In this connection Strauss cites the saying of the Jewish sage Rabbi Hanina: "But for the fear of the government, men would eat each other alive." Third, despite Cohen's anger against Spinoza—perhaps because of that anger—he failed to acknowledge his acceptance of some of Spinoza's most important legacies: the historical-critical method of reading the Bible, the critique of miracles, and so on. Cohen suffered from "defective subjectivity": in some key instances he lacked self-knowledge. In particular he failed to reflect upon the fact that he essentially took Spinoza's side in the dispute with orthodoxy:

"Cohen took for granted that Spinoza had refuted orthodoxy." But if the "old thinking"—philosophy as known to the Western tradition hitherto, including Cohen's own philosophy—had collapsed, then Cohen's critique of Spinoza was insufficient. It failed to penetrate to the fundamental question. Thus was the stage set for the question animating Strauss's Spinoza book.

The theme connecting Strauss's readings of the alternative attempts to think through a return to Judaism is thus something like "unclear premises." Rosenzweig appeals to the call or the presence of divinity, but turns out to still be under the spell of modern individualism. Heidegger calls for a resolute atheism but has borrowed essential elements of his thought from Biblical religion. Hermann Cohen reaffirms the justice of the Jewish excommunication of Spinoza but has failed to reflect upon his tacit acceptance of Spinoza's most basic premises. In each case what seems to be an inconsistent melange of positions is made possible by a lack of self-knowledge on the part of the thinker in question. In each case Strauss is enabled to expose that lack of self-knowledge by using the challenge of orthodoxy to probe the premises of post-Enlightenment thinking.

Enlightenment vs. Orthodoxy

Strauss came to think that the various harmonizations of Cohen, Rosenzweig, and others obscured more than they revealed, that it would be more honest to confront directly the original conflict between Enlightenment and orthodoxy. What can reasonably be said in the dispute between believers and the partisans of science? *Spinoza's Critique of Religion* represents his first (though not his last) attempt to take the measure of this question lurking behind the Enlightenment. As the question comes to light in the Spinoza book, the fundamental situation is an impasse. Orthodoxy cannot claim to have established the truth of its characteristic claims demonstratively, but only to believe them. But Enlightenment cannot claim to have refuted the central claims of orthodoxy: that there is a mysterious God who is omnipotent, and that He chooses when and where to reveal Himself. Accordingly, the central moment in the Spinoza book is the confrontation between Spinoza, the archetypical modern rationalist, and Calvin, the Protestant theologian. (Interestingly, Strauss chooses no Jewish thinker for the position of orthodoxy.) In that confrontation Calvin has the better of Spinoza. Neither an appeal to the principle of noncontradiction nor an appeal to experience can suffice to rule out the possibility of an omnipotent God. Science depends on the *assumption* that the world is intelligible; it does not and cannot establish that assumption.

It is one of Strauss's distinctive claims that the great thinkers who originated "modernity" were aware of this weakness, however little they wished to speak of it in public. In the absence of a more satisfying refutation on the merits, their published attacks on orthodoxy instead took the form of mockery. Mockery—still a dominant mode of critique of religion among today's avowed atheists—insinuates that religious belief is mere prejudice, mere unthinking habit that has been shed by all forward thinking persons, who cannot help but have contempt or condescending pity for those stick-in-the-mud believers. In turn, those believers cannot help but resent the evident contempt of the intellectuals. Enlightenment thus understood is necessarily divisive: even to this day in all Western democracies, believers and unbelievers confront each other with the haughtiness of contempt on the one side and an understandable resentment on the other.

Despite the passion with which some nonbelievers reject religion, however, we cannot ignore the essential weakness of the Enlightenment's substantive grounds for rejecting religion. Yet Strauss remarks that the awareness of this failure did not deter the Enlighteners from their practical project, the construction of a new world. On the contrary, precisely that awareness compelled them to forge ahead, to attack religion by another route. If orthodoxy could not be refuted on philosophical terms, then perhaps it could be circumvented or outlived. One could, for example, try to show that a clear, distinct, and adequate account of the world can be given by science; and one could try to show that the longing for religion was merely a sublimated desire for material things. Both attempts require the dedicated pursuit of the project of mastering and possessing nature or the conquering of chance in the name of rational control. Alternatively, if one could produce material plenty by means of modern technology, unsatisfied longings that had been expressed through religion and religious conflict might turn out to be satisfied by consumer goods and the like. The religious passions as religious passions might simply dry up. And that could be considered a kind of proof that those passions were never really genuinely concerned with the noble or divine in the first place. Strauss elsewhere calls this a "truly Napoleonic strategy" of forgoing a frontal attack on the enemy's fortress while conquering the country around it.[8]

Strauss goes out of his way to emphasize the negative, reactive character of this characteristically modern atheism. For this atheism does not start from a neutral point, from which it reaches a disinterested judgment on religion. Rather, its crusading, revolutionary spirit makes sense only in terms of its zealous desire to refute its opponent once and for all: "it would not rest content with dismissing the tenets of orthodoxy as not known but merely believed; having been

8. *Philosophy and Law*, 32.

impressed by the claim of these tenets, it wanted to refute them."[9] Modern science binds itself to the disinterested pursuit of truth by means of method; but the motives that lead it to do so are highly interested, indeed are generated by consciousness of inadequacy and failure. So Strauss argued at greater length in his second book, *Philosophy and Law*. "Was not the 'unique' 'world construction' of modern natural science, according to which miracles are of course unknowable, devised expressly for the very purpose that miracles be unknowable, and that thus man be defended against the grip of the omnipotent God?"[10] Strauss thereby articulates one version of what Hans Blumenberg has called the "secularization thesis," the view that modernity is dependent in an important way on the Christianity it both mimics and displaces.[11] By basing philosophy and science on the felt need to disprove the omnipotent God, the Enlightenment revealed that in the crucial respect it still *believed*; believed to the extent that it felt a moral imperative to disprove its opponent. Modern science thus conceived is not, at the deepest level, the product of the disinterested pursuit of knowledge but is motivated by a crusading spirit and a desire to disprove the claims of religion. It bears a relationship to belief in the omnipotent God rather like that of a negative to a photograph. Even at its most atheistic, Enlightenment proves to be haunted by the idea of omnipotence. Beneath the polemical attack, the Enlightenment proves to be a kind of amalgamation of philosophy and religion.

Whether this critique of the Enlightenment is successful is a very large question. Even were Strauss's account of the antitheological motives of the architects of the Enlightenment simply accurate, that mere fact would certainly not allow us to dismiss their findings. For one thing, even if their premises were faulty, their conclusions might still be true. One would have to turn away from Strauss's critique of the motives of the Enlightenment and consider the modern scientific account of nature on its merits before we could conclude that its foundations are faulty.[12] Moreover, the desire to reject religion is not the only motive of Enlightenment; it also builds on the human desires to avoid suffering and to improve one's condition, impulses that cannot be reduced to ressentiment. It is also unclear whether this judgment expresses Strauss's final

9. Ibid., 31.

10. Ibid., 32. Cf. "Preface," 12-13, 30.

11. For some prominent attempts to read early modernity along these lines, see Hans Blumenberg, *The Legitimacy of the Modern Age*, trans. Robert M. Wallace (Cambridge, Massachusetts: M.I.T. Press, 1985), and Michael Allen Gillespie, *The Theological Origins of Modernity* (Chicago: University of Chicago Press, 2008).

12. Political philosophy, it seems, succeeds but cannot dispense with natural philosophy. See Leon R. Kass, *Toward a More Natural Science: Biology and Human Affairs* (New York: Free Press, 1985).

judgment on these thinkers.[13] Suffice it to say that the modern project—in both its liberal democratic politics and its commitment to science—has proved to be remarkably durable, and its endurance is prima facie evidence that it builds on something real. To be sure, that endurance is based far more on its pragmatic successes in ameliorating undisputed human ills than on any success at providing a clear and distinct account of the whole. Nor has the attempt to dry up religious longings succeeded. Chance has not been eliminated, and the human longing for the divine has not disappeared, not even where conditions of material plenty have been achieved. Rather, the very meaning of progress has become questionable, even or especially among the beneficiaries of the real technological progress produced by modern science.

There is thus one more layer of the crisis of modernity, the crisis in the self-confidence of modernity. The Enlightenment promised material progress on the basis of human effort; the premise of that effort was the basic inhospitability of the cosmos to human beings. Since human efforts to construct a predictable world have not been wholly successful, the question arises whether facing up to the underlying truth of our bleak natural condition is not truer and more serious than taking comfort in the illusions of progress. The final wave of modernity, that of Nietzsche and Heidegger, turns this insight into the basis of its philosophy. The atheism of the original Enlighteners had made the evils and terrors of religion—most especially the fanaticism of the early modern Wars of Religion—the primary grounds for rejecting religion; the later atheists believed that we must reject religion precisely because it would be a consolation if it were true. Aware of the basic inability of the Enlightenment to refute an omnipotent God, these atheists found belief in God to be a sin against their consciences. For these thinkers, a truly morally serious life required that we look the ugly truth in the face and refuse any pleasing illusions. This new virtue, at once intellectual and moral, is a combination of fortitude and probity. It is an atheism out of conscience and on principle. Like the atheism of modern science, the new atheism is still embroiled in a complex mixture of rejection of and indebtedness to Biblical religion: "Thus it becomes clear that this atheism, compared not only with the original

13. Did Strauss change his mind about this interpretation of the reactive motives of modernity? Put differently, could he have come to think that (at least some) moderns were moved by a genuine desire to know, rather than by ressentiment against religion? The question is not easy to decide on the basis of the 1962 "Preface" because Strauss's mature views are hard to disentangle from the views he presents himself as having held in the 1920s and 30s. It is clear that Strauss in 1962 regarded the interpretation of Spinoza to be found in the Spinoza book as defective. He applies to his interpretation the same judgment he makes of Hermann Cohen: "I understood Spinoza too literally because I did not read him literally enough." Strauss uses this judgment to suggest that Cohen underestimated Spinoza's esotericism: does Strauss imply that the difference between his earlier and later interpretation of Spinoza turns on a deeper understanding of esotericism?

Epicureanism but also with the generally 'radical' atheism of the age of Enlightenment, is a descendant of the tradition grounded in the Bible: it accepts the thesis, the negation of the Enlightenment, on the basis of a way of thinking which became possible only through the Bible. . . . [I]t is itself the latest, most radical, most unassailable harmonization of these opposed positions." Late modern atheism is an indelibly post-Christian phenomenon; and while its dedication to consistency may well lead it to uncover many illusions, it cannot—according to Strauss—avoid the fact that a philosophy based on the moral imperative to conscientiousness is self-contradictory; its most fundamental premise is belief and not knowledge; and "being based on belief is fatal to any philosophy."

In Strauss's telling, all of this seems to be a working out of the willful character of modern philosophy. Spinoza and others, it seems from the vantage point of the Spinoza book, chose as an act of will to live in a world defined by the impossibility of an omnipotent God. But as an act of will, the basis of the claim is not self-evident: the modern project is a choice and not a necessity. The sneaking suspicion of an inability to refute the omnipotent God seems to be the source of motion behind the development from early modern Enlightenment to late modern existentialism. From this point of view, the unfolding of modernity might well be seen as the relentless uncovering of the moral motive behind the modern way of philosophizing, which we might call the spiritedness at the root of modernity. Let us not be afraid to acknowledge the humanly impressive, not to say terrifying, character of these late modern thinkers who both expose and exemplify the spirited roots of modernity. But an atheism based on conscience or probity is just as irrefutable and indemonstrable as is the hypothesis of the omnipotent God. Enlightenment and religion thus conceived can only confront each other as incomprehensible and uncomprehending adversaries. If, as Strauss suggests, the antagonism between Enlightenment and orthodoxy is "not theoretical but moral," it would seem to be because the antagonism is at bottom political: no further rational conversation seems possible, only the the verbal thrusts and diplomatic démarches of warring polities. The politicization of philosophy ends in the loss of the possibility of theory.

Conclusion

Strauss's "Preface" provides indispensable help in getting hold of the situation of Enlightenment—our situation. Yet the ultimate result of Strauss's inquiries remains unclear. By the end of it, all sides are compromised; every position discussed seems to be insufficient or to borrow surreptitiously from its opponents. Neither the defenders of Judaism like Rosenzweig and Cohen nor the partisans of modern Enlightenment in its various guises seem to have viable arguments. Meanwhile Strauss refrains from discussing two positions of great interest to his readers. First, orthodoxy remains an almost silent interlocutor throughout the essay. Despite the fact that orthodoxy appears at every significant turning point as the path not taken, as an ever-present alternative in whose light the defects and self-contradictions of other positions appear, Strauss never engages with it directly: no representative of orthodoxy is allowed to speak in his own name in the essay. Whatever may have been Strauss's final position on orthodoxy, he quite clearly uses it here (and elsewhere) to probe the assumptions underlying various rationalisms, to expose their unarticulated faiths and their undefended presuppositions. As such, orthodoxy is a most potent tool of the Socratic investigation of opinions. Second, the Preface is also silent in regard to Strauss's own considered judgment as of 1962; as an intellectual autobiography the essay is visibly lacking. Strauss covers the period of his life through the publication of the Spinoza book with great depth, yet merely mentions his "change of orientation" which occurred sometime in the 1930s. The mature phase of Strauss's thought, the rediscovery of classical political rationalism, appears on the horizon, but just barely. Yet these lacunae in the Preface need not mean that Strauss's treatment is of merely historical interest or only concerned with positions superseded by later events. In a dialectical fashion, we may first need to work through various inadequate positions in order to clear the way for something else. Strauss's essay is on this view a propaedeutic to further investigations, investigations for which Strauss only whets our appetite.

The initial impression that all positive positions have been discredited by the end of Strauss's essay is thus not the whole story: we readers remain "on the way" at the end of the essay, and Strauss provides rich materials for reflection on our situation. By way of conclusion, I mention three positive lessons we may learn from the essay. First, regarding *the character of politics*: Political reflection begins from the recognition of the need to act, primarily for the sake of our own self-interest, but not solely. Political responsibility requires that we be clear-sighted and hard-headed. Because we must be concerned with the long-term flourishing of ourselves and our communities, we cannot retreat into utopian moralizing. Strauss's quiet but unmistakable judgment on both Rosenzweig and Cohen is that they underestimated the power of human evil: "but for the fear of the government, men would swallow each other alive." In light of what happened in Germany between the thirties and the sixties, the significance of the point can hardly be overstated. Nevertheless, it is also true that political reflection on its own is insufficient to engage the whole human being. Politics needs a supplement; it willy-nilly looks up to something, some account of nature or the divine. Since political life is shaped, whether we intend it or not, by thoughts about what is highest, we would do well to try to see those thoughts for what they are. Better to articulate them than to allow ourselves to be unwittingly shaped by them.

Second, *the perils of religiosity*: Many of us want to have our cake and eat it too: we want the material benefits of modern science and the moral seriousness of religion. On Strauss's telling, Cohen and Rosenzweig attempted to have it both ways—not very successfully, as it turns out. Yet at least at the outset, whether or in what sense science and religion can be harmonized is very much an open question. Our attempts to put those things together often do more honor to our hopes or wishes that all good things go together than to our clear-sightedness. But as Strauss remarks elsewhere, our need or desire for a resolution to these questions does not prove that such a resolution is available.[14] That said, we must also admit that many modern atheists can be accused of an opposite confusion: being motivated by anti-Christian or anti-theological animus, they cannot see their opponents or themselves clearly. At least some of these atheists are parasitic on Christianity. In an analogous context G. K. Chesterton made the illuminating remark that such critics are largely reactive. They can neither be Christians nor leave off being anti-Christians. It would be better, as he says, to be really inside Christianity or really outside it: "It is well with a boy when he lives on his father's land; and well with him when he is far enough from it to look back on it and see it as a whole. But these people [the critics of religion] have got into an intermediate state, have fallen into an intervening valley from which they can see neither the heights beyond them nor the heights behind. . . . Now the best relation to our spiritual home is to be near enough to love it. But the next best is to be far enough away not to hate it."[15] Such a sentiment, it seems to me, is not far from Strauss's, even if made from a different point of view.

Third, *the need for anthropology or human wisdom*: Strauss's essay forces us to confront some hard questions about the nature and character of divinity and perhaps even about the nature of nature. But one need not wade into those deep waters to raise questions about the completeness of modern accounts of the human. Modern science and early modern thought more generally have proved remarkably effective in a variety of arenas; yet many later modern thinkers, from Rousseau down to our own time, bear witness to the resurgence of the human desire or need for the noble and the divine. The fact that on the political level those desires have born fruit in the variety of modern

14. Leo Strauss, *Natural Right and History* (Chicago: University of Chicago Press, 1953), 6.
15. G. K. Chesterton, *Everlasting Man* (Peabody, Massachusetts: Hendrickson, 2007), 4-5.

tyrannies and fanaticisms is all the more argument for trying to see them as they are rather than dismissing them as atavisms.[16] Prior to questions about the character of the divine or about nature, there are questions about whether we have correctly understood what has been called "the human experience of the human." Does being human involve a directedness toward the transcendent, however understood? Can an adequate account of the human be given, starting solely from the necessities of self-preservation and the like? Have we ourselves articulated and clarified our own desire or need for the noble or divine? Did certain premodern authors not possess an understanding of these questions superior to our own—superior not as a matter of metaphysics or science but of simple human self-knowledge?[17]

Strauss's essay shows why there might be a serious audience for a genuine reconsideration of the Bible in its own voice and on its own terms—the kind of inquiry to which Leon Kass's *The Beginning of Wisdom* invites us. Precisely because the giants of the Enlightenment defined themselves over and against the Bible, we inheritors of their efforts ought to try to hear and understand the Bible in its own voice, free of the polemical context of our culture wars, and uninfluenced by the dogmatic prejudice toward atheism bequeathed to us by modern science. Even more importantly, our experience of modernity, both in its undoubted successes and its great failures, compels us—as children of skeptics know all too well—to raise anew the question of how we should live. *The Beginning of Wisdom* provides an invitation to think again about that question as a real question, and to ponder the Bible's way of answering it.

But whatever substantive wisdom we may gain from that inquiry, *The Beginning of Wisdom* gives us a lesson, just as important and easily overlooked, about the way a genuinely wisdom-seeking inquiry might proceed. Such an inquiry starts neither from some orthodox presuppositions nor from a dogmatic attachment to rationalism. For us the larger danger comes from dogmatic rationalism, and its confident assertion that we know there are no miracles. But that claim is more than we know and is likely merely the expression of our desire not to be surprised, to be in control. The atheists prominent in today's culture wars often seem to be moved more by outrage at the possibility that

16. Consider Francois Furet's comment on the democratic need for utopia at *The Passing of an Illusion: The Idea of Communism in the Twentieth Century* (Chicago: University of Chicago Press, 1999), 502. As Furet remarks, the fall of the Soviet Union should by no means be taken as evidence of the end of the human desire for a more perfect life, even in liberal democracies.

17. In speaking of Hitler's Germany and Soviet Russia, Strauss remarked: "Catastrophes and horrors of a magnitude hitherto unknown, which we have seen, and through which we have lived, were better provided for, or made intelligible, by both Plato and the prophets than by the modern belief in progress." ("Jerusalem and Athens," in *Jewish Philosophy and the Crisis of Modernity*, 399.)

the world might not be fully transparent and predictable than by a thoughtful consideration of the merits of the case. A genuine openness to the world would seem to require of us both a willingness to suspend disbelief—to try things out, to hear and consider before judging—and a tenacious desire to reason things through. Reading the book of Genesis in this spirit cultivates the virtues necessary for a reader, those disciplines of the heart and head that tell us what to care about and give us the wit to recognize it when we see it. And it may well give us indispensable practice for that larger task of developing a genuine openness to the world beyond the book, or beyond any book.

The difference between that spirit and the spirit of many a modern philosopher is perhaps best illustrated by a remark of Strauss's from *Philosophy and Law*. Intellectual probity of the sort recommended by Nietzsche and Heidegger, among others, he suggests, is associated with the attempt to make atheism into a "positive, dogmatic premise." Yet if atheism is not demonstrable, the attempt to build a system on it will necessarily entail shutting off other possibilities and silencing our consciousness of our own ignorance. Strauss illustrates the difference between that intellectual probity and the love of wisdom by quoting a French scholar of ancient Greek philosophy: "This conception of probity recalls the definition of criticism: 'la critique . . . a pour essence la negation du surnaturel.' To this it was objected: 'l'essence du critique, c'est l'attention.'"[18]

18. *Philosophy and Law*, 137 n. 17.

14

The God-Seeking Animal

Eric Cohen

At the very least, they can be persuaded that the bodily position makes no difference to their prayers; for they constantly forget, what you must always remember, that they are animals and that whatever their bodies do affects their souls.

–C. S. Lewis, *The Screwtape Letters*

On the cover of *Being Human*, the anthology of writings collected by the President's Council on Bioethics under Leon Kass's stewardship in 2003, there is a picture of a ballerina. She is leaping into the air, body extended, gazing and reaching and soaring toward the heavens, looking at once so perfectly natural and so unnaturally perfect. Why this image on a book that aims to illuminate the problems and possibilities of the human condition? There are, after all, so many other possible images of being human: from the *ordinary activities of human life*, like walking or sleeping; to images of *being human together*, like conversing or embracing; from images of *human neediness and care-giving*, like the patient and the nurse, in bed and at the bedside, or the mother and child, holding and being held.

Kass would surely see rich themes to explore in these many images of the human form, and the Council's collection of readings grapples with the many faces, postures, and possibilities of the human animal. But Kass deliberately chose the ballerina to represent us—an image that celebrates our embodiment and not our rationality alone; our yearning for the beautiful and not our ordinariness alone. The ballerina embodies the graceful human animal at its best—one of us, to be sure, yet also separated from us by the heights to which she can reach, by the elevated posture she can assume, by the pleasure that she brings to those who behold her. And while we fellow humans may watch her in awe, this perfection-seeking performance seems more like her own offering to the divine, which her body seeks at the very peak of her movement.

Ovid, in his *Metamorphoses*, celebrates such heaven-gazing humans:

> And, though all other animals
> Are prone, and fix their gaze
> Upon the earth, he gave to
> Man an uplifted face
> And bade him stand
> Erect and turn his eyes
> To heaven.[1]

Perhaps the ballerina is Ovid's perfect human; her entire being—arms, eyes, "uplifted face"—reaches upward "to heaven." And perhaps this is why Kass chose her—as an image of man's heaven-seeking glimpse of perfection.

An image—but surely not the only image of the human animal seeking the divine. Consider, for a moment, the very different posture of the worshipper bowed down in prayer, prostrate rather than soaring. In those rarest moments in Jewish liturgy, coming once on Rosh Hashanah and again on Yom Kippur, the worshiping Jew lies face to the floor, hands over his eyes, in a bodily act of fear and reverence. Unlike the ballerina, the bowed worshipper's body is abject, frozen, limp, needy. Such prostrations, called for only on the holiest days of the Jewish year, are not the achievement of the graceful few but instead the practice of the God-seeking many. In fulfilling this ritual obligation, the mass of worshippers imitate the awe-filled body of Moses, who hid his face in fear when he heard the voice behind the burning bush and later fell to the ground after destroying the tablets of the law that his stiff-necked people were unworthy to receive. In a series of three further prostrations on Yom Kippur, Jewish worshippers re-enact the awed response of their ancestors, who crowded into the Temple precincts to witness the High Priest performing the annual rite of atonement and to hear him pronounce the unutterable name of the Lord.

Head up or face down, the soaring ballerina or the bent man of prayer, the human animal shows his distinctness from the other animals through the forms and activities of his body. The monkey, for all his leaping, produces no ballerinas; and the snake, cursed forever to the ground, never lies face down in reverence. To understand Kass's work, and to seek with Kass the meaning of being human, one needs to unpack the mystery of Moses and the ballerina, of Ovid and the Bible—two peaks, each divine-seeking, taking the body in opposite directions.

1. Ovid, *Metamorphoses*, trans. Frank J. Miller (London: William Heinemann, 1928), I, 8. Kass highlights this passage in *Toward a More Natural Science* (New York: Free Press, 1985), 276.

SANCTIFYING THE ANIMAL

The phrase "God-seeking animal" has three parts, best considered in reverse: The (1) animal who (2) seeks (3) God. This means we need to begin with *animality* before considering the *human* animal, and only then considering why perhaps the most distinctive truth about the human animal is that he seeks God—or, as Kass would put it, "longs" for "the divine."

I once asked Kass which piece of his own writing gave him the greatest pleasure and pride. He paused, smiled, and then directed me to a passage about a squirrel:

> What, for example, is a healthy squirrel? Not a picture of a squirrel, not really or fully the sleeping squirrel, not even the aggregate of his normal blood pressure, serum calcium, total body zinc, normal digestion, fertility, and the like. Rather, the healthy squirrel is a bushy-tailed fellow who looks and acts like a squirrel; who leaps through the trees with great daring; who gathers, buries, covers but later uncovers and recovers his acorns; who perches out on a limb cracking his nuts, sniffing the air for smells of danger, alert, cautious, with his tail beating rhythmically; who chatters and plays and courts and mates, and rears his young in large improbable-looking homes at the tops of trees; who fights with vigor and forages with cunning; who shows spiritedness, even anger, and more prudence than many human beings.[2]

It is a beautiful passage, even for those whose sensibilities (like mine) are not naturally attuned to the wonders of nature and to the aliveness of our fellow animals. (My young children, I have learned, are quite attuned, especially to squirrels.) We, too, are animals with bodies and doings—conceived and then born, nursing and then eating, crawling and then walking, babbling and then speaking, getting sick and then getting well, growing up and then giving birth, working and then resting, growing old and then shrinking, suffering and then dying. To understand our aliveness, our own being, we need to see what it means to be an animal, and then what it means to be a human animal—alike yet so unlike all the other animals.

In Kass's great work *The Hungry Soul*, he explores one of those activities—eating—that we share with the other animals. Like them, we need to eat to live. Like them, the human infant knows instinctively where—from whom—to find nourishment. Like them, we cannot take for granted the food we need in order to live; we rely upon nature's bounty for our sustenance, and

2. Kass, *Toward a More Natural Science*, 173.

the young rely upon their elders to feed them. Yet in this most animal activity, man also demonstrates his difference. For only man incorporates food into an elevated way of life. Man alone among the animals dines with old friends in fine restaurants, says grace before meals, or separates milk and meat in observance of the laws of kashrut. Man alone constrains his appetites in the name of civility or holiness. We are, in other words, not only hungry bodies but hungry bodies with hungry souls—souls that yearn for the community of friends and for the sanctification of animal life, souls that adorn animal necessity with beauty and refinement and that elevate metabolic necessity in obedience to the transcendent.

Eating is just one example of man remaining an animal while seeking to be more than an animal. Like other animals, we are born into the world, but man alone performs the *bris* and the baptism, bodily acts that symbolize the newborn's new relationship with the covenant-making and history-redeeming God. Like other animals, we die, but man alone buries the dead with rituals of remembrance, thinking beyond the lifeless body to the possibility of immortality. In one realm in particular—as sexual animals—we demonstrate both our animality and our potential transcendence of mere animality. And here, as elsewhere, there is no better guide than Kass.

In an essay explicating and appreciating his teacher Hans Jonas's *The Phenomenon of Life*, Kass suggests a deep problem with Jonas's account: Jonas forgets about sex, and in doing so portrays animal life, and especially human life, as more solitary than it is, a lonely struggle for survival in an organic world that is both the generous source of the self's being and a permanent threat (ultimately victorious) to the self's existence. This is surely true, as Kass would never deny. But it is also only part of the story. In probing the meaning of bodily life, Jonas fails to account for the very biological function that sustains life from one generation to the next: sexual attraction, leading to copulation, leading to conception, leading to reproduction. Kass, in a few pages of sympathetic criticism, thinks in Jonasian ways to turn Jonas on his head—reorienting his philosophical biology from the solitary self living against death to the united couple giving life, knowing and being known by the other, a knowing that is followed by the coming-into-being of offspring who likewise know them. He reorients our vision from mortality to natality, and from existential loneliness to marital union and inter-generational fidelity.[3]

As Kass points out, the primal layer of human sexuality is the bodily desire we share with other sexual animals. This sexual desire, like all forms of desire, is always and only felt by an individual animal: the lone wolf, the lone ape, the lone

3. Leon R. Kass, "Appreciating the Phenomenon of Life," *The Hastings Center Report* 25:6 (1995), 3-12.

man. The individual body is aroused, and the lusting animal covets both intensification and relief of that arousal. The sexual impulse drives the aroused animal toward the body of another who is like yet unlike, the complementary counterpart. This is equally true of monkeys and of men. But then comes the crucial turn, when the animal becomes the human animal. As Kass describes it, following Genesis:

> [M]an became man when he became self-conscious not of his mortality but of his sexuality, of the uncanny and mysterious doubleness in his (animal) soul. He became human—rather they became human, man and woman together—when each saw through the eyes of the other the fact (and meaning) of their nakedness. Each discovered the true meaning of being in need of the complementary other who is, in fact, not just a missing part of oneself, as the man had said (flesh of my flesh), but a genuinely independent being; each discovered the presence of unruly desires within that want something of us that we don't understand; each became aware that these infirmities are quite evident to the sexual other, from whom, therefore, each now wants not only sexual gratification but also approval and admiration. From the discovery of shame-filled nakedness comes much of civilization, beginning with the arts of concealment and beautification (the needle and the fig leaf). In turn, clothing and adornment, by means of refusal and its effects on the imagination, transform animal lust into human eros, which takes wings from the recognition that there are higher possibilities for man than the finally unfulfilling acts of bodily fusion. Among these possibilities are the establishments of long-lived familial societies, grounded in the awareness that sex means children, that human children need long-term rearing including rearing for sociality, morality, and love, and that children are indeed life's (partial) answer to mortality.[4]

Of course, Kass is only telling the elevating part of the human story. Man's sexual difference from the other animals also leads to his own unique capacity for self-degradation, and his own unique power to turn against the natural transcendence of self that comes with procreation. Human beings alone are capable of adultery and prostitution, as well as marriage. Human beings alone produce the culture of Paris Hilton and Internet pornography, as well as of Jane Austen and the Song of Songs. And human beings alone can pursue animal-like sexual pleasure without animal-like procreative consequences. The ideology of the Pill—note: not any pill, but *the* Pill—rejects the intimation of permanence embodied in the marital vow and the intimation of immortality that comes with procreation.[5] Man

4. Ibid., 12.

5. I use the phrase "ideology of the pill" quite deliberately. For there is a difference between using modern birth control to govern the spacing or number of children within marriage and seeing

sometimes chooses instead the sterile pursuit of limitless physical bliss, which typically ends in the sadness of being buried without children to mourn, or remember, or carry on.

Kass—and the Hebrew Bible from which he learns—offer a different teaching about the layers of human sexuality and the sexual ascent of man. The first layer is lust, which leads us beyond ourselves, man to woman, woman to man. For the other animals, lust is the biological driver of a natural story in which each animal plays its part—and can do no other. For men and women, lust spurs a deeper psychological and ultimately moral-theological drama: the mere animal desire for union exists alongside an awareness of our nakedness, our neediness, our incompleteness. With this awareness, two roads diverge. The pagan path—which seeks the shame-free sexual satisfactions of the other animals without the animal (procreative) consequences of sex, and which seeks erotic union with one's beloved without the burdens of progeny—is captured by the Roman poet writing to his mistress: "Let me be your one joy; you at my side, I have no need of sons to feed my pride." The path of Jerusalem—sexual modesty before the other and before God, and lust governed by the unbreakable promise of marital fidelity and the God-seeking yearning for descendents—is captured in the story of Hannah and her son: "She named him Samuel, saying, 'because I asked the Lord for him.'"[6]

From lust to nakedness, from nakedness to shame, from shame to modesty, from modesty to marriage, from marriage to children, from children to the drama of accepting one's own finitude and yearning for the transcendence of the biological self—this is God-seeking sex, the ascent of the body beyond the body. In the marital vow, husband and wife experience the intimation of permanence, of standing with *this* particular other forever and always. In the birth and rearing of children, father and mother experience the intimation of immortality, of life beyond themselves connected to *them* for eternity; and they experience the intimation of divine creation, of the God-like power of bringing new life into being out of themselves. But these intimations of the divine do not ultimately quench man's yearning for the perfect seal upon thy heart, fiercer than death. Man and woman seek, also, to be known fully by the divine—a yearning that they express, at the peak of this erotic longing, in the ecstatic language of the body. To quote the opening lines of the greatest love poem ever written:

> Oh, give me of the kisses of your mouth,
> For your love is more delightful than wine.
> Your ointments yield a sweet fragrance,

the pill as a biochemical means of sexual freedom without procreative intentions or consequences.

6. 1 Samuel 1:20.

> Your name is like finest oil—
> Therefore do maidens love you.
> Draw me after you, let us run!
> The king has brought me to his chambers.
> Let us delight and rejoice in your love,
> Savoring it more than wine.[7]

Man seeks this perfect love—but does he find it? "O you who linger in the garden, A lover is listening; Let me hear your voice. Hurry, my beloved, Swift as a gazelle or a young stag, To the hills of spices!"[8]

BENT AND STRAIGHT: THE GOD-SEEKING BODY

This image of the gazelle is itself suggestive. In human sexuality, bodily vigor and bodily submission, our powers and our neediness, are both on display. We are invigorated, yet lying down. "Swift as a gazelle" suggests a different image of bodily vigor—of the runner in stride, of the ballerina at her heights. This brings us back to where we began, and back to Kass's own reflections on the distinctive and deepest meaning of man's bodily life.

In an essay spurred by the steroid scandals plaguing professional sports, Kass explores the dehumanizing effects of biotechnological enhancement by trying to understand the meaning of distinctly human activity, in comparison with and in contrast to the bodily doings of the other animals:

> The truth and the beauty of integrated and embodied human activity are displayed and celebrated in human sport (and also in dance and musical performance). When we see an outstanding athlete in action, we do not see—as we do in horse racing—a rational agent riding or whipping a separate animal body. We see instead a body gracefully and harmoniously at work, but at work with discipline and focus, pushing its limits and displaying its powers, all the while tacitly obeying the rules and requirements of the game. We know immediately that the human athlete is engaged in deliberate and goal-directed activity, that he is not running in flight moved by fear or in pursuit moved by hunger. Yet while the human character of his bodily movements is at once obvious, the "mindedness" of the bodily activity is tacit and unobtrusive. So attuned is the body, and so harmonious is it with the heart and mind, that—in the best instance—the whole activity of the athlete appears effortlessly to flow from a unified and undivided being. At such moments

7. Song of Solomon 1:1-5.
8. Ibid., 8:13-14.

> the athlete experiences and displays something like the unity of doer and deed one observes in other animals, but with this difference: for humans, such a unity is an achievement. A great sprinter may run like a gazelle and a great boxer may fight like a tiger, but one would never mistake their harmony of body and soul for the brute instinct that spurs an animal toward flight or fight.[9]

The gazelle surely runs with more grace and arguably more beauty than most men. It is faster and more natural, surely a source of pleasure to its creator. But man alone, at his peak, performs in the knowing pursuit of perfection. Such a pursuit is dangerous indeed, and Kass has given strong moral voice to its potential dark side. In a stirring lecture at the U.S. Holocaust museum, he warns against the pagan worship of the "glass man," the idol of Weimar eugenics, which envisioned a master race of bodies engineered to perfection by the new science of genetics. Kass's lecture reminds us of the ultimate worth of mere men, not glass men—which is to say, the worth of men with imperfect, needy bodies, born messily of embodied mothers rather than conjured neatly in the laboratory.[10] But this same critic of the glass man can himself take great pleasure in the striding Olympian and choose the soaring ballerina to represent us on the cover of the Council's volume on *Being Human*. Kass thereby invites us to ponder the difference between worshipping the human body as an idol and appreciating the human being at-work as an act of gratitude for the special powers that man alone possesses—to soar like a ballerina, to run like an Olympian, to sing upward to the heavens. And so Kass ends his essay on sport with a quotation from Eric Liddell, the Scottish runner, explaining why he could not give up running—not just yet—to work as a Christian missionary in China: "I believe that God made me for a purpose, but He also made me fast, and when I run I feel His pleasure.... To give up running would be to hold Him in contempt."[11] His running, in other words, was an act of worship.

But the bodies of the runners and ballerinas will eventually decline; the voices of the singers will grow weak and off-pitch; the fingers of the violinist will lose their strength and precision; the men and women who glimpse perfection with acts of the body at their peak will one day become like the rest of us—mere imperfect mortals, submitting to man's limits, including the ultimate limit that is death, and hoping their individual lives have some ultimate

9. Leon R. Kass and Eric Cohen, "For the Love of the Game," *The New Republic*, March 26, 2008. Kass and I co-authored this essay, but the quoted section is his.

10. From an unpublished lecture delivered at the United States Holocaust Memorial Museum, March 17, 2005.

11. Leon R. Kass and Eric Cohen, "For the Love of the Game," *The New Republic*, March 26, 2008.

meaning. Even the most upright human animals cannot worship in the upright posture alone. And so they also bow their heads, and cover their faces, and cry out to the divine source of their own being in the hope that He exists, and that He cares.

There is a discussion in the Talmud about whether, on the high holidays of Rosh Hashanah and Yom Kippur, the worshipping Jew should blow a ram's horn that is straight or a ram's horn that is bent.

> On what points do [the sages] argue? One master holds that on Rosh Hashanah the more a person bows his mind, the better it is; therefore, a bent shofar is used to reflect this attitude of submission and humility. And on Yom Kippur of the Jubilee Year the more a person straightens his mind, the better it is; therefore, a straight shofar is used to reflect this attitude of freedom. But the other master maintains that on Rosh Hashanah the more a person straightens his mind, the better it is; therefore, a straight shofar is preferable. And on fast days [like Yom Kippur], the more a person bows his mind, the better it is; therefore, a bent shofar is preferred.[12]

Where these two rabbis seem to agree, however, is that man is the being who alone approaches the divine both bent and straight, assuming each God-seeking posture in its proper season.

I think it is fair to say that one of the great threads of Leon Kass's work is to understand man as the upright being who bows his head in reverence. He has illuminated, in his writings and in his very being, these two unique dimensions of our humanity—straight and bent, upright and bowing. As he wrote in his first book, the neo-Aristotelian *Toward a More Natural Science*: "We stand most upright when we gladly bow our heads." And as he writes in his most recent book, the biblical *The Beginning of Wisdom*: "The upright animal, his gaze uplifted and his heart filled with wonder and awe, begins to suspect that he may in fact stand tallest when he freely bows his head."[13] In a body of writings that spans nearly four decades and probes virtually every human subject under the sun—love, death, science, nature, men, women, progress, eternity—this image of man, upright and head-bowed, is perhaps the great anthropological continuity that binds it all together, coming into ever greater focus first for our teacher, then for all of us, his grateful students.

12. The quotation is from tract *Rosh Hashanah*, 26b of the Babylonian Talmud. I am grateful to my colleague Rabbi Yehuda Seif for illuminating this passage for me.

13. Leon R. Kass, *The Beginning of Wisdom: Reading Genesis* (New York: Free Press, 2003), 53.

15

The Traditional Animal: Leon Kass on the Wisdom of the Ages and the Perfection of Man's Nature

Yuval Levin

Many of our men of speculation, instead of exploding general prejudices, employ their sagacity to discover the latent wisdom which prevails in them. If they find what they seek, and they seldom fail, they think it more wise to continue the prejudice, with the reason involved, than to cast away the coat of prejudice, and to leave nothing but the naked reason; because prejudice, with its reason, has a motive to give action to that reason, and an affection which will give it permanence.

–Edmund Burke, *Reflections on the Revolution in France*

As the range of contributors and topics that compose this volume of appreciation helps make clear, the range of subjects to which Leon Kass has ably put his mind and pen is extraordinarily broad. From the nature of nature to the ethics of science, the meaning of the Hebrew Bible, the project of the early modern philosophers, the wisdom of Aristotle, the insights of Tolstoy, and on and on through a daunting array of humanities and sciences ancient and modern, Kass has traveled far and wide in search of understanding. We who are his students have an immense debt to acknowledge. Perhaps the most fitting way to offer some down payment on that debt is to reflect on how we understand the teachings Kass has offered, and where his wisdom and guidance have pointed us.

In my own case, the debt is very great indeed, and the question of where Kass's insights have directed me is complicated. They have surely taken me into bioethics and the philosophy of science. They have led me also to think anew and differently about the Bible, the family, and the nation, among a host of other matters. But above all, they have led me to the quandaries of tradition. Tradition is not actually a question about which Kass has said much explicitly. It of course comes up in his writings and draws his attention, but more than anything, to my mind, it rises as a consequence of the intellectual course he has charted over decades and continues still to pursue. His efforts as they have developed gesture toward an unusual and promising hybrid of philosophy and tradition—the seeking of wisdom about man's nature in his highest cultural forms, practices, and achievements—that may enrich and illuminate the study of both and reopen the path to a true anthropology long since abandoned by our sciences and increasingly ignored by our humanities as well.

An Ascent in Touch with its Beginnings

Leon Kass's professional turn to the humanities began, as he tells it, in a concern about science, or more precisely in a concern about the yawning gap "between all activities of life as lived and those activities as understood scientifically."[1] Modern science, for reasons and in ways that Kass has done much to illuminate, set itself in opposition to both ordinary human experience and speculative philosophy, and sought instead to understand the world through the rarified clarity of symbolic mathematics. This move was immensely successful, and the resulting scientific enterprise has done a world of good, but it has also turned a blind eye not only to moral questions, but to almost every question that presents itself at the level of human (and even of animal) experience: the level not of particles in motion but of organisms and phenomena, of purposes and wholes.

For Kass, the reductionism of modern science, while surely productive in its own terms, closed off some crucial paths to understanding human life in its fullness. The phenomena of life as they present themselves offer crucial insights into the nature of living things, and a natural science that ignores them is therefore grossly incomplete. As such a science grows more and more capable, moreover, it risks putting ever greater power in the hands of a populace ever more confused about its better and worse uses—a judgment, after all, that demands a sense of man's nature and his proper purposes, "a richer understanding and deeper appreciation of our humanity, necessary for facing the challenges confronting us in a biotechnological age."[2]

Kass's first book, *Toward a More Natural Science*, sought to show how a science that took greater account of the phenomena of life could lead to a deeper understanding of the natural world, and especially of the human animal. "Certain apparently superficial aspects of the body are in fact deeply revealing of

1. Leon R. Kass, *The Hungry Soul: Eating and the Perfecting of Our Nature* (Chicago: University of Chicago Press, 1999), 11.

2. The President's Council on Bioethics, *Being Human: Readings from the President's Council on Bioethics* (Washington, DC: Government Printing Office, 2003), xvii (chairman's introduction).

human being—and its irreducible perplexities," he wrote.[3] As long as we are closed off to these aspects of our humanity, Kass argues, we will fail to understand the human being, and so will fail fully to provide for our needs or to enable our flourishing. Indeed, a science that looks only at the raw material of man will be blind in particular to what makes man different from the other animals, and so to what makes the human being human. "At the center of any philosophical anthropology will be an account of the human difference, of what is peculiarly human about human nature and the human animal," he writes.[4] Without such an account—without knowing what kind of beings we are—we can have little hope of understanding how we ought to live.

In some of his earliest efforts on this front, Kass sought to address the problem by reforming our understanding of the purpose and meaning of science itself. What we lacked, he argued, was a truly scientific—truly knowledgeable—picture of the human animal in its full humanity, and so what was required was a revitalized natural science, reconnected with its classical philosophical purposes and oriented "to encourage and nurture the disposition of thoughtfulness about who we are and ought to be."[5] He worked both to demonstrate what the modern turn away from the meaningful phenomena of life had wrought, and to show how the insights left behind might be recovered without abandoning the benefits that modern science had made possible. But throughout the essays gathered in *Toward a More Natural Science*, Kass seems clearly aware that recovering the kind of anthropology he seeks would require more than reminding science of the price it has paid for its Cartesian turn. A more natural science almost certainly cannot be recovered directly, and the fuller picture of man and his nature must be looked for simultaneously in other ways.

In his ambitious sequel, *The Hungry Soul: Eating and the Perfecting of Our Nature*, Kass sought to reinforce the effort by recourse to our cultural practices and traditions, some of which, he argues, show clear evidence of having been custom-designed for precisely the kind of human being modern science now denies we are. The wisdom latent in our longstanding conventions is wisdom about human nature, and its teaching therefore *is* a more natural science. The method of *The Hungry Soul* marked a turn—a turn which in his teaching and writing Kass had long before taken—to seek after wisdom in the cultural and intellectual inheritances of our civilization on the assumption that these were forged by students of human nature confronted with the same basic questions

3. Leon R. Kass, *Toward a More Natural Science* (New York: Free Press, 1985), 13.

4. Kass, *The Hungry Soul*, xv.

5. Kass, *Toward a More Natural Science*, xii.

human beings must always confront, and that they have survived because they offer profound and in important ways also true answers to these questions.

The Hungry Soul, by taking up a subject at the nexus of the natural and the cultural, shows how this expanded search follows directly from Kass's concern about the scientific turn away from human experience. It too is directed to addressing "the gap between the ethically sterile nature studied by science and the morally freighted life lived by human beings."[6] And it too seeks to recover a mode of understanding open to a richer sense of what it is to be human. Like a forensic investigator piecing together the measurements of the missing man by studying the clothes that had fit him best,[7] Kass seeks to paint a fuller picture of the human animal by seeking wisdom latent in the cultural accoutrements that have best spoken to those aspects of ourselves ignored by our modern scientific outlook. When we consider the rituals, practices, stories, and traditions that mean the most to us and shape our lives, Kass argues, we find that we are not just matter in motion. "Our souls still crave the drama of what Tolstoy called 'real life': immediately meaningful work, genuine love and intimacy, true ties to place and persons, kinship with nature, family, and community, dignity, understanding, and an openness to the divine. But real life has become nearly impossible as we have ceased to know and honor its forms."[8]

The emphasis on forms is no coincidence. Just as in his earlier writings directed explicitly to natural science, in his writing and thinking about culture and the humanities Kass seeks to draw meaning from the *forms* of human being and doing. He makes this connection explicit in *The Hungry Soul*:

> The central thread that guides the argument in its ascent is the idea of *form*, with its multiple yet always interconnected meanings. An animal's form or organization is distinguishable (yet also inseparable) from its materials; thanks to its form an animal is distinguishable from other kinds of animals; thanks to the psychic powers that emerge with its special form or organized embodiment, many an animal—and especially the animal that bears the peculiarly upright form—can respond to and have commerce with the myriad forms of the surrounding world. These silent forms impress themselves on the imagination and receive articulate recognition in the speech of the human animal, whose rational openness to the multiform world is, paradoxically, what makes him also its great trans*former*. Yet the cultural forms that clothe his naked nature can also form him (or re-form or

6. Kass, *The Hungry Soul*, 5.

7. Kass employs this image of culture as clothing in Leon R. Kass, "Looking for an Honest Man," *National Affairs*, No. 1, Fall 2009, 176.

8. Kass, *The Hungry Soul*, xx-xxi.

> trans-form or de-form him), in the best case to conform him to the best and the highest possibilities implicit in his own unique form and embodiment.[9]

The ways we do what we do, even when we are not explicitly alert to their sources or meanings, tell us an enormous amount about who and what we human beings are. And the best and highest artifacts of our cultural traditions are those that speak to these deepest questions of meaning, and that offer us some hints of how we may conform to those highest possibilities implicit in our nature.

The search after that nature and its highest possibilities has in this way taken Kass from the study of the human animal to the study of the cultural habitat that animal has constructed for itself—but always with an eye to the true and fullest nature of the human being himself. In describing the structure of the argument of *The Hungry Soul*—which traces the meaning of eating from its biological character through the limits and constraints human beings have placed upon it, to the ways we have beautified it and turned feeding into dining, through the roles it has played in our highest religious rituals—Kass puts things this way: "The argument is thus an ascent—from nature to human nature to human nature culturally clothed by the just, then the noble, then the holy—but an ascent that remains in touch with its beginnings."[10] There in a nutshell is the arc of Kass's interests over more than four decades and counting. In search of wisdom about how human beings may flourish, he has studied nature and man's nature, and in pursuit of man's nature he has delved deeply and broadly into our cultural wisdom about justice and ethics, nobility and excellence, and then sanctity and holiness.

In his ongoing study of biology and bioethics, his teaching of great works of literature and philosophy, and his inquiry into the depths of the Bible, Kass seeks the nature of man through his ways of being and acting. In the forms of human life—the arc of the individual lifespan and the ever-repeating intergenerational shape of family life, the rituals of birth and love and marriage and mourning, the rules of courtship and worship—is the outline of the human flourishing that our modern natural science leaves out of view, but that we modern human beings desperately desire, even when we do not quite know it. "Cultural memory still holds gingerly a tattered script" for such flourishing, Kass writes, "but many of its pages are missing and the guidance it provides us is barely audible and, even then, delivered in what appears to us to be a foreign tongue."[11] Kass has worked to learn and to teach that foreign tongue, the language of human flourishing in which the

9. Ibid., 14.
10. Ibid.
11. Ibid., xx.

great cultural achievements of Western civilization are written. "An appreciation of what is given to us by nature could point us toward humanly instituted practices and beliefs that perfect our given nature," Kass writes. "If true, this would imply that some practices really are just, noble, and holy, and that we can discern or discover what they are."[12]

This is why Kass has been a student and a teacher of the humanities, in the old fashioned sense: a scholar of the best of our cultural inheritance, and so, in more ways than one, a scholar of tradition. Tradition is in many cases an enactment of implicit cultural knowledge. Its substance is often carried in its forms, so that even when it is transmitted in the form of written text it contains implicit wisdom about some fundamental human questions and lends itself well to a wisdom-seeking inquiry attuned at once to form and substance. At its best, and in the hands of inquirers intent not on exploding traditions but on discovering the wisdom they may contain, tradition offers not only a means of delivering vital teachings through practice but also a means of learning about man grounded in and tested by the human experience, and tends to address itself to precisely those questions that Kass fears our modern scientific mindset expressly ignores.

Moreover, the form of tradition itself—wisdom transmitted through instruction and practice across generations—often speaks to one of the most crucial of those human questions, and one that has been of special interest to Kass: the question of generational continuity and family life. The family sits at the core of any true anthropology. The family, not the state, is the first essential arena of human fulfillment and flourishing. Any human endeavor intended to last more than one generation must be advanced or reinforced through the family, and any attempt at a radical overthrow of traditional cultural, social, and political practices must contend first and foremost with the family, and will often find it an implacable foe—as the smartest radicals and revolutionaries have always understood. Beginning from the natural character of the human drive to reproduce clothed by the just, the noble, and the holy, the family is a crucial means by which the human animal perfects its nature, and it is both the means and the end of a great portion of our cultural traditions.

For all these reasons, the kind of revitalized anthropology (or more natural science) that Leon Kass seeks has made him a student and a teacher of the best and highest of our cultural traditions. He seeks in them both evidence of the character of the human animal, and guidance from the greatest students of human nature through the ages, and so he engages our traditions neither as a detached and skeptical debunker of myths nor as a pious and unquestioning follower of

12. Ibid., xiv.

instruction, but as a seeker of wisdom, aiming "to cast fresh light on the sensible and the familiar" with the aim of better understanding it and so ourselves.[13]

This philosophical contention with the forms and substance of tradition has become very rare in our time, for precisely the reasons that moved Kass to pursue it. His engagement with the humanities in search of the human therefore helps illuminate not only the question of human nature that Kass is after, but also some of the deepest and most difficult questions regarding tradition itself, and the challenges it confronts in the modern age. Kass has not generally taken up these challenges explicitly, but a brief exploration of their character will help us to see how his work clearly speaks to them.

THE CASE FOR TRADITION

Traditionalists in our time confront a simple but difficult question: Why? We live in an age of progress, when knowledge grows from more to more and every generation is ever bombarded with reasons to imagine itself an improvement upon its predecessors. The means of our material progress seem decidedly untraditional in character, and largely uninterested in the kind of understanding carried by our cultural traditions. Everything around us compels us to look forward, and only through great acts of cultural exertion can we look backward with a meaningful regard for what we find there. Such exertions are possible, of course. Indeed, they remain still quite common. But why are they worthwhile? Why do our traditions deserve our allegiance?

Our answers to this question tend to coalesce into two views that stand in some tension with one another. One argues that we ought to abide by tradition because it draws upon an authoritative original source that commands our assent as it has that of prior generations; and the other argues that we ought to follow our traditions because they represent an evolved understanding of some important truths that has been built up arduously over time and that we may further build upon. In practice, these are not necessarily mutually exclusive approaches to tradition—they can and do coexist up to a point. But they draw upon and feed very different approaches to the past and the future and to social and political change.

The first view is of course now especially (though not exclusively) identified with the Biblical religions in the West. In this view, roughly speaking, we do as our parents did because we, like them, are commanded by a source of authority that preceded us all and informed by teachings and rules that began in the beginning. We resort to tradition for an understanding of these teachings because we no

13. Kass, *Toward a More Natural Science*, xii.

longer have direct access to them, as a few selected people in the distant past once did, and so we strive to approach through learning and to emulate by faithful practice those ancient authorities. We see ourselves living out teachings and truths that were once better understood than they are today, and so we see human history as something of a decline, even if we believe that in the long run—perhaps helped along by our fidelity to tradition and the ancient teachings—some redemption will bring us nearer than ever to the right path, and the human story might end in ultimate triumph. There is of course a tradition of interpretation that we hope may be bringing us closer over time to understanding the sources and meanings of our ancient faith, but in the final analysis time takes us further from the source, and we must strain ever harder to hold fast to traditional practices and the truths they convey. In this view, then, tradition is our link to the beginning, and the beginning is the crucial source of insight and authority.

This cultural originalism is perhaps what we first imagine when we think of traditionalism, but it actually presents some difficult challenges to intergenerational fidelity and transmission. Because its goal is an allegiance to a distant source, and not to the prior generation, it always runs the risk of fundamentalist purism—of an effort to connect directly with the source and so to abandon the built-up residue of generations of interpretation, approximation, and compromise. Religious communities deal with this danger in various ways—emphasizing practice and ritual, for instance, or empowering institutions with interpretive authority. The Hebrew Bible in places seems also to make generational continuity itself a religious obligation commanded directly by God, defining the place of each individual in a chain reaching back to the origin and dependent on the strength of each link, and thus making traditionalism a function of fidelity to the divine source. When the hapless King Ahab demands that his subject Naboth trade him his vineyard for a better one in the first Book of Kings, the steadfast farmer refuses on the extraordinary grounds that "The Lord forbids that I should give over the inheritance of my fathers."[14] Many modern traditionalists approach their cultural inheritance with the same loyalty and piety.

But in our time, and in our liberal regime, the most serious obstacle this approach to traditionalism confronts in making its case is its reliance on original authority, which most often means also divine authority. This is its great strength as well, to be sure, and religious believers will always be the most reliable and capable traditionalists. But without a common faith in the divine character of the original source, and so a reason to believe that our distant ancestors had access to transcendent truths that we cannot hope to grasp directly,

14. 1 Kings 21:3.

it becomes difficult to make this case for tradition in our skeptical age, and so to show our fellow modern liberal democrats what they might learn from books and practices whose premise they reject on what they take to be firm modern grounds. Indeed, one need not be a skeptic (or a modern) to raise doubts about the notion that the men of the past possessed unique insights that we cannot hope to access. Aristotle, in the *Politics*, expressed his own doubt of such traditionalism:

> It is likely that the first humans, whether they were born from the earth or survived some calamity, were like any chance person of our time or were simpletons (as indeed is said of primitives). It would be a strange thing, therefore, to abide by their opinions.[15]

The superior wisdom of our ancestors cannot simply stand unexamined as a case for tradition, Aristotle argues. If their ways were wise, we ought to be able to see them as such on the merits. And if they were not, then the only real case for sustaining them—for leaving unchanged the laws they enacted if we have reason to find fault with them—is that changes in the law carry costs of their own. "It is a base thing to get accustomed to reckless dissolution of the laws," he writes, so "some faults of past legislators and rulers should be left alone, if the gain resulting from the change will not be as great as the harm of getting used to disobeying the rulers."[16] This is surely a sorry case for tradition.

But sheer inertia and habit is of course not the only alternative to the case from original authority. The real alternative, and the second and more modern sort of traditionalism, argues instead that we ought to persist in the ways of our forefathers because those ways have been immensely successful, and we are hardly equipped to construct better ones from scratch on our own. It argues that tradition represents not so much a remnant of the original authoritative source but rather a process of gradual cultural development and evolution which offers a proven means of sustainable human thriving and advancement across generations. Tradition in this sense builds on what is good about the given world to address what is bad about it. It is a body of practice formed over countless iterations of serious engagement with the basic human questions and with the facts of human nature.

This kind of traditionalism approaches the ways of the past with reverence and respect and seeks to draw wisdom from them that might be applied to the problems of the present, on the assumption that those ways that have survived the test of time possess some insights we might learn from. Tradition in this

15. Aristotle, *Politics* 1269a.
16. Ibid.

sense draws its authority not from its origin but from its longstanding use. It is valued not because it began ages ago but because it has evolved for ages; not because it is ancient but because it is advanced, and so the means by which it has slowly developed—means that begin from a respect for the given—are deemed to merit protection and honor. These means harness the wisdom of many generations, and so their products, our traditions, are taken to possess more wisdom than any individual or even any generation can separately employ. Radical change that disrupts the continuity of tradition is likely to harm us more than it helps us, by severing our links to this chain of experience and insight. Change must instead come gradually and in continuity with longstanding practice; and change does not necessarily point in any one direction but rather responds to the needs of the moment in ways that draw understanding from the experience of the past. Because of this slow cultural evolution, the present is in many respects better than the past, and the future can be better still, provided we do not break with our traditions or abandon the achievements of our civilization, but rather build on them.

This mode of traditionalism is nowhere better exemplified and articulated than in the work of Edmund Burke, the late-eighteenth-century British statesman and writer, and a father of modern conservatism. Burke did not call himself a traditionalist. Indeed, he almost never uses the word "tradition" at all. But he thought through the logic of this approach to the past and its implications and makes an exceptional case for it. Burke explicitly rejects the appeal to beginnings as sources of authority and wisdom. The beginnings of any human society, he argues, are almost certain to involve some form of barbarism, but over time, by slow reform in response to circumstantial exigencies, societies develop more mature forms—a process that, as Burke puts it, "mellows into legality governments that were violent in their commencement."[17] Rather than seek out an original wisdom, he argues that earliest beginnings should be kept obscure while the process of cultural and social development—a process of slow change responsive to circumstances and respectful of longstanding practices—should be guarded and revered. Burke equates this process with the inheritance of property, which each generation gratefully receives from the last and seeks responsibly to improve and enhance for the benefit of the next. It is an approach to the past and the future in line with the forms of human nature and human life. In their politics and culture, Burke writes, the English have always sought "to derive all we possess as an inheritance from our forefathers."[18] This attitude, he later states, "appears to me to

17. Edmund Burke, "Reflections on the Revolution in France," in *The Writings and Speeches of Edmund Burke*, ed. Paul Langford (Oxford: Oxford University Press, 1988), VIII: 213.

18. Ibid., 81.

be the result of profound reflection, or rather the happy effect of following nature, which is wisdom without reflection, and above it."[19] In an extraordinary passage in the *Reflections on the Revolution in France*, Burke lays out most fully this appeal to the natural example, which is crucial to his larger view of political life:

> By a constitutional policy, working after the pattern of nature, we receive, we hold, we transmit our government and our privileges, in the same manner in which we enjoy and transmit our property and our lives. The institutions of policy, the goods of fortune, the gifts of providence, are handed down to us, and from us, in the same course and order. Our political system is placed in a just correspondence and symmetry with the order of the world, and with the mode of existence decreed to a permanent body composed of transitory parts; wherein, by the disposition of a stupendous wisdom, molding together the great mysterious incorporation of the human race, the whole at one time is never old, or middle-aged, or young, but in a condition of unchangeable constancy, moves on through the varied tenor of perpetual decay, fall, renovation, and progression. Thus, by preserving the method of nature in the conduct of the state, in what we improve, we are never wholly new; in what we retain, we are never wholly obsolete. By adhering in this manner and on those principles to our forefathers, we are guided not by the superstition of antiquarians, but by the spirit of philosophic analogy. In this choice of inheritance, we have given to our frame of polity the image of a relation in blood; binding up the constitution of our country with our dearest domestic ties; adopting our fundamental laws into the bosom of our family affections.[20]

In an important respect, this kind of traditionalism begins not from veneration of the old (that "superstition of antiquarians") but from humility about the capacity of human reason to invent new forms. There is more to the human animal than we can readily discern immediately and individually, and so we must learn about it from the ways that have enabled it to thrive in the past, and not just from what we find by direct applications of reason. "We are afraid to put men to live and trade each on his own private stock of reason," Burke writes, "because we suspect that this stock in each man is small, and that the individuals would do better to avail themselves of the general bank and capital of nations, and of ages."[21] We ought to trust that there is wisdom in that common stock on the evidence of its having enriched human lives for generations, even if we do not readily perceive it. Burke makes this case explicitly, and in terms that begin

19. Ibid., 83.
20. Ibid., 84.
21. Ibid., 138.

to turn us back to Leon Kass's search for wisdom about human nature in great works of the past. In his *Appeal from the New to the Old Whigs*, Burke writes:

> If ever we should find ourselves disposed not to admire those writers or artists, Livy and Virgil for instance, Raphael or Michelangelo, whom all the learned had admired, [we ought] not to follow our own fancies, but to study them until we know how and what we ought to admire; and if we cannot arrive at this combination of admiration with knowledge, rather to believe that we are dull, than that the rest of the world has been imposed on.[22]

This is traditionalism in search of wisdom in past examples of excellence, and inclined to assume the relative superiority of longstanding practice and judgment over present reason alone. It argues for venerating and continuing beliefs and practices that have for ages offered wisdom on the fundamental human questions, and that therefore seem to point toward some coherent anthropology that we ought not to ignore.

Like Leon Kass, Burke arrived at this approach by reflecting on the barren and emaciated notion of humanity at the heart of the modern project, which "endeavor[s] to persuade the people that they are no better than beasts"—and especially at its absence of any appreciation for human sentiment, familial attachment, and generational continuity.[23] As a young man, Burke jotted in a notebook his concern about "that philosophy which would strip [our nature] naked. . . . Of such sort is the wisdom of those who talk of the love, the sentiment and the thousand little dalliances that pass between the sexes, in the gross way of mere procreation. They value themselves as having made a mighty discovery; and turn all pretence to delicacy into ridicule."[24] Such disregard for man's real nature and the cultural forms that clothe it, Burke thought, caused some to disparage their very humanity and to wish to overcome it, which he took to be a profoundly misguided aim:

> There is no part of our condition but we ought to submit to with cheerfulness. Why should I desire to be more than man? I have too much reverence for our nature to wish myself divested of even the weak parts of it. I would not wish, as I have heard some do, that I could live without eating or sleeping. I rather thank

22. Edmund Burke, "An Appeal from the New to the Old Whigs," in *Further Reflections on the Revolutions in France*, ed. Daniel Ritchie (Indianapolis: Liberty Fund, 1992), 199.

23. Edmund Burke, "Letters on a Regicide Peace," in *The Writings and Speeches of Edmund Burke*, ed. Paul Langford (Oxford: Oxford University Press, 1988), IX: 246.

24. Edmund Burke, *A Note-Book of Edmund Burke*, ed. H. V. F. Somerset (Cambridge: Cambridge University Press, 1957), 91.

> providence that has so happily united the subsistence of my body with its satisfaction. When we go into another State we shall have means fitted to it, with equal wisdom no doubt. At the present we ought to make the best of our condition; and improve our very necessities, our wants, and imperfections, into elegancies—if possible into virtues.[25]

Burke and Kass both appeal to a modern traditionalism for similar reasons: a search for a comprehensive vision of human nature in the face of a philosophy that ignores its forms and aspirations; a sense that much latent wisdom on that subject may be found in cultural practices and products that have endured by speaking to the needs of countless generations; and a regard for generational transmission as both a means and an end of human flourishing.

But because Burke is a statesman first and foremost—concerned for social peace and effective government—he employs his traditionalism above all in defense of the political sphere from intrusions by reckless metaphysics. "Politics ought to be adjusted not to human reasonings, but to human nature, of which the reason is but a part, and by no means the greatest part," Burke writes.[26] The search for human nature is for him a search for guidance on political matters in the face of thinkers who would look for such guidance in abstract reason alone, and so he seeks only some general boundaries, and not a detailed anthropology. He is less concerned with completing our picture of human nature than with defending a social order he believes essential to the happiness of future generations.

Kass is much more a student of human nature itself—a seeker after wisdom about what we are and how we ought to live. His interests are therefore less expressly political and more truly anthropological, which helps him avoid one of the great problems of Burkean traditionalism.

PHILOSOPHY AND TRADITION

If a resort to tradition that values the end more than the beginning—or evident success more than authoritative origin—is largely immune to the dangers of fundamentalism, it is very vulnerable to the charge of utilitarianism. If our culture does not answer to an authoritative original code but has rather come over time to its practices and beliefs, how can we tell the difference between what

25. Ibid., 92.

26. Edmund Burke, "Observations on a Late Publication entitled The Present State of the Nation," in *The Writings and Speeches of Edmund Burke*, ed. Paul Langford (Oxford: Oxford University Press, 1988), II: 196.

is right and what is merely effective? Is all that matters just that change be carried out in a gradual way, or are some changes for the better and others for the worse? As Burke himself puts it, there is a danger that such a view might "make the success of villainy the standard of innocence."[27]

Burke's defense against this charge is, roughly stated, that the shape that the political and social institutions of a successful regime assume over a great span of time offers a sense of the shape of the higher justice that lies beyond them. We do not have direct access to that higher justice by pure reasoning, but we may gain indirect access to it by the very experience of political and social life. Through long-term trial and error, society effectively rubs up against that higher justice and so comes to assume something of its form. Thus longstanding forms and practices come to offer a sense of how to distinguish positive reform from harmful innovation. The forms of the English constitution, Burke argues, offer a test of proposed reforms and innovations: those in line with the character of the constitution—those that make society what it already is but more so—may be judged worthwhile reforms, while those that would break in a decisive way with the forms and patterns of the past are to be carefully avoided. A society in this way comes to establish some general boundaries within which it carries out its political life, a life of bounded but constant change and flux. Within these boundaries political questions can be safely resolved by appealing to prudence, rather than to abstract principle or higher justice. It is only when politics breaks these bounds—as Burke believed was the case, for instance, in the British mistreatment of the natives of India and the Catholics of Ireland—that an extraordinary appeal to political principles grounded in human nature and even divine justice is called for. And it is only when politics threatens to break with the very allegiance to the model of gradual change that has made progress possible (which Burke believed was happening in France) that all-out resistance was called for.

This view puts Burke somewhere between a utilitarianism that would judge what is right by what is effective and a natural law theology that holds practical judgment to a transcendent standard that draws on a divine authoritative origin. It is a view that may well do for the practical needs of political life, but that nonetheless leaves Burke's political traditionalism open to the charge that it confuses what is with what is right.

Leon Kass's related but less political traditionalism offers an interesting correction to this weakness in Burke's case, a correction that suggests that anthropology and politics are not simply two sides of the same coin. Kass, like Burke, believes there is likely to be more wisdom in our great cultural artifacts

27. Burke, "An Appeal from the New to the Old Whigs," 176-77.

and practices than is readily evident on the surface, so that an exploration of these is well worth our while and likely to uncover useful insight. But he pursues this insight with the purpose of better understanding the human animal, so that this understanding could then be applied to our personal, social, and political life. Rather than seeing in social forms a simulacrum of higher justice, he sees in them (as in other great works and longstanding traditions) clues as to the character of man. Such clues might well inform the study of justice or political order, but they do not stand in for it. Burke is fundamentally a student of political change, while Kass is fundamentally a student of human nature—which does not change. He seeks after the prerequisites for human flourishing, some of which are political, but most of which are familial and cultural. Like Burke, he is most alert to dangers to the means of continuity—which for Burke translates above all to a vehement opposition to radical transformations of society and politics but for Kass translates above all to a vehement opposition to radical transformations of the family.

There is of course still some danger in Kass's project of mistaking what is for what should be, but the danger is greatly mitigated by the fundamentally philosophical rather than political (that is, wisdom-seeking rather than rule-making) character of his efforts.[28] He has championed the use of politics and law in the defense of crucial human goods, to be sure, but only in cases when he has judged that the essential prerequisites to human flourishing, and especially the family, are at risk. For the most part, even in bioethics, Kass's efforts are a search for understanding of the human animal, which might inform the efforts of his students and his readers to live well. He argues neither *from* nor *for* authority, even when expounding on the meaning of the Ten Commandments, or when arguing for laws that would prohibit human cloning.

This is actually most evident in the portion of Kass's work that might be thought both most inclined to authoritative rulemaking and most reliant on the authority of origin, but which turns out to be neither: his study of the Hebrew Bible. His reading of Genesis does not lean on the authority of the text's claim to divine origin, but on the premise that the text offers teachings that, once unpacked, will help show why the practices they enjoin contain latent but persuasive wisdom. Such ways of reading, offered with "thoughtful children of

28. A further danger, that of undermining the wisdom implicit in our cultural traditions by the very act of making that wisdom explicit, is of course a concern for both, and a profound and complex dilemma of modern conservatism. It too is a far greater concern for Burke than for Kass because of the political character of his enterprise, as the danger of demystifying myths is above all a danger to the polity. Burke is surely of two minds on the question of whether it is finally possible to discover the latent wisdom that prevails in general prejudices without exploding them, but he knows we can have no choice but to try.

skeptics" especially in mind,[29] leave us both wiser and more confident of our traditional practices—and suggest that the books of origin speak directly to us, but speak in terms that, once properly understood, offer reasons to persist, beyond proof of success. They thus go some way toward bridging the gap between the two modes of traditionalism, and also offer a counter-example to the approach of modern skeptics to traditional texts. Kass seeks for the roots of our traditions without seeking to uproot them. He believes that properly understood our traditions and the highest accomplishments of our culture speak to a fuller understanding of human nature that can help us see what we are, and therefore how we might make the most of ourselves.

In this way, Leon Kass's work offers a model of the philosophical study of tradition—a humanism sadly out of style today. It is grounded in the desire to understand more fully the nature of the human being, and in the assumption that men and women have been pursuing such understanding for countless generations, so that the efforts they have undertaken—and especially those that have spoken to generations of readers and followers—have something to say to us today, and will have something to say to human beings for as long as such beings exist. It is an attitude that approaches the past not with unswerving piety and not with arrogant doubt, but with openness and, above all, with gratitude: gratitude for our nature, and gratitude for what our predecessors have made of it.

Wisdom-seeking gratitude is the dominant flavor of every page of Kass's work, and more than any particular insight it is that passion that we students of his ought to strive to learn and emulate. In this sense, too, we may hope that essays of appreciation for his work are not only well deserved but also a truly fitting tribute.

29. Leon R. Kass, *The Beginning of Wisdom: Reading Genesis* (New York: Free Press, 2003), 1.

Courses Taught by Leon R. Kass

St. John's College

Sophomore Laboratory (Biology)
Freshman Seminar (Great Books, Greeks)
Preceptorials on: Aristotle, *De Anima*
Darwin, *Origin of Species*
Aristotle, *Nicomachean Ethics*

Georgetown University

Philosophy of Nature: The Organism

The National Endowment for the Humanities: Humanities Seminars for Health Professionals

Human Being and Citizen
Man, Nature, and Morality

University of Chicago

Aristotle, *Nicomachean Ethics*
Plato, *Symposium*
Philosophy of Nature: The Organism
Philosophy of Nature: Lucretius
The Human Passions
Science and Society: Knowledge, Morals, and Power
Human Being and Citizen
Rousseau, *Discourse on the Origin of Inequality*
Philosophy of Nature: Purpose and Form
Genesis (also, graduate tutorial)

Aristotle, *De Anima* (graduate seminar)
The Meaning of Darwinism
Human Beginnings: *Genesis* and Rousseau
Science and Inquiry: Descartes and Plato
Descartes, *Discourse on the Method*
Nature: Aristotle and Descartes (graduate seminar)
Classical Geometry and Its Transformations
Tolstoy, *War and Peace* (with Amy A. Kass)
Ethics of Everyday Life: Courtship (with Amy A. Kass)
Law and Legislator: *Exodus* (graduate seminar)
Science and Morals: Friends or Foes?
Plato, *Meno* (graduate seminar)
Biotechnology and the Human Future

Published Writings of Leon R. Kass

Books

Toward a More Natural Science: Biology and Human Affairs, New York: The Free Press, 1985. (Paperback edition, 1988.)

The Hungry Soul: Eating and the Perfecting of Our Nature, New York: The Free Press, 1994. (Second edition, with a new Foreword, Chicago: University of Chicago Press, 1999.)

(With James Q. Wilson) *The Ethics of Human Cloning*, Washington, DC: The American Enterprise Institute, 1998.

(With Amy A. Kass) *Wing to Wing, Oar to Oar: Readings on Courting and Marrying*, Notre Dame, Indiana: University of Notre Dame Press, 2000. (Part of a five-volume series on the Ethics of Everyday Life.)

Life, Liberty, and the Defense of Dignity: The Challenge for Bioethics, San Francisco: Encounter Books, 2002. (Paperback edition, 2004.)

The Beginning of Wisdom: Reading Genesis, New York: The Free Press, 2003. (Paperback edition, Chicago: University of Chicago Press, 2006.)

Scientific Articles

Kass, L. R., Brock, D. J. H., and Bloch, K. ß-Hydroxydecanoyl-Thioester Dehydrase. I. Purification and properties. *J. Biol. Chem.* 242:4418-31, 1967.

Brock, D. J. H., Kass, L. R., and Bloch, K. ß-Hydroxydecanoyl-Thioester Dehydrase. II. Modes of action. *J. Biol. Chem.* 242:4432-40, 1967.

Kass, L. R., and Bloch, K. On the enzymatic synthesis of unsaturated fatty acids in Escherichia coli. Proc. *Natl. Acad. Sci. USA* 58:1168-73, 1967.

Kass, L. R. The antibacterial activity of 3-Decynoyl-N-Acetylcysteamine: Inhibition in vivo of ß-Hydroxydecanoyl-Thioester Dehydrase. *J. Biol. Chem.* 243:3323-28, 1968.

Rosner, J. L., Kass, L. R., and Yarmolinsky, M. B. Parallel behavior of F and Pl in causing induction of lysogenic bacteria. *Cold Spr. Harb. Symp. Quant. Biol.* 33:785-89, 1968.

Kass, L. R. ß-Hydroxydecanoyl-Thioester Dehydrase from Escherichia coli. *Methods in Enzymology*, Vol. XVI:73-80, 1969.

Kass, L. R., and Brock, D. J. H. Synthesis of Thioesters of N-Acetylcysteamine. *Methods in Enzymology*, Vol. XVI:696-98, 1969.

Kass, L. R., and Yarmolinsky, M. B. Segregation of Functional Sex Factor into Minicells. Proc. *Natl. Acad. Sci. USA* 66:815-22, 1970.

ARTICLES IN BIOMEDICAL ETHICS, SCIENCE AND HUMAN AFFAIRS, AND SOCIAL THOUGHT

"A Caveat on Transplants," Outlook, *The Washington Post*, January 14, 1968.

"Problems in the Meaning of Death," *Science* 170:1235-36, 1970.

"What Price the Perfect Baby?" *Science* 173:103, 1971 (Letter).

Review of *Fabricated Man* by Paul Ramsey, *Theology Today* 28:105-107, 1971.

"Death as an Event: A Commentary on Robert Morison," *Science* 173:698-702, 1971.

"The New Biology: What Price Relieving Man's Estate?" *Science* 174:779-88, 1971.

"Babies by Means of In Vitro Fertilization: Unethical Experiments on the Unborn?" *New England Journal of Medicine* 285:1174-79, 1971.

"Man's Right to Die," *The Pharos of Alpha Omega Alpha* 35 (2):73-77, 1972.

"Making Babies—The New Biology and the 'Old' Morality," *The Public Interest*, Number 26:18-56, Winter, 1972.

"New Beginnings in Life," in *The New Genetics and the Future of Man*, M. P. Hamilton, ed., Grand Rapids, Michigan: Eerdmans, 1972, 13-63.

"Refinements in Criteria for the Determination of Death" (with colleagues from Task Force on Death and Dying), *Journal of the American Medical Association* 221:4853, 1972.

"A Statutory Definition of the Standards for Determining Human Death: An Appraisal and a Proposal," (with Alexander M. Capron), *University of Pennsylvania Law Review* 121:87-118, 1972.

"Ethical Implications of Pre-Natal Diagnosis for the Human Right to Life," in *Ethical Issues in Human Genetics*, Bruce Hilton, et al., eds., New York: Plenum Press, 1973, 185-99.

"The Future of Man, the Organism: The New Biology," an essay published in 1974 in many newspapers as part of the National Endowment for the Humanities sponsored program, "America and the Future of Man: Courses by Newspaper."

"Averting One's Eyes or Facing the Music?—On Dignity and Death," *Hastings Center Studies* 2:67-80, 1974.

"Regarding the End of Medicine and the Pursuit of Health," *The Public Interest*, Number 40:11-42, Summer, 1975.

"Determining Death and Viability in Fetuses and Abortuses," *Research on the Fetus, Appendix*, The National Commission for the Protection of Human Subjects of Biomedical and Behavioral Research, U.S. Department of Health, Education, and Welfare Publication Number (OS) 76-128, 1975.

"Teleology and Darwin's *The Origin of the Species*: Beyond Chance and Necessity?" in Stuart F. Spicker, ed., *Organism, Medicine, and Metaphysics*, Dordrecht, Holland: D. Reidel, 97-120, 1978.

"Ethical Issues in Human In Vitro Fertilization, Embryo Culture and Research, and Embryo Transfer," *In Vitro Fertilization, Appendix*, Ethics Advisory Board, U.S. Department of Health, Education and Welfare, May 4, 1979.

"'Making Babies' Revisited," *The Public Interest*, Number 54:32-60, Winter, 1979.

"A Conversation with Dr. Leon Kass: The Ethical Dimensions of In Vitro Fertilization," an occasional paper published by the American Enterprise Institute for Public Policy Research, Washington, DC: AEI Studies 242, 1979.

"Ethical Dilemmas in the Care of the Ill," *Journal of the American Medical As-*

sociation 244:1811-16 (Part I: "What Is the Physician's Service?") and 244:1946-49 (Part II: "What Is the Patient's Good?"), 1980.

"Ethical problems of the new biology," (Review of *Life Manipulation: From Test-tube Babies to Aging* by David G. Lygre), *Chemical & Engineering News*, September 15, 1980, 47-48.

"Defining Healthy Functioning," *Proceedings of the Institute of Medicine of Chicago* 33 (4), (1980).

"Patenting Life," *Commentary*, December, 1981, 45-57.

"Change and Permanence: Reflections on the Ethical-Social Contract of Science in the Public Interest," *In Vitro* 17:1091-99, 1981.

"Professing Ethically: On the Place of Ethics in Defining Medicine," *Journal of the American Medical Association* 249:1305-10, 1983.

"The Case for Mortality," *The American Scholar* 52 (2):173-91, 1983.

"Darwinism and Ethics: A Response to Antony Flew," in Arthur L. Caplan and Bruce Jennings, eds., *Darwin, Marx and Freud: Their Influence on Moral Theory*, New York: Plenum Press, 47-66, 1984.

"Modern Science and Ethics: Time for a Re-examination?" *The University of Chicago Magazine*, Summer, 1984, 24-30.

"Thinking About the Body," *The Hastings Center Report* 15 (1):20-30, February, 1985.

"The Academic Vocation Revisited," (A Symposium on Teaching, Learning, and Publishing) *The Cresset* (Valparaiso University), September, 1985, 5-8.

(With W. Gaylin, E. D. Pellegrino, and M. Siegler), "Doctors Must Not Kill," *Journal of the American Medical Association* 259:2139-40, April 8, 1988.

"Citizens with Mental Retardation and the Good Community," in Lawrence A. Kane, Phyllis Brown, and Julius S. Cohen, eds., *The Legal Rights of Citizens With Mental Retardation*, Lanham, Maryland: University Press of America, 1988, 7-23.

"Evolution and the Bible: Genesis I Revisited," *Commentary,* November, 1988, 29-39. (Response to Letters, *Commentary*, April, 1989, 8-10.)

"What's Wrong With Babel?" *The American Scholar* 58 (1):41-60, Winter, 1989.

"Neither for Love Nor Money: Why Doctors Must Not Kill," *The Public Interest*, Number 94:25-46, Winter, 1989. (A somewhat revised version was later published as "'I Will Give No Deadly Drug': Why Doctors Must Not Kill," *American College of Surgeons Bulletin*, Vol. 17, No. 3, March 1992, 6-17.)

"Medicine: Profession or Trade?" *Medicine on the Midway*, Spring, 1989, 8-11.

"Do Institutional Guidelines Help in Termination of Treatment Decision Making?", Point/Counterpoint column in *Decisions Near the End of Life, Vol. 2: Working with the Law*, Newton, Massachusetts: Education Development Center, 1989, 4-5.

"Practicing Ethics: Where's the Action?", *The Hastings Center Report* 20 (1):5-12, January/February, 1990.

"Death with Dignity and the Sanctity of Life," *Commentary*, March, 1990, 33-43. (Response to Letters, *Commentary*, August, 1990, 5-6.)

"New Technologies and Ethical Choice," *Barnard* (Alumnae Magazine), Winter, 1990, 2-4, and 24.

"The Care of the Doctor," *Perspectives in Biology and Medicine* 34 (4):553-60, Summer, 1991.

"Death with Dignity and the Sanctity of Life," in *A Time to Be Born and a Time to Die*, Barry Kogan, ed., Aldine-DeGruyter, 1991, 117-45.

"Why Doctors Must Not Kill," *Commonweal*, August 9, 1991, 472-76.

"A Woman for All Seasons," *Commentary*, September, 1991, 30-35. (Response to Letters, *Commentary*, January, 1992, 8.)

"Man and Woman: An Old Story," *First Things*, Number 17:14-26, November, 1991.

"Suicide Made Easy: The Evil of 'Rational' Humaneness," *Commentary*, December, 1991, 19-24. (Response to Letters, *Commentary*, May, 1992, 13-15.)

"Regarding Daughters and Sisters: The Rape of Dinah," *Commentary*, April, 1992, 29-38. (Response to Letters, *Commentary*, July, 1992, 12-13.)

"Organs for Sale? Propriety, Property, and the Price of Progress," *The Public Interest*, Number 107:65-86, Spring, 1992.

"Seeing the Nakedness of His Father," *Commentary*, June, 1992, 41-47. (Response to Letters, *Commentary*, October, 1992, 5-7.)

"Death on the California Ballot," *The American Enterprise*, September/October, 1992, 44-51.

"Is There a Right to Die?", *Hastings Center Report* 23 (1):34-43, January/February, 1993. A slightly different version appears in Robert A. Licht, ed., *Old Rights and New*, Washington, DC: AEI Press, 1993, 75-95.

"The Problem of Technology," in Arthur Melzer, Jerry Weinberger, and M. Richard Zinman, eds., *Technology and the Western Political Tradition*, Ithaca, New York: Cornell University Press, 1993, 1-24.

"The Path Not Taken," (Review of *Assimilation versus Separation: Joseph the Administrator and the Politics of Religion in Biblical Israel* by Aaron Wildavsky), *Commentary*, September, 1993, 58-61.

"Why the Dietary Laws?", *Commentary*, June, 1994, 42-48. (Response to Letters, *Commentary*, October, 1994, 10-16.)

"Educating Father Abraham: The Meaning of Wife," *First Things*, Number 47:16-26, November, 1994.

"Educating Father Abraham: The Meaning of Fatherhood," *First Things*, Number 48:32-43, December, 1994.

"Am I My (Foolish) Brother's Keeper?" *The American Enterprise*, November/December, 1994, 16-27.

"The Need for Piety and Law: A Kristol-Clear Case," in Christopher De Muth and William Kristol, eds., *The Neoconservative Imagination: Essays in Honor of Irving Kristol*. Washington, DC: AEI Press, 1995, 112-33.

"Comment on *The Giving Tree*" (Contribution to Symposium), *First Things*, Number 49:42-43, January, 1995.

"Intelligence and the Social Scientist," *The Public Interest*, Number 120:64-78, Summer, 1995.

(With Amy A. Kass) "What's Your Name?" *First Things*, Number 57:14-25,

November, 1995.

"The Permanent Limitations of Biology," in William A. Rusher, ed., *The Ambiguous Legacy of the Enlightenment*, Lanham, Maryland: University Press of America, 1995, 120-41.

"Appreciating The Phenomenon of Life," *Hastings Center Report* 25 (7):3-12, Special Issue on Hans Jonas, 1995.

"Farmers, Founders, and Fratricide: The Story of Cain and Abel." *First Things,* Number 62:19-26, April, 1996.

"A Genealogy of Justice." *Commentary*, July, 1996, 44-51. (Response to Letters, *Commentary*, November, 1996, 16-18)

"Dehumanization Triumphant," *First Things*, Number 65:15-16, August/September, 1996. Reprinted in *Connecticut Medicine* 60 (10):619-20, 1996.

"Whither Medicine? Marginal Musings About Central Questions," *Proceedings of the National Meeting on M.D./Ph.D. Education and Research in the Humanities and the Social Sciences,* Chicago: The University of Chicago, 1996, 23-39.

"Charity and the Confines of Compassion," *Philanthropy* X (2): 5-7 & 28-31, Spring, 1996.

"The Akedah as Final Examination: Abraham, *Summa cum Laude*," *Sources: The Chicago Journal of Jewish Studies*, Number II, Spring, 1996, 24-31.

(with Nelson Lund) "Physician-Assisted Suicide, Medical Ethics, and the Future of the Medical Profession," *Duquesne Law Review* 35 (1):395-425, 1996.

(with Nelson Lund) "Courting Death: Assisted Suicide, Doctors, and the Law," *Commentary,* December, 1996, 17-29. (A somewhat altered version of the previous item.) (Response to Letters, *Commentary,* April, 1997, 3-7.)

"The Troubled Dream of Nature as a Moral Guide," *Hastings Center Report* 26 (6):22-24, November/December, 1996.

"The End of Courtship," *The Public Interest,* Number 126:39-63, Winter, 1997.

"The Wisdom of Repugnance: Why We Should Ban the Cloning of Human Beings," *The New Republic*, June 2, 1997, 17-26.

"The Aims of Liberal Education," in *The Aims of Education*, ed. John Boyer, The University of Chicago, 1997, 81-106.

"Beyond Biology," (Review of *Brave New Worlds: Staying Human in the Genetic Future* by Bryan Appleyard), *The New York Times Book Review*, August 23, 1998, 7-8.

"Love of Woman and Love of God: The Case of Jacob," *Commentary*, March, 1999, 46-54.

(With Amy A. Kass) "Proposing Courtship," *First Things*, Number 96:32-41, October, 1999.

"The Moral Meaning of Genetic Technology," *Commentary*, September, 1999, 32-38. (Response to Letters, *Commentary*, December, 1999, 5-8.)

"Why We Should Ban the Cloning of Human Beings," *Texas Review of Law & Politics*, 4 (1):41-49, Fall, 1999.

"On Aldous Huxley's Brave New World," *First Things*, Number 101:51-52, March, 2000.

"Am I My Foolish Brother's Keeper? Justice, Compassion, and the Mission of Philanthropy," in *The Ethics of Giving and Receiving: Am I My Foolish Brother's Keeper?*, ed. William F. May and A. Lewis Soens, Jr., Dallas, Texas: The Cary M. Maguire Center for Ethics and Public Responsibility and Southern Methodist University Press, 2000, 1-16. Also, "A Response to [critics] Curran, Lovin, and Sverdlik," 42-53.

"The Humanist Dream: Babel Then and Now," *Gregorianum* 81 (4):633-657, 2000.

"Triumph or Tragedy? The Moral Meaning of Genetic Technology," *The American Journal of Jurisprudence*, 45:1-16, 2000.

"Preventing a Brave New World: Why We Should Ban Human Cloning Now," *The New Republic*, May 21, 2001, 30-39.

"L'Chaim and Its Limits: Why Not Immortality?" *First Things*, May, 2001, 17-24.

(with Daniel Callahan) "Ban Stand," *The New Republic*, August 6, 2001.

"'I Will Give No Deadly Drug': Why Doctors Must Not Kill," in *The Case Against*

Assisted Suicide, ed. Kathleen Foley, M.D. and Herbert Hendin, M.D., Johns Hopkins University Press, 2002, 17-40. (An updated version of the 1989 and 1992 essay, see supra.)

"Brave New Biology: The Challenge for Human Dignity," London: The Institute of United States Studies, 2002.

"The Right to Life and Human Dignity," in Kenneth L. Vaux, Sara Vaux, and Mark Stenberg, eds., *Covenants of Life: Contemporary Medical Ethics in Light of the Thought of Paul Ramsey*, Dordrecht: Kluwer Academic Publishers, 2002, 57-69. (A revised version was published in Svetozar Minkov, ed., *Enlightening Revolutions: Essays in Honor of Ralph Lerner*, Lanham, Maryland: Lexington Books, 2006, 127-41, and a further revised version in *The New Atlantis*, Number 16, Spring 2007, 23-40.)

"Biotechnology: A House Divided," (a symposium), *The Public Interest*, Number 150:38-41, 58-62, Winter, 2003.

"Ageless Bodies, Happy Souls: Biotechnology and the Pursuit of Perfection," *The New Atlantis*, Number 1, Spring, 2003, 9-28.

"Reflections on Public Bioethics: A View from the Trenches," *Kennedy Institute of Ethics Journal* 15 (3):221-50, 2005.

(with Eric Cohen) "Cast Me Not Off in Old Age," *Commentary*, January, 2006, 32-39. (Response to letters, *Commentary*, April 2006, 12-16.)

"Science, Religion, and the Human Future," *Commentary*, April, 2007, 36-48. (Response to letters, *Commentary*, July-August 2007, 16-22.)

"The Follies of Freedom and Reason: An Old Story," in Richard Velkley, ed., *Freedom and the Human Person*, Washington: DC, Catholic University of America Press, 2007.

"Defending Human Dignity," *Commentary*, December 2007, 53-61.

"How Brave a New World?" *Society* Vol. 45, No. 1, February 2008, 5-8. (Originally the 2007 Convocation Address, St. John's College, Annapolis, Maryland.)

"Defending Life and Dignity: How, Finally, to Ban Human Cloning," *The Weekly Standard*, February 25, 2008, 30-33.

(with Eric Cohen) "For the Love of the Game: Against the Adulteration of American Sport," *The New Republic*, March 26, 2008, 34-42.

"Keeping Life Human: Science, Religion, and the Soul," *Azure*, Number 32, Spring 2008, 31-46. (Originally the 2007 Wriston Lecture at the Manhattan Institute for Public Policy Research.)

"A Truer Humanism," *Azure*, Number 34, Autumn 2008, 36-47. (A response to Prof. David Heyd's critique of the previous essay.)

"Permanent Tensions, Transcendent Prospects," in Christopher DeMuth and Yuval Levin, eds., *Religion and the American Future*, Washington, DC: AEI Press, 2008, 83-117.

"Defending Human Dignity," in *Human Dignity and Bioethics: Essays Commissioned by the President's Council on Bioethics*, Washington, DC: Government Printing Office, 2008, 297-331. (Reissued in 2009 by the University of Notre Dame Press.)

"The (Super?)Human Roots of Law and Justice: Lessons from the Book of Genesis," *The American Journal of Jurisprudence*, 53:1-22, 2008.

"Biotechnology and Our Human Future: Some General Reflections," in Sean D. Sutton, ed., *Biotechnology, Our Future as Human Beings and Citizens*, SUNY Series in Philosophy and Biology, David Edward Shaner, gen. ed., SUNY Press, 2009.

"Forbidding Science: Some Beginning Reflections," *Science and Engineering Ethics*, Vol. 15, No. 3, September 2009, 271-82.

PUBLICATIONS OF THE PRESIDENT'S COUNCIL ON BIOETHICS UNDER LEON KASS'S CHAIRMANSHIP

Human Cloning and Human Dignity: An Ethical Inquiry (A Report by The President's Council on Bioethics), Washington, DC: July 2002. (A commercial edition, with a new Foreword by Dr. Kass, was published as *Human Cloning and Human Dignity: The Report of the President's Council on Bioethics*, New York: Public Affairs, 2002.)

Beyond Therapy: Biotechnology and the Pursuit of Happiness (A Report by The President's Council on Bioethics), Washington, DC: October 2003. (Two commercial editions, under the same title but each with a new and different Foreword by Dr. Kass, were published in 2003: one by Regan Books/Harper Collins, one by the Dana Press.)

Being Human: Readings from the President's Council on Bioethics, Washington,

DC: January 2004. (A commercial edition, with a new Foreword by Dr. Kass, was published as *Being Human: Core Reading in the Humanities*, New York: W. W. Norton, 2004.)

Monitoring Stem Cell Research (A Report by The President's Council on Bioethics), Washington, DC: January 2004.

Reproduction and Responsibility: The Regulation of New Biotechnologies (A Report by The President's Council on Bioethics), Washington, DC: March 2004.

Alternative Sources of Human Pluripotent Stem Cells: A White Paper (A Report by The President's Council on Bioethics), Washington, DC: May 2005.

Taking Care: Ethical Caregiving in Our Aging Society (A Report by The President's Council on Bioethics), Washington, DC: September 2005.

Index

Apples of Gold in Pictures of Silver

About the Contributors

Amy A. Kass is a Senior Fellow at the Hudson Institute in Washington, DC.

Ralph Lerner is the Benjamin Franklin Professor Emeritus in the College and Professor Emeritus of Social Thought at the University of Chicago.

Gilbert Meilaender is the Richard and Phyllis Duesenberg Professor of Christian Ethics at Valparaiso University and was a member of the President's Council on Bioethics.

Harvey C. Mansfield is the William R. Kenan, Jr., Professor of Government at Harvard University.

Harvey Flaumenhaft is a Tutor and former Dean of St. John's College, Annapolis.

Michael Fishbane is the Nathan Cummings Professor of Jewish Studies in the Divinity School, the Committee for Jewish Studies, and the College at the University of Chicago.

Paul McHugh is the University Distinguished Professor of Psychiatry at the Johns Hopkins University School of Medicine.

Rebecca Dresser is the Daniel Noyes Kirby Professor of Law and Professor of Ethics in Medicine at Washington University in St. Louis and was a member of the President's Council on Bioethics.

Nelson Lund is the Patrick Henry Professor of Constitutional Law and the Second Amendment at the George Mason University School of Law.

Adam Schulman is a Tutor at St. John's College, Annapolis, and was a Senior Research Consultant at the President's Council on Bioethics.

Diana J. Schaub is a Professor of Political Science at Loyola College in Maryland and a member of the Hoover Institution Task Force on the Virtues of a Free Society and was a member of the President's Council on Bioethics.

Paul W. Ludwig is a Tutor at St. John's College, Annapolis.

Thomas W. Merrill is an Assistant Professor of Government at American University in Washington, DC, and was a senior research analyst at the President's Council on Bioethics.

Eric Cohen is the Executive Director of the Tikvah Fund and editor-at-large of *The New Atlantis*.

Yuval Levin is the editor of *National Affairs* and a fellow at the Ethics and Public Policy Center in Washington, DC.

Breinigsville, PA USA
07 May 2010
237528BV00003B/5/P

9 780739 141595